Janet Wilkie.

Principles of
Clinical Measurement

Principles of
Clinical Measurement

M. K. SYKES
MA, MB, BChir, DA,

FFARCS, FFARACS(Hon)

Nuffield Professor of Anaesthetics,
University of Oxford

M. D. VICKERS
MB, BS, MRCS, LRCP, DA,

FFARCS, FFARACS(Hon)

Professor of Anaesthetics,
Welsh National School of Medicine, Cardiff

C. J. HULL
MB, BS(London), FFARCS

Senior Lecturer in Anaesthetics,
University of Newcastle on Tyne

With an additional chapter by
P. J. WINTERBURN
BSc, PhD

Lecturer in Biochemistry,
University College, Cardiff

**BLACKWELL
SCIENTIFIC PUBLICATIONS**
OXFORD LONDON EDINBURGH
BOSTON MELBOURNE

© 1970, 1981 by
Blackwell Scientific Publications
Editorial offices:
Osney Mead, Oxford, OX2 0EL
8 John Street, London, WC1N 2ES
9 Forrest Road, Edinburgh, EH1 2QH
52 Beacon Street, Boston,
    Massachusetts 02108, USA
214 Berkeley Street, Carlton
    Victoria 3053, Australia

First published 1970 (entitled
*Principles of Measurement
for Anaesthetists*)
Reprinted 1973
Second edition 1981

Printed and bound in
Great Britain by
Billing & Sons Ltd and
Kemp Hall Bindery
Guildford, London, Oxford,
Worcester

DISTRIBUTORS

USA
  Blackwell Mosby Book Distributors
  11830 Westline Industrial Drive
  St Louis, Missouri 63141

Canada
  Blackwell Mosby Book Distributors
  120, Melford Drive,
  Scarborough
  Ontario M1B 2X4

Australia
  Blackwell Scientific Book
  Distributors
  214 Berkeley Street, Carlton
  Victoria 3053

British Library
Cataloguing in Publication Data

Sykes, M K
  Principles of clinical measurement.
  1. Human physiology—Measurement
  I. Title   II. Vickers, M D   III. Hull, C J
  612   QP34.5

  ISBN 0-632-00044-9

Contents

Preface to Second Edition

The first edition of this book was entitled *Principles of Measurement for Anaesthetists*. Its aim was to acquaint the anaesthetist with the basic principles of measurement techniques which could be applied to clinical practice. At that time the importance of the subject to anaesthetists had been recognized by its inclusion in the Primary FFARCS examination, but the practice of clinical measurement was mostly restricted to specialized centres. During the past ten years measurement technology has steadily improved and the use of sophisticated instruments has spread from the cardiac catheter laboratory and operating theatre to the intensive care unit, premature baby unit and obstetric unit. Furthermore, techniques which were at one time mainly the province of the cardiologist, respiratory physiologist or anaesthetist are now increasingly being used by all disciplines, whilst long-term monitoring is frequently practised on the general wards. In preparing a second edition it therefore seemed reasonable to broaden the coverage and to try and provide a simple text which would be of use not only to anaesthetists, but also to physicians, surgeons, paediatricians and obstetricians. Although aimed primarily at doctors, it is hoped that the text will also be of use to technicians and nurses concerned with clinical measurement or monitoring. The basic plan of the first edition has been retained. The general principles used in measurement are outlined in the first part, specific measurements are described in the second part and the handling of the data so obtained is considered in the third part.

Because of the wider scope of this edition, we have felt it necessary to seek the help of additional contributors with special expertise. Dr C. J. Hull has concentrated particularly on the electronically-orientated material, but because of his wide experience, we have been grateful to him for becoming a joint author. Dr P. J. Winterburn has written Chapter 8, concerned with measurements using electromagnetic radiations, and we should like to pay tribute to the skill with which he has blended with the other material and matched our style.

In this respect, we have retained the same simple, if dogmatic, approach and have assumed that the reader has only an elementary knowledge of mathematics and physics. We have avoided technical jargon whenever possible and have described the electronic devices in the simplest possible terms. We have tried to avoid referring to specific apparatus and have not included detailed instructions for the performance of individual measurements, for these can be obtained by reading the references provided or, in some cases, by referring to the operating manual provided by the manufacturer. It is our hope that this approach will dispel the mysteries associated with clinical measurement and will provide a sound basis for the understanding of future developments in the subject.

M. K. Sykes
M. D. Vickers

Introduction

Acute, life-threatening illness can only be treated effectively if the abnormality can be diagnosed and the magnitude of the disturbance quantified simply and quickly. Although the physical signs derived from clinical examination provide a rapid means of assessing the patient's condition, they are of limited value and open to subjective error. For this reason they are usually supplemented by simple clinical measurements such as blood pressure or urine flow. Unfortunately, such measurements provide only a rough guide to the condition of the patient, for they are not directly related to the basic functions which should be measured. Blood pressure, for example, depends on both cardiac output and peripheral resistance, whilst urine output may be affected by many factors besides renal blood flow. To manage a patient with severe hypotension the clinician must know whether the filling pressures of the heart are adequate, whether the heart muscle is functioning properly and whether the peripheral resistance is normal. Metabolic derangements commonly complicate primary organ failure but may also cause derangements in other systems, so that repeated clinical and biochemical measurements are now an essential part of the management of the acutely ill patient.

The first essential in the making of any measurement is that the operator should understand the principle on which the measurement is based and should know what other factors may affect the measurement. For example, radioisotope measurements of lung blood flow may be affected by radioactivity in the chest wall, whilst dye dilution measurements of cardiac output may be rendered inaccurate by the presence of intracardiac shunts. The second essential is that the measurement must be referred to an internationally agreed standard, so that the units of measurement are comparable. The third essential is that the accuracy of the measurement must be known, not only in terms of the accuracy possible with a given instrument, but also in terms of the accuracy obtained in the hands of the user. The last essential is that the normal range of the measurement should be established so that its biological significance can be correctly assessed.

This book deals mainly with the first two requirements, namely the principles of measurement and the standards by which such measurements are judged. The third requirement, accuracy, depends largely on the choice of method, available instrumentation and the ability of the user: it can therefore only be discussed in general terms. The last requirement, the establishment of a normal range of values, is more properly the province of physiologists and clinicians and the reader is referred to other texts for information on the interpretation of the measurements herein described.

With the development of microprocessors the level of sophistication is rising rapidly, so that measurement systems can now monitor their own performance and reject obviously erroneous information. Unlike humans, machines will pay attention all the time, and will, if necessary, provide a permanent and unbiased record which can be studied at leisure. Sophisticated calculating facilities can provide complex derivatives from the original data with such speed that this secondary information can readily be applied to patient management. If continuous monitoring really is of demonstrable benefit to sick patients, there is no doubt that only electronic devices can now supply it. Nevertheless, it is still timely to issue a word of warning. The results obtained from even the most impressive instrumental systems are only as good as the person who operates them; they must therefore be used to confirm or extend our clinical observation of the patient rather than to act as a substitute for it. Only when instrumentation systems can match the efficiency of the human brain in the perception and interpretation of the data obtainable from the patient will one dare to rely on them. When that stage is reached this book will no longer be necessary.

Part 1
General Principles
and Instruments

Chapter 1
General Principles of Measurement

Basic components of a measurement system

Successful medical treatment depends on accurate diagnosis. Diagnosis is, in turn, based on the history and on the elicitation of physical signs. Simple instruments, such as the stethoscope, facilitate the detection of physical signs. Other instruments, such as the thermometer, increase the accuracy with which changes can be measured. More complicated instruments, such as the electrocardiograph, enable changes outside the range of human perception to be charted.

Instruments are therefore used in medicine either to display or record signals which can be appreciated by the human senses, or to detect, display and record signals which are outside the range of human perception. In either event the system must consist of a detector, which senses the signal, and some form of display. The signal may be transferred directly from detector to display or may be altered in some way to make it more suitable for display. Finally the signal may be used to actuate a warning device, or even to set in motion a mechanism which reacts back upon the patient and controls some aspect of function. This plan is summarized in Fig. 1.1.

SENSING DEVICES

The body takes in food and converts the chemical energy contained therein into electrical, mechanical, heat and sound energy. Electrical energy may be sensed by *electrodes* and then processed by standard electronic techniques. Mechanical energy may be sensed directly by connecting the recording devices to the body with a thread or lever but, more commonly, it is transformed into electrical energy in order to facilitate measurement. Heat and sound energy are also usually changed into electrical energy before being measured, although transformations into other types of energy are sometimes used for convenience. Any instrument which is used to change one form of energy to another is known as a *transducer*. Although this term is commonly associated with the measurement of pressure, it will become apparent that it has a more widespread application in the measurement field.

Electrodes

Certain aspects of bodily function (nerve, muscle or sense organ activity) are accompanied by electrical changes which can be sensed by electrodes placed on the active tissue or on the body surface. One of the

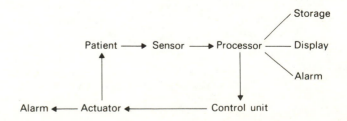

Fig. 1.1. The essential components of a clinical measurement system.

difficulties in recording from such sites is that electrodes tend to become polarized (i.e. develop a high resistance) when placed in contact with tissues (p. 49). The recording of potentials from the skin surface introduces additional problems because of the very high electrical resistance of the skin. Since the changes in electrical potential within the body are usually small (of the order of millivolts) it is important to minimize such resistances if satisfactory recordings are to be obtained.

When the signals are very small, for example in electroencephalography, it may be necessary to place a *pre-amplifier* close to the recording site so that the signal strength is increased to a level which ensures that there is minimal electrical interference during its transmission to the main processing unit.

Transducers

The main types of transducers used in medical applications are listed in Table 1.1. Displacement measurements can be processed to provide signals related to velocity or acceleration whilst force or weight can be measured by the displacement of the free end of a fixed spring. Similarly the displace-

ment of a flexible diaphragm or a liquid manometer can be used to indicate pressure. Measurements of flow may utilize some property of the liquid or gas (e.g. thermal conductivity, viscosity, density) or may be based on a mechanical device which directly meters the volume passing a given point in unit time. Temperature transducers measure a change in some property of a substance induced by heat (e.g. thermal expansion or chemical change) whilst thermographic techniques measure the quantity of heat radiated from the skin. Chemical reactions may also produce electrical energy. A common example is the electric battery but similar reactions form the basis of the galvanic cell for oxygen measurement and the various electrode techniques for measuring pH or blood–gases.

PROCESSING DEVICES

In a few simple instruments the signal is transmitted directly to the recorder or display unit without intermediate processing. Obvious examples are the measurement and display of temperature by the mercury-in-glass thermometer, or the sensing of pressure by a tambour directly linked by a

Table 1.1. Transducers for medical applications.

	Quantity measured	Transduction method
1	Displacement (velocity, acceleration) force, weight (spring) pressure (diaphragm)	Resistive, capacitive, inductive, piezo-electric, photoelectric, electromagnetic, ultrasonic.
2	Flow (volume)	Electromagnetic, ultrasonic, thermal, optical, mechanical.
3	Sound	Piezo-electric, capacitive, resistive, inductive.
4	Heat	Thermal expansion, thermo-chemical, thermoelectric, resistive, thermographic.
5	Light	Photoelectric (photovoltaic cell, photodiode, photoconductor, phototransistor).
6	Gases, blood-gases, pH	Galvanic cell, electrodes.
7	Humidity	Capacitive

thread to a pen writing on a rotating drum (Fig. 1.2a). However, if the tambour is connected to the pen by a lever and the fulcrum of the lever is placed closer to the tambour than to the drum, then the amplitude of the pen excursion will exceed that of the tambour so that the signal is *amplified* (Fig. 1.2b). This primitive technique is the simplest example of signal processing.

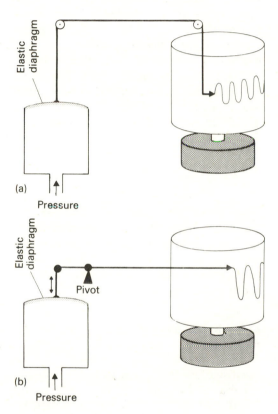

Fig. 1.2a. Simple pressure transducer diaphragm directly connected to a pen writing on a drum. b. The movement of the diaphragm is amplified by placing the pivot of the writing arm nearer the diaphragm.

Amplification is usually required because the signal from the electrode or transducer is inadequate to drive a display or recorder. Amplification is most commonly accomplished by first changing the signal into electrical energy. This energy can then be amplified to a degree which would be quite impossible by the use of mechanical methods. Most processing units are more complex and modify the signal in some other way. For example, a flow signal from a pneumotachograph may be *integrated* to give a signal proportional to volume; or a volume signal *differentiated* to yield flow; impulses from a nerve fibre may be *counted*, and their frequency displayed; or a non-linear output from a rapid gas analyser may be *rendered linear* before being displayed or recorded. Many instruments now incorporate much more complicated processing units which may be classified as *microcomputers*. For example the processor in an automated blood–gas analyser not only controls the whole process of calibrating the electrodes, measuring the electrical output from the electrodes and instigating regular wash and calibration cycles, but also continually checks the functioning of the machine and calculates and prints out the results. A cardiac output computer similarly analyses the indicator dilution curve, applies calibration factors and displays the results in digital form.

DISPLAY SYSTEMS

The design of data display units has been neglected in the past. As the volume of data increases and the time allowed for digestion of the data decreases (e.g. in avionics), display has been subjected to closer study. Unfortunately, progress in methods of display has been only slowly assimilated into the medical field.

In some instruments the measurement is displayed directly on a graduated scale as in the gas meter or in the mercury thermometer. However, in most measurement systems the processor delivers an *analogue* signal to the display unit. The characteristic of such a signal is that the signal is represented by a continuous output of a voltage or current which varies directly with the magnitude of the input signal. The output may be displayed as a *trace* on a cathode-ray tube with the amplitude of the signal on the *y*-axis, and time or some other variable on the *x*-axis. Alternatively the magnitude of the signal may be displayed on a graduated *scale*. In some applications the output may be represented by *lights* of varying intensity, colour or size, whilst in diagnostic instruments using ultrasound, radioisotopes or thermography *grey scale* or *colour images* may be produced. In some types of apparatus there is no specific display unit, this being replaced by a trace or image on a recorder, the so-called *hard copy* display.

The increasing use of digital processing has encouraged the use of *digital* forms of display in which the data is presented in the form of alphanumeric characters (alphabetical characters or numbers). This form of display is only suitable for relatively stable signals but such signals can often be derived from rapidly changing signals by suitable processing. Thus a microcomputer can be programmed to measure systolic, diastolic and mean blood pressures at each heart beat and then to display the average reading over, say, the preceding ten heart beats.

RECORDERS

Recorders may be broadly classified as *direct-writing*, *photographic*, and *magnetic*. In the first type the signal is inscribed directly onto paper. In the second type a display is photographed or a trace is recorded by moving a light spot across light-sensitive paper or film. In the third type signals are recorded on magnetic tape or in a computer 'store' for subsequent playback or recording. Recorders are dealt with more fully in Chapter 7.

CONTROL SYSTEMS

Control systems are widely used in industrial automation but their use in medicine is still limited. Part of the reason has been the high cost of developing safe and reliable systems. However, although the advent of the microprocessor has greatly simplified the instrumental problems there are still major difficulties in securing a reliable patient-sensor interface. These difficulties can, to some extent, be overcome by the use of complicated artefact-rejection systems, alarms and fail-safe mechanisms but the incorporation of such devices greatly increases the cost of the apparatus, and no control system can function in the absence of a signal from the patient.

Early examples of control systems were the control of the depth of intravenous anaesthesia from EEG signals (Kiersey, Faulconer & Bickford 1954) and the mechanical control of ventilation from the end-tidal P_{CO_2} (Frumin 1957). The latter technique was even developed to the stage where a further injection of suxamethonium was given whenever the patient attempted to breathe spontaneously! Other examples of control systems include the demand pacemaker, which is switched on when the heart rate falls below a pre-set level, and the neonatal temperature controller, which regulates the heat supplied by an infrared source to maintain a constant abdominal skin temperature. Attempts have also been made to control fluid replacement on the basis of measured blood loss and vascular pressures (Sheppard *et al.* 1968).

Essential requirements for a measurement system

A satisfactory measurement system must be capable of isolating the signal of interest from other unwanted signals and then reproducing this signal with consistent accuracy despite normal environmental variations. This requirement can only be satisfied by ensuring that a high signal-to-noise ratio is maintained throughout the system and by using instruments that have good zero and gain stability, minimal amplitude nonlinearity and hysteresis, and an adequate frequency response.

SIGNAL-TO-NOISE RATIO

When a biological signal is detected, amplified and recorded, it will be more or less obscured by a variety of unwanted signals, which are collectively described as *noise*. At its source, the signal can be considered to be 'clean', but progressively contaminated by noise as it passes through the various stages in the data pathway.

The most critical stage is the first, since most biological signals are very small, and are therefore easily obscured. For instance, an electrocardiograph (ECG) signal may be mixed with intercostal electromyograph (EMG) signals of equal amplitude, and with wideband noise (i.e. of many frequencies) generated by electrochemical activity at the skin–electrode interface. As the signal travels along a wire to the amplifier, electrostatic and electromagnetic linkage with mains cables and mains-powered devices may add noise which will be predominantly 50 Hz (and its harmonics). Radiofrequency noise may also be added at this stage, from sources such as surgical diathermy, staff-paging systems, or nearby radiotransmitters. Physical disturbance of the cable, by minutely altering its capacitance, may add low frequency noise (microphony) to the signals. As the signal is amplified, it is joined by thermal noise generated within the electronic components themselves. Thermal noise may be a major problem when detecting signals in the microvolt range (such as those recorded by the electroencephalograph), so that special 'low noise' input stages are required. As the signal grows larger, thermal noise is still added by each component, but being of relatively constant amplitude, makes very little contribution to the overall noise level. When the signal is transmitted to another location or recorded on magnetic tape, it is often closely associated with other physiological signals undergoing similar treatment. Each signal is usually referred to as a *channel*, and may acquire some signal from an adjacent channel (crosstalk) which must now be considered to be noise.

Successful recording of a signal therefore depends upon isolating the signal, not only from unwanted biological signals, but also from electronic noise sources. The efficiency with which a signal can be isolated is thus defined by the signal:noise ratio. Since signal:noise ratios may vary widely, the logarithmic bel scale is often used to define them. Thus 1 bel is a ratio of 10:1, whilst 2 bels represents a ratio of 100:1. For convenience bels are usually multiplied by 10 to yield decibels, so that 10:1 = 10 dB whilst 100:1 = 20 dB. If, therefore an instrument claims a signal:noise ratio of 45 dB, a ratio of 31 623:1 is implied.

A low signal:noise ratio can often be improved by selective *filtering* (rejecting unwanted frequencies), by employing amplifiers with a *high common mode rejection ratio* (p. 41) and by the use of special techniques such as *signal averaging*.

ACCURATE REPRODUCTION OF THE INPUT SIGNAL

The second requirement of any system of instrumentation is that it should provide an accurate display or record of the input signal. Most instrumentation systems are inherently unstable, their performance being affected by temperature, mains voltage and frequency, ageing of components, etc. When considering the accuracy of any system one must consider the zero stability, the gain stability, the linearity and the frequency response. The latter includes a consideration of damping and phase shift.

Zero stability

The first aspect to be assessed is zero stability *ie* the ability to maintain a zero reading on the display unit or recorder when the input signal is zero. A certain amount of zero instability can usually be tolerated, but, obviously, the degree of stability required will vary with the application. For example, slight zero instability will prove less of a disadvantage when recording blood pressures during cardiac catheterization than when recording blood pressures over prolonged periods of days or weeks.

Zero drift may vary around a mean or

the signal may drift progressively in one direction. In either case it may be regarded as noise of very low frequency. Progressive drift is extremely important in long-term measurements because of its inherently cumulative nature. Furthermore, in some types of apparatus, zero drift may be amplified or integrated thus affecting the gain stability.

Gain stability

The sensitivity of the processing device can usually be adjusted to vary the ratio between input and output signals by means of one or more 'gain' controls. There should always be ample reserve gain in the instrument and, once set, the degree of gain should remain constant over a period which is adequate for the purpose in hand.

Amplitude linearity

The degree of amplification of the signal should be equal throughout the whole range of signal strengths likely to be encountered. If this is not so the system is said to be nonlinear. Figure 1.3 illustrates nonlinearity in a blood pressure transducer–amplifier–recorder system which occurred only in the higher range of pressure.

Normally the linearity of an instrument or system is specified in such terms as 'better than 1 per cent'. This means that the reading on the display unit should never be in error by more than ±1 per cent of

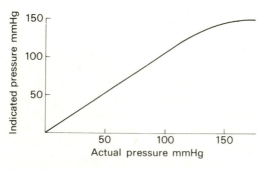

Fig. 1.3. Nonlinearity in a blood pressure measuring system in the higher ranges of pressure.

the actual reading throughout the range of the instrument. Unfortunately, this statement sometimes only applies to part of the range and this may not be made clear in the literature provided by the manufacturer. It is most important to assess the linearity of the complete system, since minimal non-linearity in each component may prove additive and so lead to a greater error in the recorded signal.

Certain instruments such as thermistors and humidity sensors may display _hysteresis_. This means that the signal produced by a given temperature or humidity is different when the input is rising than when it is falling. A hysteresis loop is thus produced (Fig. 1.4). This is another cause of nonlinearity.

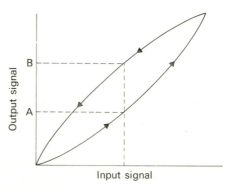

Fig. 1.4. A hysteresis loop. A given input signal produces an output signal 'A' when the signal is rising and an output signal 'B' when it is falling.

Frequency response

Most signals follow a complicated pattern or waveform. Fourier showed mathematically that any complex waveform could be constructed by taking a simple sine wave of the same frequency as the slowest component (called the fundamental frequency) and adding to it a number of sine waves, the frequency of which bore a simple whole-number relationship to the fundamental (Fig. 1.5). These higher-frequency components are called harmonics of the fundamental frequency. Electrical and mechanical systems which transmit wave-

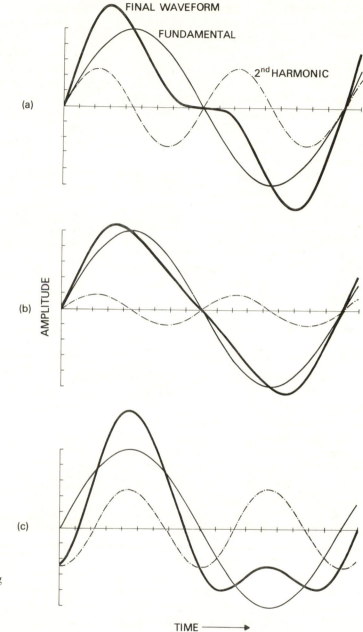

Fig. 1.5. Fourier analysis. A complex waveform can be resolved into the fundamental waveform and a series of harmonics. Variations in the shape of a complex wave (bold line) are due to differences in the amplitude and phase of the harmonics present. a. Fundamental (first harmonic) plus second harmonic. b. Effect of reducing amplitude of harmonic. c. Effect of changing phase of harmonic.

forms behave as though all the components of a complex wave are really separate. To reproduce a complex wave accurately, therefore, the system must be able to handle all the component frequencies in the waveform in a similar manner. This implies equal amplification of each frequency (i.e. no *amplitude* distortion), and, if any delay occurs in the system, there must be no alteration in the relative positions of the various components of the wave (i.e. no *phase* distortion). Although this is the ideal solution, for many purposes it is sufficient if the system reproduces accurately up to the tenth harmonic, that is up to ten times the fundamental frequency. However, if one is particularly concerned with the high-frequency components, then a higher frequency response would be necessary.

Matching

A complete instrumentation system consists of a number of units each of which has special characteristics. The efficiency of the complete system depends, not only on the behaviour of the components, but also the way they are matched to each other. Such matching must take account, not only of the strength and character of the signals fed from one unit to another, but of the way in which each part interacts with the other.

In complete systems this is properly taken care of by the maker, but when systems are constructed of separate 'black boxes' it is necessary to match both the current or voltage and the input and output impedances (see Chapter 3). If this is not done the characteristics of one part of the system may be considerably altered by the other. A false record may also be obtained by adding a recorder to a device which normally only feeds a meter. A recorder may create a shunt across the meter and provide a path for part of the signal. Both the recorder and the meter will then give a lower reading from a standard signal than would have been shown on the meter with the recorder unconnected.

It will be apparent from the above discussion that a large number of factors have to be taken into account when considering any system of measurement. Before a choice of instrumentation is made it is necessary to consider the degree of accuracy required and the manner in which the system is to be used. When these fundamentals have been decided detailed planning of the complete system becomes possible. If they are ignored the system may prove inadequate or unnecessarily expensive.

MONITORING SYSTEMS

This text deals mainly with the physical principles which are used in measurement apparatus. The other important aspect of the subject, the application of measurements to the clinical situation, is evolving with equal rapidity. Many monitoring systems, which appeared to be well designed, have failed in the clinical situation, whilst others have stood the test of time. For good reviews of the current practice of monitoring readers are referred to Cooper (1973); Symposium on Monitoring (1976); Rolfe (1976); Steer (1977); Stott (1977); Miller (1978); Poole-Wilson (1978); Saidman & Smith (1978).

References

COOPER R. (1973) The measurement of intracranial pressure. *British Journal of Hospital Medicine: Equipment Supplement*, **10**, 18.

FRUMIN M.J. (1957) Clinical use of physiological respirator producing N_2O amnesia-analgesia. *Anesthesiology*, **18**, 290.

KIERSEY D.K., FAULCONER A. & BICKFORD R.G. (1954) Automatic electro-encephalographic control of thiopental anesthesia. *Anesthesiology*, **15**, 356.

MILLER T.D. (1978) Intracranial pressure monitoring. *British Journal of Hospital Medicine*, **19**, 497.

POOLE-WILSON P.A. (1978) Clinical physiology: interpretation of haemodynamic measurements. *British Journal of Hospital Medicine*, **20**, 371.

ROLFE P. (1976) Monitoring equipment for the neonate. *British Journal of Clinical Equipment*, **1**, 189.

SAIDMAN L.J. & SMITH N.T. (1978) *Monitoring in anesthesia.* New York: John Wiley and Sons.

SHEPPARD L.C., KOUCHOUKOS N.T., KURTTS M.A. & KIRKLIN J.W. (1968) Automated treatment of critically ill patients following operation. *Annals of Surgery*, **168**, 596.

STEER P.J. (1977) Monitoring in labour. *British Journal of Hospital Medicine*, **17**, 219.

STOTT F.D. (1977) Ambulatory monitoring. *British Journal of Clinical Equipment*, **2**, 61.

Symposium on Monitoring (1976) *Anesthesiology*, **45**, 113–259.

Further reading

BELVILLE J.W. & WEAVER C.S. (1969) Techniques in clinical physiology. *A survey of techniques in anesthesiology.* London: Collier-Macmillan.

DEWHURST D.J. (1966) *Physical instrumentation in medicine and biology.* Oxford: Pergamon Press Ltd.

GEDDES L.A. & BAKER L.E. (1975) *Principles of applied biomedical instrumentation, 2nd ed.* London: John Wiley and Sons.

HILL D.W. (1973) *Electronic measurement techniques in anaesthesia and surgery,* 2nd ed. London: Butterworth.

HILL D.W. & DOLAN A.M. (1976) *Intensive care instrumentation.* London: Academic Press.

MCMULLAN J.T. (1977) *Physical techniques in medicine Vol. 1.* London: John Wiley and Sons.

ROLFE P. (1979) *Non-invasive physiological measurements. Vol. 1.* London: Academic Press.

Chapter 2
Units of Measurement and Basic Mathematical Concepts

Measurement became necessary when human beings began to exchange one commodity for another. Initially, measurements were related to commonly available objects. Thus in early Egyptian times length was related to the width of the finger (the digit) or to the distance from the elbow to the fingertips (the cubit). The fathom, equivalent to the 6-foot span of the arms, is still used for measuring the depth of the sea and the hand (4 inches) is still used for measuring the height of a horse. Later, an attempt was made to rationalize the measurements so that individual variation did not affect the comparisons. For example, the Egyptians standardized on the cubit and ordered that all other measurements should be fractions or multiples of a cubit. Thus the digit became one twenty-eighth of a cubit, and the fathom 4 cubits.

Even greater exactitude became possible when standards were adopted. Thus, even in Anglo–Saxon times, there was a standard yard, in the form of an iron bar kept at Winchester. A similar standard was maintained at Westminster until 1959, but after that date both the pound and the yard were related to the kilogram and the metre.

Metric standards were first developed in France at the end of the 18th century. Initially the metre was supposed to be a distance equal to one ten-millionth of the distance along the earth's surface between the pole and equator, and the litre and kilogram were defined from this primary standard. In 1875 an International Bureau of Weights and Measures was established at Sèvres, a suburb of Paris, and new standards of the metre and kilogram were set up and sent to a number of countries. Later this International Bureau concerned itself with other standards. As the need for greater and greater accuracy has become apparent the Bureau has increasingly turned towards standards present in natural phenomena, since these can be measured by scientists anywhere in the world. Thus the standard metre (a bar made of platinum and iridium and kept at Sèvres) was discarded in 1960 in favour of a standard related to the wavelength of the orange light given off by krypton-86 and, in 1967, time was related to atomic vibrational frequency.

For many years, therefore, two main systems of measurement have existed alongside each other: the metric and the imperial. Because of its decimal basis the metric system has always been more attractive for scientific use. It greatly simplifies calculations and has progressively replaced the imperial system. The metric system based on the centimetre, gram and second (CGS) was initially replaced by the MKS system (metre, kilogram, second). Further refinement and extension of this became the Système Internationale d'Unités (SI), the principle difference being the creation of a nongravitationally-derived unit for force.

The replacement of the imperial by the metric system has proceeded at different rates for different applications and in different countries. In the United Kingdom, imperial units of length (yard, mile) are still frequently employed, whereas pounds are slowly giving way to kilograms and pints and gallons to litres in some trades and industries. The last imperial unit in medicine (grains in drug dosage) was officially abandoned on 1 January 1971.

The change to SI is likewise patchy. SI units were made mandatory in any new legislation in EEC countries from 21 April

1978; from December, 1977 many imperial and non-SI metric units 'ceased to be authorised' (a term which has no prohibiting effect in itself). The remaining non-SI units ceased to be authorized from December, 1979 (*Official Journal of the European Communities*, 1976).

Scientists in many countries around the world have not uniformly adopted SI units, nor indeed have all clinicians in the UK. Since the principal difference relates to the definition of force, it is pressure measurements (force per unit area) which show the greatest diversity. There are in routine use at present, units of pressure based on non-gravitational definitions in the CGS system (e.g. the bar) as well as the SI system (the Pascal) and gravitationally-based definitions in metric terms (kilograms and kiloponds per square metre, Torr, standard atmosphere, mmHg, cmH$_2$O) and in imperial terms (inch of water, lb/sq.in.). Throughout this text SI units are used, conversion factors and explanations being provided where necessary in the relevant chapters.

SI units

SI is an extension of the traditional metric system. There are seven base units from which all the other units are derived (Table 2.1). The exact definition of these units is set out in Table 2.2 but the physical basis for the standards is as follows:

The metre (m) is defined in terms of the wavelength in a vacuum of a specified emission from the krypton-86 atom. The vacuum wavelengths of specified emissions from other atoms, such as ^{198}Hg and ^{144}Cd, are precisely related to the primary standard and can therefore be used as secondary standards.

The second (s) was originally related to the rotation of the earth, but since 1967 it has been defined in terms of the frequency of structure transitions in the atoms of

Table 2.1. SI base units and supplementary units.

Quantity	Unit Name	Symbol
Base units		
Length	metre	m
Mass	kilogram	kg
Time	second	s
Electric current	ampère	A
Thermodynamic temperature	kelvin	K
Amount of substance	mole	mol
Luminous intensity	candela	cd
Supplementary units		
Plane angle	radian	rad
Solid angle	steradian	sr

Table 2.2. Definition of SI base units.

The metre is the length equal to 1 650 763.73 wavelengths in vacuum of the radiation corresponding to the transition between the levels $2p_{10}$ and $5d_5$ of the krypton-86 atom.

The kilogram is the unit of mass; it is equal to the mass of the international prototype of the kilogram.

The second is the duration of 9 192 631 770 periods of the radiation corresponding to the transition between the two hyperfine levels of the ground state of the caesium-133 atom.

The ampère is that constant current which, if maintained in two straight parallel conductors of infinite length, of negligible circular cross-section and placed one metre apart in a vacuum, would produce between these conductors a force equal to 2×10^{-7} newtons per metre of length.

The kelvin, the unit of thermodynamic temperature, is the fraction 1/273.16 of the thermodynamic temperature of the triple point of water.

The mole is the amount of substance of a system which contains as many elementary entities as there are atoms in 0.012 kg of carbon 12. When the mole is used the elementary entities must be specified and may be atoms, molecules, ions, electrons, and other particles or specified groups of such particles.

The candela is the luminous intensity, in the perpendicular direction, of a surface of 1/600 000m^2 of a black body at the temperature of freezing platinum under a pressure of 101 325 newtons per square metre.

caesium-133. With present instruments the time difference between two caesium atomic clocks amounts to less than 1 s in 30 000 years!

The kilogram (kg), the unit of mass, is equal to the mass of the international prototype kilogram, a platinum–iridium cylinder preserved at the International Bureau of Weights and Measures at Sèvres, France. The platinum–iridium alloy is used because it has a thermal coefficient of expansion close to zero.

The ampère (A) is the unit of electric current and is defined as the amount of current which would have to flow down each of two parallel conductors of infinite length and negligible circular cross-section in a vacuum to generate a given force between them.

The kelvin (K) the unit of temperature, is 1/273.16 of the temperature of the triple point of water (the point at which solid, liquid and gaseous phases are in equilibrium). The 'degree Kelvin' was rendered obsolete in December 1977 and is replaced by the kelvin. A difference in temperature may be expressed in kelvins or in degrees Celsius (°C) for $1K = 1°C$.

The candela is the unit of luminous intensity and is defined in terms of the brightness (looked at perpendicularly) of a small area of molten platinum at a given temperature and pressure (see p. 16).

SUPPLEMENTARY SI UNITS

These are used in the definition of derived units, but are not regarded as base units since they have no dimensions. They are the unit of plane angle (radian) and solid angle (steradian) and are defined as follows:

The radian is the plane angle between two radii which, on the circumference of a circle, cut an arc equal in length to the radius. (Since 2π radians $= 360°$, 1 radian $= 57.296°$ —see Fig. 2.1).

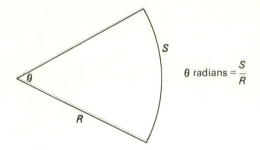

$$\theta \text{ radians} = \frac{S}{R}$$

Fig. 2.1. An angle of 1 radian (rad) is subtended by an arc of a circle (S) equal in length to the length to the radius R. Hence θ rad $= \dfrac{S}{R}$ and 2π rad $= 360°$.

The steradian is the solid angle which has its apex at the centre of a sphere and which describes on the surface of the sphere an area equal to that of a square having its side as the radius of the sphere (see Fig. 2.2).

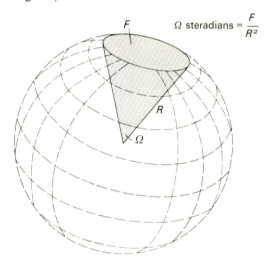

$$\Omega \text{ steradians} = \frac{F}{R^2}$$

Fig. 2.2. One steradian (*sr*) is subtended at the centre of a sphere of radius R by a portion of its surface of area R^2.
Hence Ω *sr* $= \dfrac{F}{R^2}$ and 1 sphere $= 4\pi$ *sr*.

DECIMAL MULTIPLES AND SUBMULTIPLES

The approved prefixes and their symbols are given in Table 2.3. These are normally attached to the appropriate unit, e.g. milli-

Table 2.3. Prefixes and their symbols used to designate certain decimal multiples and submultiples.

Factor	Prefix	Symbol	Factor	Prefix	Symbol
10^{18}	exa	E	10^{-1}	deci	d
10^{15}	peta	P	10^{-2}	centi	c
10^{12}	tera	T	10^{-3}	milli	m
10^{9}	giga	G	10^{-6}	micro	μ
10^{6}	mega	M	10^{-9}	nano	n
10^{3}	kilo	k	10^{-12}	pico	P
10^{2}	hecto	h	10^{-15}	femto	f
10^{1}	deca	da	10^{-18}	atto	a

second (ms or s $\times$ 10^{-3}), kilometre (km or m $\times$ 10^{3}). In the case of mass, however, the adoption of the kilogram as the base unit would lead to millikilogram to indicate a gram. Accordingly in the case of mass, the prefixes are attached to gram and to the symbol 'g', e.g. mg (milligram) and μg (microgram).

When a derived unit is expressed as a function (e.g. 1000 ohms per metre) it is permissible to apply the prefix to the numerator (1 kilohm per metre), to the denominator (1 ohm per millimetre) or to both if appropriate (1 megohm per kilometre). Compound prefixes (millimicrometre) are not permitted.

Note that some prefixes use the same letter as some units: thus m is used for both milli and metre. To clarify the meaning it is necessary to observe the convention that the prefix precedes the unit symbol without space or punctuation. Thus ms indicates millisecond, μm micrometre and MHz megahertz. To denote the product of two symbols the symbols are separated by a space or by a central point. Thus metre $\times$ second in m s or m·s whilst metre per second is m s^{-1} or m·s^{-1}.

DERIVED SI UNITS

Almost all of the units required in scientific work can be derived from the nine base and supplementary units listed in Table 2.1.

Derived units are expressed as algebraic expressions in the form of products of powers of the base and supplementary units. For example, the unit of pressure, the pascal (Pa), can be represented in base units as m^{-1}·kg·s^{-2}, and electric resistance (Ω) by m^2·kg·s^{-3}·A^{-2}. This may not strike the reader as self-evident unless some algebraic rules are recalled.

Consider the series:

$$10^3 \quad 10^2 \quad 10^1 \quad 10^0 \quad 10^{-1} \quad 10^{-2}$$

These are equivalent to:

1000.0 100.0 10.0 1.0 0.1 0.01

It can be observed that the second row of figures is the same set of numerals repeated six times but with the decimal point moving one place to the left on each occasion. Note that 10^{-1} or 0.1, is also 1/10 which could be regarded as one out of ten, or one *per* ten. Using minus powers such as 10^{-1} is therefore a convenient way of expressing fractions or ratios. In the same way, m^{-1} means 'per metre', s^{-1} means 'per second' and kg^{-1} means 'per kilogram'. A velocity of 25 metres per second can therefore be simply expressed as 25 m·s^{-1}. An acceleration of 6 metres per second per second is likewise 6 m·s^{-2}. Read like this, it does not matter if one can visualize a negative square second or not, or indeed if such an entity exists. These are just the mathematical dimensions of the measurement.

In Table 2.4 are listed those derived SI units which have officially been accorded special names (eponyms): the third column expresses each quantity by reference to others from which it is most simply derived. For example, a pascal is a newton per square metre (N·m^{-2}), a joule is a newton metre (N·m) a watt is a joule per second (J·s^{-1}), a volt is a watt per ampere (watts = volts $\times$ amps; therefore. V = W/A or W·A^{-1}), an ohm is a volt per ampere (V·A^{-1}) and so on. In the fourth column the dimensions are given in their most fundamental form in terms of the base and supplementary units.

Many other quantities can be derived directly from the base and supplementary units but have not yet been given a special name. Some common ones are listed in Table 2.5.

Table 2.4. Derived SI units having names and symbols.

Quantity	Unit		Expression	
	Name	Symbol	In other SI units	In terms of base or supplementary SI units
Frequency	hertz	Hz		s^{-1}
Force	newton	N		$m \cdot kg \cdot s^{-2}$
Pressure, stress	pascal	Pa	$N \cdot m^{-2}$	$m^{-1} \cdot kg \cdot s^{-2}$
Energy, work, quantity of heat	joule	J	$N \cdot m$	$m^2 \cdot kg \cdot s^{-2}$
Power	watt	W	$J \cdot s^{-1}$	$m^2 \cdot kg \cdot s^{-3}$
Quantity of electricity, electric charge	coulomb	C		$s \cdot A$
Electric tension, electric potential, electromotive force	volt	V	$W \cdot A^{-1}$	$m^2 \cdot kg \cdot s^{-3} \cdot A^{-1}$
Electric resistance	ohm	Ω	$V \cdot A^{-1}$	$m^2 \cdot kg \cdot s^{-3} \cdot A^{-2}$
Electric conductance	siemens	S	$A \cdot V^{-1}$	$m^{-2} \cdot kg^{-1} \cdot s^3 \cdot A^2$
Electric capacitance	farad	F	$C \cdot V^{-1}$	$m^{-2} \cdot kg^{-1} \cdot s^4 \cdot A^2$
Magnetic flux	weber	Wb	$V \cdot s$	$m^2 \cdot kg \cdot^{-2} \cdot A^{-1}$
Magnetic flux density	tesla	T	$Wb \cdot m^{-2}$	$kg \cdot s^{-2} \cdot A^{-1}$
Electric inductance	henry	H	$Wb \cdot A^{-1}$	$m^2 \cdot kg \cdot s^{-2} \cdot A^{-2}$
Luminous flux	lumen	lm		$cd \cdot sr$
Illuminance	lux	lx	$lm \cdot m^{-2}$	$m^{-2} \cdot cd \cdot sr$
Activity	becquerel	Bq		s^{-1}
Absorbed dose*	gray	Gy	$J \cdot kg^{-1}$	$m^2 \cdot s^{-2}$

*And other quantities of ionizing radiations of the same dimensions.

A special word of explanation may be helpful concerning luminous flux and illuminance which invoke the steradian. The base unit of luminous intensity, the candela, is defined in terms of brightness in the perpendicular direction of an emitting surface, slightly larger than a square milli-metre. The luminous flux in lumens (lm) which is being emitted depends on the brightness and the angle in space through which the light is distributed. The unit of angle in space, the steradian (sr), is the angle at the point of a cone whose apex is at the centre of a sphere and whose base has

Table 2.5. Examples of other derived SI units.

Physical quantity	SI unit	Symbol for unit
Area	square metre	m^2
Volume	cubic metre	m^3
Density	kilogram per cubic metre	$kg \cdot m^{-3}$
Velocity	metre per second	$m \cdot s^{-1}$
Angular velocity	radian per second	$rad \cdot s^{-1}$
Acceleration	meter per second squared	$m \cdot s^{-2}$
Kinematic viscosity diffusion coefficient	square metre per second	$m^2 \cdot s^{-1}$
Dynamic viscosity	newton second per square metre, i.e. (Pascal second)	$N \cdot s \cdot m^{-2}$ or $Pa \cdot s$
Surface tension	newton per metre	$N \cdot m^{-1}$

an area equal to the square of the radius of that sphere (see Fig. 2.2). Luminous flux therefore has the dimensions of cd · sr. The amount of light actually shining on a surface, illuminance (lx), is further dependent on the area of the surface. Illuminance therefore has the dimensions of lm · m^{-2}, or cd · sr · m^{-2}.

SPECIALLY-AUTHORIZED NAMES AND SYMBOLS

SI allows the retention of some quantities which, although they can be defined in terms of the base units, are not decimal multiples or submultiples of them (see Table 2.6). The

101.325 Pa) and the wavelength unit, the angstrom (1 A = 10^{10} m). Also temporarily retained are some CGS units which are familiar in medicine such as the *poise* (P) for dynamic viscosity (1P = 10^{-1} Pa · s) and the *stokes* (St) for kinematic viscosity (1 St = 10^{-4} m^2 · s^{-1}).

Definitions and standards

With some quantities, the standard can be 'defined' in a way which is reproducible by any competent scientist who is suitably motivated. For such quantities, definitions have been developed which involve sub-

Table 2.6. Special authorized names and symbols.

Quantity	Unit		
	Name	Symbol	Value
Volume	litre	l	1 l = 1 dm^3 = 10^{-3} m^3
Mass	metric ton	t	1 t = 1 Mg = 10^3 kg
Pressure, stress	bar	bar	1 bar = 10^5 Pa

litre is a necessary convenience in medicine or we would find ourselves measuring cardiac output, for example, in cubic metres per second. The *bar* is a pressure close to atmospheric pressure and is useful in meteorology and in the gas industry. The unified *atomic mass* unit is one twelfth of the mass of an atom of ^{12}C. It is approximately equivalent to 1.660 565 5 × 10^{-27} kg. The *electronvolt* is the kinetic energy acquired by an electron passing in a vacuum from one point to another whose potential is one volt higher. 1 eV is approximately equal to 1.602 189 × 10^{-19} J.

NON-SI UNITS TEMPORARILY RETAINED

Several non-SI units have been retained, but will be reconsidered in the future. Of interest in medicine are the millimetre of mercury (1 mmHg = 133.322 Pa) for blood pressure, the standard atmosphere (1 atm =

stances which are universally available. For example time and length are now defined in terms of physical phenomena (atomic vibration of a particular atom and wavelength of a certain light), which are reproducible anywhere in the world. In practice, of course, an acknowledged authority provides a secondary standard, such as Greenwich for time or the National Physical Laboratory for temperature, and this is trusted to be as accurate as is humanly possible.

With regard to mass, however, such an approach is not at present possible. The definition of mass, as can be seen from page 14, is quite circular; a kilogram is equal to the mass of a lump of metal which we have chosen to say has a mass of a kilogram. If a lighter piece of metal were to be secretly substituted all other masses would, *by definition*, now be greater than they were! There is no external reference which would prove that the earth and all its works had not got more massive, although commonsense could be invoked in favour of the alternative explanation.

Several important quantities involve mass in their definition, in particular the newton and pascal. The newton is the force which would give a frictionless mass of one kilogram an acceleration of one metre per second per second, in a vacuum. It would be impossible to create such conditions terrestrially and quite difficult even in an orbiting satellite. The pascal is derived from the definition of the newton. Such definitions cannot, therefore, be used as standards for calibration.

For such purposes, the gravitational effect of the earth on mass has to be invoked so that columns of fluids of known density are still needed as standards for calibration even though they do not serve as a definition. Thus for the calibration of blood pressure manometers, columns of mercury will always be required. It can be argued that if blood pressure is being both calibrated and measured in millimetres of mercury it is only logical to express it in these units. (The fact that the marks on a sphygmomanometer are not exactly millimetres apart, due to the need to compensate for the change in level in the reservoir, is not relevant to this argument: although the marks are not millimetres apart, the pressure *is* in millimetres of mercury).

The case for abandoning such units and adopting pascals is not, therefore, related to a more universally available standard or to a more precise definition, but is concerned with providing a single measurement quantity for *all* pressure measurements. This is of particular importance in anaesthesia, for a doctor may be involved with pressure in a cylinder (labelled in atmospheres, lb/in^2, or kg/m^2), pressure in pipelines (labelled in kPa, bars, atmospheres or lb/in^2), airway or ventilator pressures (in cm of H_2O), blood pressure (in mmHg), central venous pressures (in mmHg with transducers or cmH$_2$O with U-tube manometers), pneumotachograph pressure manometers (in mmH$_2$O) and blood–gases in

kilopascals. The universal adoption of SI would help to clarify the magnitude of these pressures in relation to one another and would prevent a great deal of unnecessary confusion. Until then it is necessary to use the greatest care when converting one unit of measurement into another. This is particularly important in pressure measurement (see Table 12.1). Not only is it very easy to confuse the factor for conversion from old to new and vice versa, but a small error in a conversion factor when applied to a large number may result in a considerable absolute error. Suitable conversion factors for respiratory, cardiovascular and biochemical measurements are given in Tables 2.7 and 2.8.

Basic mathematical concepts

Most clinical measurement systems can be operated satisfactorily by persons with no mathematical knowledge. However, the principles on which measurement techniques are based can only be understood by those with some knowledge of basic mathematical concepts such as differentiation, integration, exponential and trigonometrical functions, and logarithms. This section attempts to provide a simple introduction to these concepts.

SYMBOLS AND FUNCTIONS

Mathematical statements are usually expressed as equations which are abbreviated by the use of symbols. These symbols may confuse those with a nonmathematical mind but can usually be rendered clearer by translating the statement into English. Thus $P \times V = k$ (Boyle's law) means that pressure (P) times volume (V) always equals a constant value (k) or that pressure must be inversely proportional to volume. In this equation P and V are *variables* and k is a *constant*.

If two variables are related in such a way that the value of one of them can only be determined when the other is known, the

Table 2.7. Conversion factors for units used in respiratory and cardiac physiology.

Quantity	Traditional units (x)	SI unit or multiple (y) Name	Symbol or units	Conversion factors (f) Old to SI $y = fx$	SI to old $x = fy$
Force	dyne	newton	N	1×10^{-5}	1×10^{5}
	kilopond kilogram-force }	newton	N	9.806	0.102
Pressure	mmHg or Torr }			0·133	7.501
	cmH$_2$O	kilopascal	kPa	0.098	10.197
	atmosphere }			101.325	0.010
	lb/square inch }			6.895	0.145
Energy	kilocalorie	joule	J	4.184	0.239
Work	kilopond metre/min	watt	W	9.806	0.102
Flow	litres/min	l/sec	$l \cdot s^{-1}$	0.017	60
Resistance—gas	cmH$_2$O/l/sec	kPa/l/sec	$kPa \cdot l^{-1} \cdot s$	0.098	10.197
—liquid	mmHg/l/min	kPa/l/sec	$kPa \cdot l^{-1} \cdot s$	7.999	0.125
Conductance	l/sec/cmH$_2$O	l/sec/kPa	$l \cdot s^{-1} kPa^{-1}$	10.197	0.098
Compliance	l/cmH$_2$O	l/kPa	$l \cdot kPa^{-1}$	10.197	0.098
Elastance	cmH$_2$O/l	kPa/l	$kPa \cdot l^{-1}$	0.098	10.197
O$_2$ consumption	ml/min STPD	mmol/min	$mmol \cdot min^{-1}$	0.045	22.40
CO$_2$ output	ml/min STPD	mmol/min	$mmol \cdot min^{-1}$	0.045	22.26*
O$_2$ concentration	vols per cent	mmol/l	$mmol \cdot l^{-1}$	0.446	2.240
CO$_2$ concentration	vols per cent	mmol/l	$mmol \cdot l^{-1}$	0.449	2.226*
Transfer coefficient	ml/min/mmHg	mmol/min/kPa	$mmol \cdot min^{-1} \cdot kPa^{-1}$	0.335	2.985

*Non-ideal gas.

Table 2.8. Conversion factors for blood chemistry and haematology.

Measurement	Traditional Unit (x)	SI Unit (y)	Conversion factors Old to SI $y = fx$	SI to old $x = fy$
Blood-gases	mmHg, Torr	kPa	0.133	7.501
Standard bicarbonate Base excess }	mEq/l	mmol/l	1.0	1.0
Calcium	mg/100 ml	mmol/l	0.25	4.0
Chloride	mEq/l	mmol/l	1.0	1.0
Cholesterol	mg/100 ml	mmol/l	0.026	38.7
Cortisol	μg/100 ml	nmol/l	27.6	0.036
Creatinine	mg/100 ml	μmol/l	88.4	0.011
Glucose	mg/100 ml	mmol/l	0.056	18.0
Magnesium	mg/100 ml	mmol/l	0.411	2.43
Potassium	mEq/l	mmol/l	1.0	1.0
Sodium	mEq/l	mmol/l	1.0	1.0
Urea	mg/100 ml	mmol/l	0.167	6.0
Hb	g/100 ml	g/dl	1.0	1.0
RBC WBC Platelets }	cells/mm^3	cells/l	10^6	10^{-6}

first variable is said to be a *function* of the second. The mathematical statement of this is that $y = f(x)$. The values of x and y which correspond with each other can be regarded as the *co-ordinates* of a point on an ordinary two-dimensional graph.

When plotted in this way $y = f(x)$ yields a straight line with a slope which is determined by f (Fig. 2.3). The line passes through zero on both x and y axes for if x is zero, f(x) is also zero. A slightly more complicated relationship is $y = f(x) + b$. In this case the slope of the line is the same but there is an intercept on the y axis: when x is zero $y = (f \times o) + b$ or $y = b$. Still more complicated equations yield graphs with different shapes. For example, the function $y = x^2$ yields a parabola which passes through zero (since zero squared is zero) whilst the function $y = x^2 + 5$ produces a similar parabola which has a y intercept at $+5$ (Fig. 2.4).

In these examples y varies in a manner which is proportional to the change of x. Therefore y is said to be the *dependent* variable and x the *independent* variable. f and b are *constants* which are fixed for

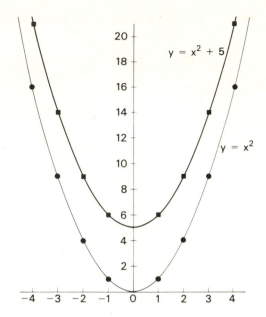

Fig. 2.4. Graphs of the two functions $y = x^2$ and $y = x^2 + 5$.

a particular set of conditions but may have a different value if conditions change. They are therefore called *parameters*.

SIMPLE TRIGONOMETRY

A knowledge of this topic is essential for an understanding of wave motion and biological signals. The functions to be considered are those relating to any triangle which contains one right angle (90°). It does not matter how large or small such a triangle is for when the size of one angle has been specified, the ratios of the lengths of the sides to each other are constant for all triangles in which that angle is the same. There are three pairs of sides and therefore three primary ratios (Fig. 2.5a). The side opposite the right angle is called the hypotenuse. The ratio of the length of the side opposite the defined angle (θ) to the length of the hypotenuse (BC ÷ AB) is called the *sine* of the angle θ. When the angle is very small the sine of the angle is itself very small (Fig. 2.5b). When the angle is close to 90° (Fig. 2.5c) the ratio approaches unity. The ratio of the adjacent side to the

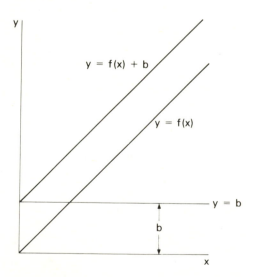

Fig. 2.3. Graphs of the three functions $y = b$, $y = f(x)$ and $y = f(x) + b$. x is the *independent* variable, y is the *dependent* variable, f is a *parameter* (the slope of the line) and b is a *parameter* (the y intercept).

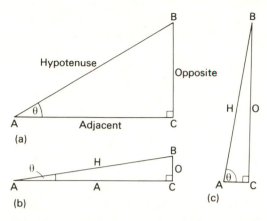

Fig. 2.5. a. A right-angled triangle. b. The sine of the angle is very small when θ is small. c. The sine approaches 1 when θ approaches 90°.

hypotenuse is called the *cosine*, so named because the cosine of the angle added to the sine of the *co*mplimentary angle opposite must add up to unity. The remaining ratio 'opposite divided by adjacent' is called the *tangent*.

The sine wave

Figure 2.6a represents a point (A) rotating around the circumference of a circle at constant velocity in the direction shown by the arrow. If the *amplitude* of displacement of point (A) from the axis (B–C) is plotted on the y co-ordinate and time on the x co-ordinate the graph shown in Fig. 2.6b is obtained. At each point in the cycle (A, A', A'') the displacement is given by $\sin \theta$, $\sin \theta'$ and $\sin \theta''$, so that the resultant shape is called a *sine wave*. Since the point is moving at constant velocity, the time axis can be calibrated in degrees, radians or time. Each complete revolution is termed a *cycle* and the number of complete cycles per second is the *frequency* of the wave in Hertz. The use of angular displacement as a measure of timing is particularly valuable when comparing phase differences between waves. Thus a second sine wave of identical characteristics starting at point X in Fig. 2.6b would be 90° out of phase with the original wave.

Physical quantities which vary in a sinusoidal fashion are legion. The generation of mains electricity is accomplished by rotating a coil in a magnetic field. The voltage generated is therefore sinusoidal in character. Oscillating systems oscillate in a sinusoidal fashion: the position of a weight, moving up and down on the end of a spring describes such a motion. Wave motion, e.g. light, is also sinusoidal. The important

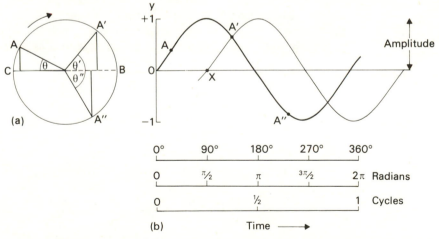

Fig. 2.6. a. The relationship of the sine wave to uniform motion in a circle. As the point (A) rotates at constant velocity its projection moves as in the graph on the right (Fig. 2.6b). Points A, A', A'', correspond with the points in the circle A, A', A''. The y value on the graph is equal to $\sin \theta$ and time can be measured in degrees of rotation or in cycles.

relationship to appreciate is that the relative magnitude of the y-axis at any particular instant can be derived by knowing the x value solely in terms of an angle.

The tangent

The tangent (opposite ÷ adjacent) is another trigonometrical ratio which is often involved in measurement. The tangent is a number which expresses the commonly understood notion of slope. A hill which rises one metre in a horizontal distance of two metres has a slope of one in two ($\frac{1}{2}$) or 0.5. Drawn on paper (Fig. 2.7a) such a slope is found when the angle is 30°. Tan 30° is therefore 0.5. Tan 45° can be seen to equal one when both sides equal 1 (Fig. 2.7b). In fact, between 0° and 90° the value of the tangent goes from zero to infinity.

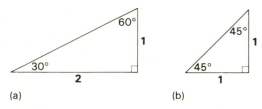

(a)   (b)

Fig. 2.7. Two right-angled triangles: tan 30° = $\frac{1}{2}$ = 0.5 (tan 60° = 2, tan 45° = 1).

The slope of the line which is climbing at 30° to the horizontal can equally be viewed in terms of an increase in the value of y for a given change of x, when the line is plotted on a traditional graph, i.e.

$$\text{slope} = \frac{y'' - y'}{x'' - x''},$$

where x', y', and x'', y'', are two points which lie on the line in Fig. 2.8. Since tan 30° = 0.5 it is not difficult to see that when $y'' - y' = 1$, $x'' - x'$ must equal 2. This relationship is equally described by the equation $2y = x$ or $y = 0.5x$. Thus the value which multiplies x in the straight line relationship between x and y is the value of the *slope*. In statistics the quantity measuring the slope is called the *regression coefficient* (p. 301).

In the first example, slope must have its natural meaning of a change of vertical distance per change of horizontal distance. Obviously, any such relationship when plotted, has a slope, even though the quantities themselves are unrelated to the notion of slope. For example, velocity (loosely equated with speed in common parlance), can be thought of as the slope of a line relating distance travelled to time. Thus, a graph showing the progress of a person walking one mile in 2 hours would look exactly the same as Fig. 2.8, the y-axis representing distance and the x-axis representing time. Distance divided by time, i.e. miles per hour, is velocity; this is represented on the graph by the slope, tan 30° or 0.5. If this idea is extended so

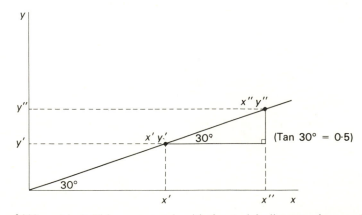

Fig. 2.8. A slope of 30°, or 1 in 2. This corresponds with the straight line equation $y = 0.5x$.

that y represents velocity and x represents time, the graph will show how velocity increases with time. The rate of change of velocity with time is now represented by the slope and so indicates acceleration.

DIFFERENTIALS

There are, of course, numerous occasions on which quantities do not change linearly with respect to time or with respect to any other variable. When a relationship between y and x is a complex function the result is usually a curve. For example the trigonometric function $y = \sin x$ results in an oscillating wave, the slope of which is constantly changing (Fig. 2.6). At the height of the peak and the bottom of the trough y is, for an instant, *not* changing and at these points the slope is zero. Likewise one can see that the slope is steepest as the line passes through the x-axis. There is no easy way of seeing, from the formula, what the slope is at any given moment. However, if one imagines that one could greatly enlarge a very, very short segment of the line (Fig. 2.9) at the point of interest, it would *seem* to be almost straight. The slope would

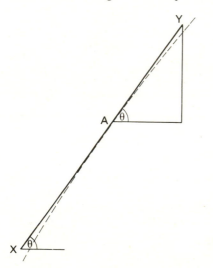

Fig. 2.9. An enlargement of a very short section of the curve of $y = \sin(x)$ from Fig. 2.6. θ is the angle between the straight line X–Y and the horizontal and instantaneously also between the curve and the horizontal at the point (A).

still be change of y for change in x, i.e. the tangent of the angle θ at point (A). The solid line, which is straight, just touches the curve at one point only; because the tangent of the angle at that point is the slope, it is not surprising that the solid line is said to touch the curve 'tangentially'.

In point of fact, a graphical solution is not sufficiently accurate or efficient. By using *calculus* (which is a form of mathematical manipulation which considers what the situation will be when one takes curves in infinitely small bits) one can calculate the slope at any required value of x. This is done by the mathematical process of *differentiating* the equation of the slope and substituting the required value of x. The differential of y which is thus obtained is the slope: in consequence velocity is often said to be the differential of distance with respect to time, and acceleration is the differential of velocity with respect to time. Acceleration may therefore be called the second differential of distance with respect to time. The word differential indicates the underlying concept: it is the actual difference in y for an infinitely small change in x.

INTEGRALS

The slope is not the only secondary function of a curve which may be of interest in measurement. The area between the curve and the x-axis between defined values of x is often required because of the quantity it represents. Again, it is simplest to start with a straight line example. Figure 2.10a represents the record which would be obtained when a flow of gas is turned on, allowed to flow at a constant rate for a given time, and then switched off. The record shows that a flow of five litres per minute flowed for six minutes. It is obvious that the total volume that passed was 30 litres. This answer has been obtained by multiplying the y and x values and is thus represented by the area between the line and the x-axis. (In dimensional terms, we have L^3T^{-1} (flow) $\times$ T (time) $= L^3$ (volume)).

Even if the volume had changed from

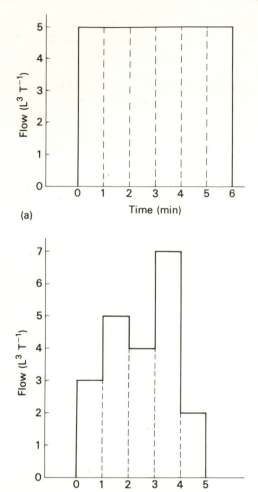

(a)

(b)

Fig. 2.10. a. Representation of a flow (constant) of 5 litres per minute running for 6 min. b. An irregular flow varying between 2 and 7 litres per minute changing each minute. Total volume (a) 30 litres, (b) 21 litres.

minute-to-minute as in Fig. 2.10b the same principle could be applied by adding up the separate columns. In this example the total volume would be 21 litres. However, when the line varies rapidly the application of this method is not so easy. Under such circumstances the total area could only be obtained by dividing the area under the curve into an infinite number of small strips and adding their areas (see Fig. 2.11). This technique is employed by the calculus and is termed *integration*.

The area under a curve is usually related to the total quantity of the substance: the area under a flow–time curve is a volume; flow is therefore integrated to give volume. The area under a concentration curve plotted against time gives quantity and is used in the calculation of cardiac output by the dye dilution method (see p. 211). Similarly the area under the peak of a gas chromatogram represents the total quantity of the substance present.

Both differentiation and integration are easily performed by electronic means. Integration may also be performed mechanically, either by cutting out the area of the curve and relating the weight of the paper to the weight of a known area of paper or by using an instrument such as a *planimeter* which mechanically integrates the area as a small wheel is moved around the line delineating the curve.

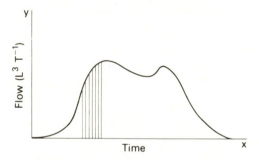

Fig. 2.11. A varying flow plotted against time. Again the area can be discovered by summating columns under the curve to give the total area.

POWER FUNCTIONS AND LOGARITHMS

The notion of powers is a commonplace one and, in its simplest form, easily comprehended. The notation 10^2, may be read as 'ten squared' or 'ten to the (power) two'. The arithmetic solution is the number ten, multiplied by itself, i.e. 10×10, or one hundred. At the practical level, it gives the area of the square, the length of whose sides is ten units. In the same way it is fairly easy to visualize the practical meaning of 10^3, i.e. ten cubed or 1000, which is the volume of a cube whose sides are each 10 units long. However, such a concrete view is not helpful when one considers 10^4 and higher powers, even though the mathematical answer ($10^4 = 10\,000$, $10^5 = 100\,000$) is but a simple extension of the same idea.

The figure 5 in 10^5 is termed the *index* or *exponent* and signifies that five tens are to be multiplied together to get $100\,000$ or that ten is to be raised to the power of five. The 5 may also be referred to as the *logarithm* of $100\,000$ to the *base* ten. In mathematical notation this is written $\log_{10}(100\,000) = 5$. Thus the logarithmic notation is another way of expressing exponential relationships.

It will be apparent that all the numbers between 10 and 100, or between $10\,000$ and $100\,000$ can be characterized by exponents between 1 and 2, or between 4 and 5. These can be derived from tables of common logarithms or from an electronic calculator. Thus the logarithm of 10 is 1, and the logarithm of 20 is 1.301, whilst the logarithms of $10\,000$ and $20\,000$ are 4 and 4.301. Similar (antilog) tables are available to change logarithms back to natural numbers. *A logarithm, then, is the power to which a fixed number (the base) must be raised to produce a given number.* Note that since $\log 1 = 0$ the logarithm of any number below 1 must be a negative quantity. Furthermore it is not possible to have a logarithm of a negative number.

Logarithms have several useful properties. Thus two numbers may be multiplied together by adding the logarithms of the numbers. Division is achieved by subtracting one logarithm from another and a number can be raised to a given power by multiplying the logarithm of the number by that power. In all these manipulations the answer is obtained by taking the antilog of the result. Table 2.9 summarizes these calculations in both logarithmic and exponential notation.

Logarithms are also used to compress a numerical scale. Thus the normal hydrogen-ion concentration is $0.000\,000\,04$ grams per litre (i.e. 4 out of $100\,000\,000$) or $4 \times 10^{-8}\,\text{g} \cdot 1^{-1}$. Since $\text{pH} = -\log[\text{H}^+]$ we may rewrite this as

$$-\text{pH} = \log(4) + \log(10^{-8})$$
$$= 0.6 - 8 = -7.4$$

or $\quad \text{pH} = 7.4$.

Since pH $7.0 = 100$ and pH $8.0 = 10$ one pH unit represents a tenfold change in $[\text{H}^+]$ (see Table 18.1).

Logarithmic changes are of importance in biology for many input–output functions are related logarithmically. Thus a ten-fold increase in drug concentration is often required to double the effect whilst a ten-fold increase in energy input is required to make a light appear twice as bright. Logarithmic units are also used when comparing amounts of power. The relevant unit is the *bel* (*B*), two amounts of power P_1 and P_2 differing by N bels when:

$$N = \log\left(\frac{P_2}{P_1}\right).$$

Table 2.9. Methods of calculation using logarithmic and exponential notations.

Logarithmic	Exponential
$\log(M \cdot N) = \log(M) + \log(N)$	$B^m \cdot B^n = B^{m+n}$
$\log\dfrac{M}{N} = \log(M) - \log(N)$	$\dfrac{B^m}{B^n} = B^{m-n}$
$\log(M^n) = n \cdot \log(M)$	$(B^m)^n = B^{m \cdot n}$
$\log\sqrt[n]{M} = \log(M^{1/n}) = \dfrac{1}{n}\log(M)$	$\sqrt[n]{B^m} = (B^m)^{1/n} = B^{m \cdot n}$

For example if $P_2 = 1000\,\text{W}$ and $P_1 = 10\,\text{W}$, then $P_2/P_1 = 100$, $\log 100 = 2$, so that the ratio is 2 bels.

Thus 1 bel represents a ten-fold alteration in power, 2 bels a hundred-fold and so on.

In electronic apparatus power comparisons are usually made in *decibels* (*dB*). These units are one tenth of a bel so that:

$$N = 10 \cdot \log_{10}\left(\frac{P_2}{P_1}\right) \text{dB}.$$

One decibel represents an alteration in sound intensity of about 26 per cent, which is about the smallest change that the ear can detect.

Other bases

Logarithms to the base 10 are termed *common* or *Briggsian* logarithms after the Englishman who invented them nearly four centuries ago. Their convenience lies in the fact that common logarithms of numbers with the same significant figures differ by a whole number, the difference depending on the relative positions of the decimal point in the numbers. Thus $\log 3.650 = 0.5623$ whilst $\log 365.0 = 2.5623$. However, there is no reason why we should not use some other base such as 2. Then since $2^2 = 4$, 2 is the logarithm of 4, but this time *to the base* 2. This base is used in binary arithmetic (p. 62). Strangely enough the most common base other than 10 is an *irrational* number, a nonterminating decimal denoted by the symbol e. It has a value of 2.71828. . . . This number and the constant π ($= 3.14159 \ldots$) are the two most widely-used constants in mathematics.

Logarithms to the base e are variously known as *natural, Naperian* or, less commonly, as *hyperbolic* logarithms. They offer none of the computational conveniences of common logarithms, their importance being related to the function e^x, which is very relevant to growth and decay processes in biology and medicine. In modern terminology $\log_e(x)$ is usually written $\ln(x)$ or $\ln x$ (the natural logarithm

of x), whereas $\log_{10}(x)$ is often written $\log(x)$.

It is important to realize that the special characteristics of a logarithmic pattern of change are not affected by the base used for the logarithms simply differ by a proportionality factor. Conversions between common and natural logarithms are effected by using the equations:

$$\ln x = 2.302585 \cdot \log x$$
$$\log x = 0.434294 \cdot \ln x$$

In order to grasp the significance of e it is now necessary to consider the exponential function.

THE EXPONENTIAL FUNCTION

This is a function which arises so often in physics and in physiology that it requires a special mention. A number of processes increase or decrease in a way in which the *rate* at which the process is proceeding is proportional either to how far it has gone, or to how far it still has to go. Such processes are termed *exponential functions*. Compound interest is an example of a process in which one's money increases at a progressively faster rate if the interest is continuously reinvested. The passive emptying of the lung is a process in which the rate slows down as it approaches a final figure because the difference between the recoil pressure of the lung and the atmospheric pressure becomes progressively smaller as the lung empties. The filling of the lungs in response to the application of a constant positive pressure to the airway is an example of the same process in reverse. These phenomena are typified by the three curves in Fig. 2.12–2.14 and are known respectively as breakaway, wash-out and wash-in curves. Why is e the basis of such curves? It is easiest to grasp the concept by considering compound interest, which is an example of the simple *breakaway function* $y = e^x$. Suppose one was lucky enough to invest £100 at 100% per annum (or expressed as a fraction, × 1 per annum). If the interest were calculated and paid at the end

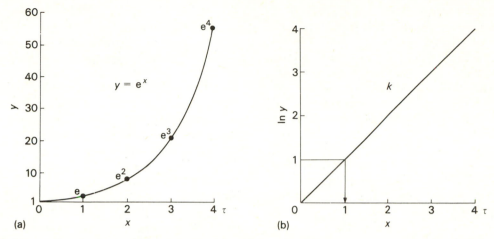

Fig. 2.12. a. The breakaway function $y = e^x$. This would describe the pattern of growth associated with compound interest. b. The logarithmic replot of (a). k = rate constant. τ = time constant.

of every complete year one would possess £200 at the end of the first year. Suppose however, that the interest were calculated every six months and immediately re-invested. At the end of the first six months one's investment would be worth £150. During the second six months the interest would be calculated on £150 rather than the original sum, so that £75 would be earned instead of £50. The total at the end of the year would now be £225, which is £25 more than with the single calculation day. One would need to be an inept investor not to suggest even more frequent calculation points! If one tries successively three, four, five...eight, ten times a year one can calculate that the year end sum would be respectively, £237, £244, £248,...£256,... £259. Clearly the gain from more and more divisions is not getting very much greater. Ultimately if one calculated daily, hourly, by the minute, or infinitely frequently, the 'best' one can ever do is to get the sum up to £271.83. The original sum has thus been increased by a factor of 2.7183 which is an approximation to the value of e. Expressed mathematically,

$$\frac{\text{final sum}}{\text{starting sum}} = e.$$

If the interest rate were set at 200%, or ×2,

the effect of compound growth would be even more startling, for the investment would not yield £300 (simple interest) but £729. The above equation can now be written

$$\frac{\text{final sum}}{\text{starting sum}} = 8.29 = e^2.$$

It can now be seen that raising e to the *power* of the interest rate (as a fraction), yields the growth of the starting sum over a single time period. To calculate for several years, the exponent (2 in this case) is simply multiplied by the number of time periods. Thus $y = e^{kt}$, where k is the *rate*, and t the number of periods. After 5 years at 50% interest, the investor would therefore have

$$100 \times e^{0.5 \times 5} = 100 \times e^{2.5} = £1218.25.$$

Now if the natural logarithms are taken of both sides of the equation $y = e^{kt}$, the result is $\ln y = kt$, or $\ln y/t = k$ (because the natural logarithm of a number is the power to which e must be raised to yield that number). A graph of $\ln y$ against t will therefore be a straight line of gradient k (Fig. 2.12b).

From this graph a fundamental property of exponential change can be deduced. The time taken for any value of y to increase by a factor of 2.718 (i.e. 1 on the natural log. scale since ln 2.718 = 1) is constant and is the reciprocal of the rate k. Thus if it takes 1 year the slope is 1, but if it takes 2 years it is 0.5. Since kt is the exponent in the equation $y = e^{kt}$, the ratio of final to starting value can be solved for any value of t. For example if the accrued sum were found to be £271.83 after 0.5 years, $k = 1/0.5 = 2$, or 200%. If on the other hand it took 10 years to accrue, $k = \frac{1}{10} = 0.1$, or 10% interest. The time to rise by a factor of 2.718... is called the time constant, and given the greek letter τ (tau). k is termed the rate constant, and since it is $1/\tau$, has the dimension of reciprocal time, i.e. hours^{-1} or, in this example, years^{-1}.

It will now be evident that given a starting value and either τ or k, the value at any time can easily be calculated.

If a process is exponential and some values at different times are known, then a plot of ln y against time will be most useful, since the slope k can be determined graphically.

If logarithms are not readily available, a less precise alternative is to plot the values of y on graph paper whose vertical axis is printed at logarithmic intervals. This method demonstrates the linear relationship, but does not help us to calculate k.

The log of one variable plotted against a second variable is called a semilogarithmic or log–linear plot as opposed to a log–log plot in which both axes are on logarithmic scales. Semilog plots are very useful in that they both demonstrate the exponential relationship and enable extrapolation or interpolation to other parts of the time scale (e.g. computation of cardiac output from part of the dilution curve).

The washout, or exponential decay function is mathematically very similar to the breakaway function, except that the rate constant is negative. Thus the ratio of 'new' to 'starting value' (y) is an exponentially decaying system is characterized by $y = e^{-kt}$ (see Fig. 2.13). This yields a straight line on a semilog plot of gradient $-k$. The decay of charge as a capacitor discharges through a resistor is a simple example of washout exponential decay. It is also exemplified by the change in concentration of a gas in the lung when replaced by a second gas, by the change of lung volume during a passive expiration or by the downslope of a dye-dilution curve. In all these circumstances, the quantity under consideration decreases at a rate which is proportional to the amount still present. (The similarity with the breakaway function should now be

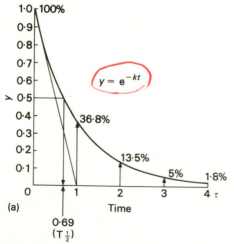
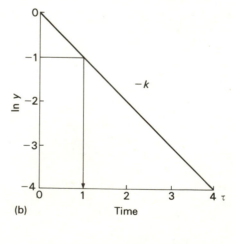

Fig. 2.13. a. The washout curve $y = e^{-kt}$. This would describe the discharging of a capacitor or the passive emptying of the lungs. Time expressed in terms of time constants. $T_{\frac{1}{2}}$ is seen to be 0.69 of a time constant b. The logarithmic replot of (a). k = the rate constant.

clear, since in both cases the rate of growth or decay is directly proportional to the amount present). If the *initial* decay rate is extrapolated (Fig. 2.13) it reaches zero after l time constant (τ). During 1 time constant, the value in fact decays to $1/e$ of its initial value (i.e. $1/2.718 = 36.8\%$).

In a second similar period, the value will again fall by the same proportion, but during the decay over two time constants, it will fall to $1/e^2 = 1/7.389 = 13.54\%$. Over four time constants it decays to $1/e^4 = 1/54.60 = 1.83\%$ of the original value. As the decay proceeds, it approaches zero at an ever decreasing rate, and theoretically reaches it at time infinity.

Exponential decays are often characterized by a parameter known as the half-life ($T_{\frac{1}{2}}$). This is the time taken for the value to halve, and is, of course, constant throughout the decay. Since $\tau = 1/k$, the value of t when $y/y_0 = 0.5$ will be; $\ln 0.5 = -t/\tau$, so $t = 0.698\,\tau$. The half-life is thus a simple fraction of the time constant.

The time constant is determined by the characteristics of the system. For example, the rate of emptying of the lungs depends on the compliance of the lungs (C) and the resistance of the airways (R) so that $\tau = CR$. Hence if compliance is increased

(i.e. there is a smaller recoil pressure for a given volume) or resistance is increased, the rate of emptying will be reduced because of the increased time constant.

The wash-in exponential function is different from the other two, in that the variable rises to a final value (called the asymptote) at an ever-decreasing rate (Fig. 2.14). The ratio of present to final volume (y) is characterized by the expression $y = 1 - e^{-kt}$. The rate constant is negative since this is really an exponential *decay* although the function is rising. The wash-in function is exemplified by the increase in volume of the lung resulting from the application of a constant pressure to the airway, by the change in gas concentration in a lung after it is suddenly switched to a new gas mixture or by the increase in blood P_{CO_2} after a step reduction in ventilation.

As in the other functions, it is possible to obtain a straight line by a logarithmic transform, but not directly, since $-e^{-kt}$ has no logarithm. The equation is instead rearranged to $1 - y = e^{-kt}$, and then transformed to $\ln(1 - y)/t = -k$.

The linear transforms of an exponential function can be displayed graphically on a semilogarithmic plot, i.e. the log of the variable (or its ratio with starting or finishing

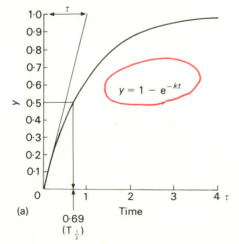

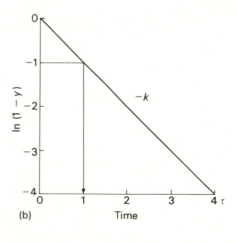

Fig. 2.14. a. The wash-in curve $y = 1 - e^{-kt}$. This would describe the pattern of charging of a capacitor or the filling of the lungs in response to the application of a constant pressure to the airway. $\tau =$ time constant. b. Logarithmic replot of (a). $k =$ rate constant.

values) plotted on the ordinate, and time on the abscissa. The rate constants can then be derived immediately from the slopes of the straight lines.

The recognition that there is a logarithmic relationship between two variables greatly facilitates data handling in many measurement applications. For example, the downslope of the dye-dilution curve in cardiac output measurement is known to be exponential but the lower part of this curve is altered by the occurrence of recirculation of the indicator. By establishing the rate constant from a semilog plot of the early part of the downslope it is possible to predict the shape of the lower part of the curve and so establish the area under the curve (p. 211). Another example is provided by the analysis of washout curves which represent a composite of two or more exponential processes (e.g. the washout of slow and fast compartments in the lung, or the washout of a radioactive tracer from the grey and white matter in the brain). Replotting of the washout data on semilog paper permits the two processes to be separated by manual exponential stripping of the curves (p. 216) so that the contribution of each process can be defined. Many biological mechanisms respond logarithmically to a stimulus. Thus the output of biological receptor systems such as touch, hearing and sight varies as the logarithm of the stimulus whilst many responses to drugs are also related to the logarithm of drug dose. Thus if the response is plotted against the logarithm of the stimulus or drug dose a straight line is obtained. This greatly facilitates subsequent statistical processing of the results.

The breakaway curve of compound growth is commonly encountered in biology and medicine but has little application in measurement. The build-up and die-away curves are, however, ubiquitous. Light decreases in intensity exponentially as it passes through a coloured solution:

voltages build up and discharge from capacitors exponentially: lungs empty, drip rates fall, drug concentrations fall, radioactivity decreases, all exponentially.

It is unlikely that a doctor undertaking clinical measurement will need to be able to work out any particular exponential function. However, it is not difficult, and anyone wishing to acquire the simple mathematical skills involved is recommended to read Waters & Mapleson (1964), Franklin & Newman (1973), Hogben (1974), Duffin (1976) and Nunn (1978).

References

UNITS

BARRON D.N., BROUGHTON P.M.G., COHEN M., LANSLEY T.S., LEWIS S.M. & SHINTON N.K. (1974) The use of SI units in reporting results obtained in hospital laboratories. *Journal of Clinical Pathology*, **27**, 590.

Official Journal of the European Communities (1976) **19**, No. 1262 (Legislation).

PADMORE G.R.A. & NUNN J.F. (1974) S.I. Units in relation to anaesthesia. *British Journal of Anaesthesia*, **46**, 236.

Statutory Instruments (1976). *Weights & measures. The Units of Measurement Regulations, 1976, No. 1674*, H.M.S.O. London.

(1977) *Units, Symbols and Abbreviations. A guide for biological and medical editors and authors.* London: Royal Society of Medicine.

MATHEMATICS

DUFFIN J. (1976) *Physics for anaesthetists*. Springfield, Illinois: C.C. Thomas.

FRANKLIN D.A. & NEWMAN G.B. (1973) *A guide to medical mathematics*. Oxford: Blackwell Scientific Publications.

HOGBEN L. (1974) *Mathematics for the million*. London: Allen & Unwin Ltd.

NUNN J.F. (1978) *Applied respiratory physiology*. London: Butterworth.

WATERS D.J. & MAPLESON W.W. (1964) Exponentials and the anaesthetist. *Anaesthesia*, **19**, 274.

Chapter 3
Simple Electronics

Although most of the apparatus used in clinical measurement can now be operated by personnel who have no knowledge of electronics, some understanding of basic electronic principles is necessary for those who wish to use their equipment to the fullest advantage. This chapter deals with the fundamental concepts which are referred to in later sections of the text and again assumes that the reader has no previous knowledge of the subject.

DIRECT CURRENT

When a potential difference exists between two points on a conductor, a current will flow. The relationship between the current and potential difference is contained in Ohm's law:

> *The potential difference between two points on a conductor through which a current is flowing is proportional to the current, provided that physical conditions remain constant.*

This relationship can be expressed mathematically:

$$\frac{E}{I} = k \qquad \left(\frac{V}{I} = R\right)$$

where E = potential difference (volts), I = current (amperes) and k is a constant which has the dimension of resistance, and can thus be expressed in ohms. If R symbolizes resistance then $E/I = R$, and by rearrangement, $E = IR$ and $I = E/R$. The use of this relationship is illustrated in Fig. 3.1a. If two

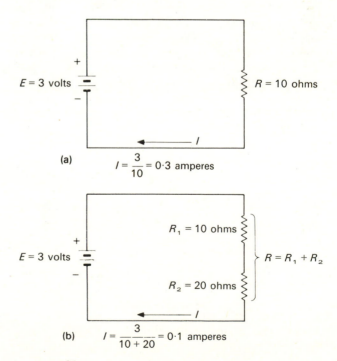

(a) E = 3 volts R = 10 ohms

$$I = \frac{3}{10} = 0.3 \text{ amperes}$$

(b) E = 3 volts R_1 = 10 ohms R_2 = 20 ohms $R = R_1 + R_2$

$$I = \frac{3}{10 + 20} = 0.1 \text{ amperes}$$

Fig. 3.1. Ohm's law is used to calculate the current (I) (a) in a simple resistive circuit, and (b) in a circuit with two resistances in series.

31

resistors are connected in series the total resistance presented by the combination is simply the sum of the two (Fig. 3.1b). If, on the other hand, the same two resistors are connected in parallel (Fig. 3.2), the combined resistance is determined by the expression:

$$\frac{1}{R} = \frac{1}{R_1} + \frac{1}{R_2}$$

When a current passes through a resistance, work is done and heat generated. The <u>rate at which work is done is power, i.e. energy per unit time.</u> Thus <u>1 joule (energy)</u> expended in <u>1 second</u> is <u>1 watt</u> of power. Power in this context is the product of the current through the resistor and the voltage across it. Thus in Fig. 3.1a, 0.3 amperes and 3 volts produce a power dissipation of 0.9 watts, or 900 mW.

It is, of course possible to derive expressions for power for all Ohm's law variables. For example:

$$W = E \times I \quad \text{so} \quad W = \frac{E^2}{R} \quad \text{and} \quad W = I^2R.$$

Power calculations are basic to even the simplest circuit design, as all components must be capable of dissipating the heat generated. (If, for instance we take a 100-ohm resistor rated at 5 watts, and pass 0.5 amperes through it, the power dissipation will be $0.5^2 \times 100 = 25$ watts, so that it will promptly explode!)

ALTERNATING CURRENT

Faraday's Law of electromagnetic induction states that '*when the flux-linkage between a coil and a magnetic field is varying, an induced electromotive force (e.m.f.) is set up in the coil proportionate to the rate of change of the flux-linkage*'. (In very simple terms, the rate of change of flux linkage between a wire and a magnetic field can be considered to be the rate at which it crosses the magnetic lines of force.) If a loop of wire is rotated between the poles of a permanent magnet, the flux-linkage will change continuously, inducing an e.m.f. which reverses in polarity after every 180° of rotation, i.e. an alternating e.m.f. The rate of change of flux-linkage is proportional to the sine of the angle through which the loop has turned, and so produces an e.m.f. whose magnitude is also proportional to the sine of the angle (Fig. 3.3). Thus if we designate the peak current during the cycle as $I_{\max}$ and the rotational angle of the coil θ, the current I at any point in the cycle will be $I_{\max} \sin \theta$. For this reason, the current waveform is called a *sine-wave*. When an alternating current passes through a resistor, the potential across it always obeys Ohm's law, and therefore has an identical sinusoidal appearance ($E = E_{\max} \sin \theta$) and is precisely in phase with the current. The *frequency* of the alternating current is the number of complete cycles per sec, and is expressed in Hertz (Hz). Mains electricity

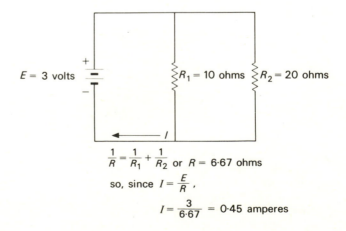

$E = 3$ volts

$R_1 = 10$ ohms $R_2 = 20$ ohms

$$\frac{1}{R} = \frac{1}{R_1} + \frac{1}{R_2} \quad \text{or} \quad R = 6.67 \text{ ohms}$$

so, since $I = \frac{E}{R}$,

$$I = \frac{3}{6.67} = 0.45 \text{ amperes}$$

Fig. 3.2. Ohm's law applied to two resistances (R_1 and R_2) in parallel.

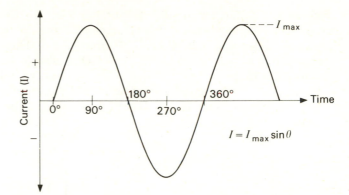

Fig. 3.3. Alternating current produced by the rotation of a coil in a magnetic field. The horizontal axis represents *time*, and is therefore related to the angular position of the coil as it turns (θ).

is supplied at 50 Hz in Britain but at 60 Hz in the USA.

Now if we pass an alternating current through a resistor, work will be done, and heat generated. Since both current and voltage are constantly changing, there is no conveniently static way of calculating 'watts', so that we must go back to first principles. Since the power dissipation is determined by $W = I^2 R$, it is evident that we need a value for I^2.

Figure 3.4 shows the sinusoidal current, and a continuously computed line representing I^2. (This will always be positive irrespective of the sign for I.) The heat dissipated will be related to the *mean* value of I^2, averaged over the whole cycle, so that the mean of the I^2 wave form can be inserted directly into the power equation above. *The effective* value for I is the square root of this 'mean I^2', value, and as such can be used in other Ohm's law equations.

This Root Mean Square current (r.m.s.) is the form in which amperes are expressed in a.c. circuits. When considering volts, we have a precisely analogous situation so that a.c. volts are also expressed in r.m.s. terms.

Thus the domestic mains supply voltage of 240 volts is actually 240 V. r.m.s., the instantaneous voltage alternating between $+339$ volts and -339 volts, 50 times per second.

CAPACITANCE

If two conductors (plates) are separated by an insulator (dielectric) a capacitor is formed. In its simplest form, this consists of two metal plates separated by a thin layer of air. When connected to a battery as in Fig. 3.5a (with S_1 closed) a current flows. The current flowing into the capacitor cannot escape from the other plate, but is stored as a static charge in the dielectric. If the potential of this charge were measured, it would be seen to rise progressively to the same voltage as the source (E) and then stop (Fig. 3.5b).

The size of a capacitor determines the quantity of electricity it can absorb for a given rise of charge potential, and depends upon the surface area of the plates, the thickness of the dielectric, and its ability to store charge (permittivity). The unit of

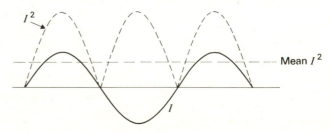

Fig. 3.4. R.m.s. current.

capacitance is the Farad (F).* 1 coulomb of electricity (which passes when 1 ampere flows for 1 second) will charge a 1 farad capacitor to a potential of 1 volt. Thus if Q coulombs charge C Farads, $E = Q/C$. It follows that if a capacitor is charged by a constant current, the potential will rise at a constant rate.

and so on. Thus as the capacitor discharges, the current decreases progressively (Fig. 3.6). This behaviour can be described by the simple exponential expression $V_t = E \cdot e^{-kt}$, where V_t is the voltage across the capacitor at t seconds, E the initial charge (10 volts) and k the rate constant (see Chapter 2).

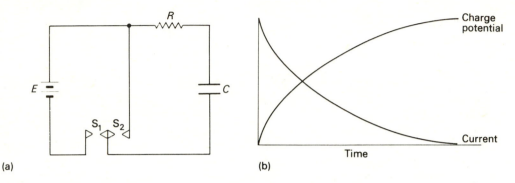

(a)   (b)

Fig. 3.5. a. Circuit containing resistance (R) and capacitance (C). If S_1 is closed, the capacitor charges; if S_2 is closed it discharges. b. The current and voltage waveforms following closure of the switch (S_1).

If the capacitor in Fig. 3.5a is charged to 10 volts (by closing S_1 for a few seconds) and then allowed to discharge through the resistor (by closing S_2) the initial current will be $E/R = \frac{10}{10} = 1$ ampere. As soon as this initial current flows, the charge on the capacitor is reduced. When it is reduced to, say 9 volts, the discharge current will fall to 0.9 amperes; when 5 volts to 0.5 amperes

If the initial discharge current were continued, and did not decline progressively, it would reach zero at τ seconds, this symbol being called the *time constant*. Since $\tau = 1/k$ and is expressed in seconds, k has the dimension of reciprocal seconds or s^{-1}. In any circuit analogous to that shown in Fig. 3.5a the time constant (seconds) is the product of the resistance (ohms) and capacitance (farads), i.e. $\underline{\tau = R \times C}$ seconds. The behaviour of the circuit can now be fully expressed as:

$$V_t = E \cdot e^{-t/R \cdot C}$$

* In practice, a 1F capacitor is very large, so that the microfarad (μF $= 10^{-6}$F) or picofarad (pF $= 10^{-12}$F) are more usual units.

Fig. 3.6. Exponential decay of current during the discharge of a capacitor through a resistor. τ is the time constant, during which the current falls to $\frac{1}{e}$ of its initial value (i.e. 37%).

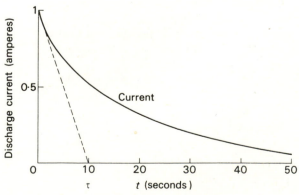

so that, knowing the values for R and C, V_t can be calculated at any time. In this case, $\tau = R \times C = 10$ seconds, so that the equation becomes:

$$V_t = E \cdot e^{-t/10}$$

Thus after 10 seconds (1τ),

$$V_t = E \cdot e^{-1} = 10 \times \frac{1}{e} = 10 \times 0.37$$

$$= 3.7 \text{ volts.}$$

If a capacitor is placed in an alternating current circuit (Fig. 3.7a) a more complex situation arises. It will be recalled that when a direct voltage is applied to a capacitor,

leads the voltage by 90°. This is illustrated in Fig. 3.7b which shows that when the current has reached its peak at 360°, the voltage has risen only to zero.

It will be apparent that the current 'through' a capacitor is <u>proportional</u> to the <u>*rate of change* of</u> the applied voltage. Thus a rise in frequency (which increases the rate of change of current) will result in an increased current; and a decrease in frequency, a reduced current. The variation in current with frequency implies a proportionate variation in the 'opposition to current flow' presented by the capacitor. Since this 'opposition' varies with frequency, it cannot be termed resistance, and so is

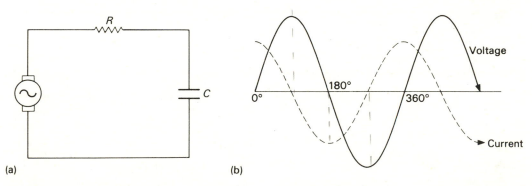

Fig. 3.7. a. An a.c. circuit containing resistance (R) and capacitance (C) in series. b. Current through, and voltage across the capacitor.

the current rapidly falls to zero, and the charge potential rapidly rises to that of the source (Fig. 3.5b). In an <u>a.c. circuit,</u> the <u>applied voltage is constantly changing</u> in opposite directions, so that the <u>current and voltage *never reach* the steady-state</u> conditions, but follow sinusoidal waveforms of the same frequency as the source. Figure 3.5b shows that the voltage on the capacitor and the current do not change in direct proportion (as would be the case for a resistor), and Fig. 3.7b shows that they are, in fact, <u>90° out of phase</u>, for the <u>current is maximal when the voltage is changing fastest</u> (i.e. passing through <u>zero</u>), and <u>minimal</u> when the <u>voltage is not changing</u> at all (i.e. <u>at peak values</u>). The phase difference is such that the current waveform

given the special term 'reactance'. The reactance of a capacitor (X_c) may be calculated from the formula

$$X_c = \frac{1}{2\pi f C} \text{ ohms,}$$

where f is the frequency (Hz). Although the <u>units of reactance are *ohms*</u> they cannot be inserted directly into Ohm's law equations because of the phase difference between current and voltage in a capacitative circuit. We must instead consider both resistive and <u>reactive</u> 'ohms' present in the circuit, and calculate the <u>overall opposition</u> to current flow (the *impedance*) at the frequency required, taking the phase differences into account. Only then can Ohm's law be used to compute current, etc.

The resulting 'impedance Ohms' *can* be used directly in Ohm's law equations, but *cannot* be added directly to other resistances or reactances, for all the resistance and capacitance in the circuit must be taken into account to yield an effective value for impedance. If there is more than one capacitor, the nett capacitance must first be found. Capacitors in parallel are simply summed but capacitors in series are calculated:

$$\frac{1}{C} = \frac{1}{C_1} + \frac{1}{C_2} + \frac{1}{C_3} \dots$$

(This is of course the same calculation as for resistors in parallel.)

INDUCTANCE

An *inductor* is a circuit element consisting of a number of turns of wire wound in the form of a coil. The centre space of the coil may contain only air, or a *core* of magnetic material. When a steady current flows through the inductor, it is impeded only by the relatively small resistance of the wire forming the coil. However, a change in current produces a change in the magnetic field induced by the current. This change in magnetic field induces an e.m.f. in the coil which opposes the change in current which produced it (the so-called back-e.m.f.). The effect of the inductor is thus like a brake, since it slows down any change of current, irrespective of whether the current is increasing or decreasing. When, in Fig. 3.8a, the switch is closed the current rises rapidly, but is 'braked' by the back-e.m.f., so that it only slowly reaches its final value (Fig. 3.8b). Similarly, the voltage across the inductor is maximal when the switch is first closed, and the rate of change of current maximal; it then decays to zero as the current settles to a steady value. Current and voltage are thus 90° out of phase, but in a different manner to that of a capacitor. In the capacitor, the charge potential is maximal and current zero when a steady e.m.f. is applied, whereas in the inductor,

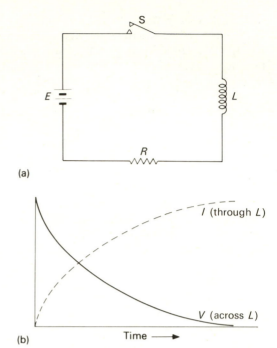

(a)

(b)   Time ⟶

Fig. 3.8. a. A circuit containing a resistance (R) and inductance (L) in series. b. Voltage and current waveforms following closure of switch S.

the current is maximal and the voltage across it zero under the same conditions.

The unit of inductance is the *henry* (H). When the current through a coil changes at a rate of 1 ampere per second, a 1 henry coil will induce a back-e.m.f. of 1 volt. The voltage across the inductor in Fig. 3.8a will, in fact decay exponentially, in an exactly analogous fashion to the decay of current in a capacitor, so

$$V_t = E \cdot e^{-Rt/L}$$

where the time constant is now L/R seconds.

If, in a steady state, the switch is suddenly opened, a reverse situation exists, in that the current now tends to stop, but the collapsing magnetic field induces an e.m.f. which attempts to maintain the current. Since the 'resistance' of the circuit is now infinite, the continuing current may raise the voltage to a very high level, until the current sparks across the switch con-

$(V = I \cdot R)$

$R \doteq \infty$

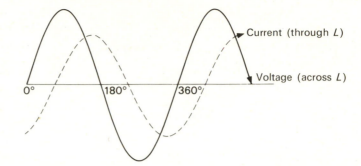

Fig. 3.9. Voltage and current waveforms in an inductive circuit.

tacts. (Switches controlling heavy inductive loads have to be protected against this eventuality, as it may lead to the switch contacts welding together.)

There is always a resistive element in an inductive circuit, due to the resistance of the wire from which the coil is wound, so that a perfect inductor is unattainable. The efficiency of an inductor is indicated by the ratio of the inductance to its resistance, and is greatly increased by the presence of a magnetic core (i.e. ferrite).

If an inductor is placed in an a.c. circuit the current and voltage follow sinusoidal waveforms as in the case of the capacitor, but with different phase relationships. Since the current in the a.c. circuit is constantly changing, the back e.m.f. will also change constantly, and will be related to the rate of change of the applied current. Thus the voltage across the inductor is greatest when the current is changing most rapidly (i.e. crossing zero) (Fig. 3.9). At 90° the voltage has reached its peak, but the current has only just risen to zero, so that the current now lags behind the voltage by 90°. An inductor has a reactance to an a.c. current, which, since the opposition rises as the rate of change of current increases, will increase linearly with frequency, according to the expression:

$$X_L = 2\pi f L$$

where L is the inductance in henrys. The impedance in an inductive circuit can be calculated by a method similar to that used for capacitance.

We may now consider a circuit in which

inductance, capacitance and resistance are all present in the same circuit (Fig. 3.10). The combined reactances of the capacitor and inductor are not simply additive, since we have just shown that the voltages across the two are 180° out of phase (i.e. directly opposing), and will tend to cancel out.

Consider the variation of reactance (X_C) and inductance (X_L) with frequency (Fig. 3.10b). There is a frequency (f_r) at which X_C and X_L are identical, so that they will cancel

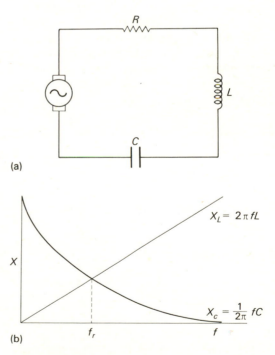

Fig. 3.10. a. An a.c. circuit containing resistance (R), inductance (L) and capacitance (C) in series. b. Variation of reactance (x) with frequency (f).

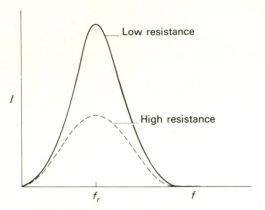

Fig. 3.11. The selectivity of the circuit in Fig. 3.10 depends upon the series resistance.

out, resistance presenting the only opposition to the current. This frequency is called the *resonant frequency*, and by definition, reactance is zero at this point. Figure 3.11 shows that since the reactance at f_r is zero, the circuit current will be at a maximum at this point. At all other frequencies the reactance will be higher and will therefore hinder current flow. This is the basis of a passive 'band-pass' filter. The selectivity of such a filter depends upon the resistance in the circuit, for if this is low the reactance becomes the major factor controlling current flow.

Figure 3.12a shows the inductance and capacitance in parallel. In this arrangement, the effect of resonance is to greatly increase the reactance so that a 'band-reject' passive filter has been formed (Fig. 3.12b). Filters are widely used in measuring equipment to select frequencies of interest and to reject interference, e.g. from muscular movement.

MUTUAL INDUCTANCE

If two coils A and B are placed close together and a current is passed through coil A, then some of the electromagnetic flux from A will also link with B, so that a current will be induced there also. The flux-linkage with B due to current in A is called the *mutual inductance*, and is measured in henrys. The flux-linkage, and therefore the mutual inductance depends upon (a) the size and number of turns of the two coils; (b) the proximity and orientation of the coils, and (c) the magnetic permeability of the material within the coils. (If they are wound onto an iron core, the mutual inductance will be many times greater than if on a plastic former.)

The a.c. transformer is a good example of the application of mutual inductance. In Fig. 3.13a two coils are wound onto an iron core, and an alternating current passed

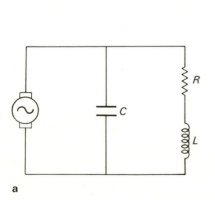

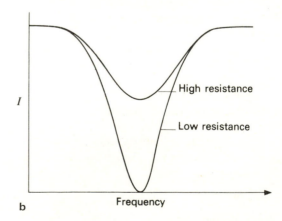

Fig. 3.12. a. A.c. circuit containing capacitance (*C*) and inductance (*L*) in parallel. b. The relationship between current (*I*) and frequency (*f*). As in the series circuit, the selectivity of a parallel-tuned circuit depends upon the resistance 'in series', with the inductance. This circuit operates as a 'band reject' filter.

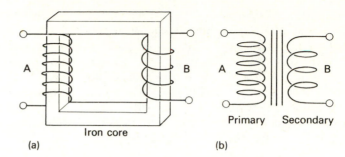

Fig. 3.13. a. A mutual inductance: the transformer. b. Symbolic representation of a step-down transformer.

Iron core

(a)   Primary   Secondary

(b)

through A. Mutual inductance will induce an alternating e.m.f. in B, whose voltage will relate to that in A by the ratio of the number of turns in each coil. Thus if A = 100 turns and B = 10 turns the voltage in B will be 10 times smaller than that in A. Power transmission through a simple *transformer* of this type will be poor, since eddy currents will be induced in the iron core, which will then heat up; the heat dissipated representing loss of efficiency. By constructing the core of laminated sheets of iron, the eddy currents are minimized, so that a practical transformer can be constructed to have a high efficiency, in which the only significant heating effect is by the passage of current through the ohmic resistance of the coils. Transformers are widely used in modern electronics, but appear most frequently in *power supplies*, where the mains voltage is stepped down to low voltages for transistor circuits (Fig. 3.13b). The low voltage output from the secondary winding is rectified and smoothed using a large capacitor to produce a relatively steady d.c. voltage. The power supplies for instrumentation circuits need very precise voltage regulators, so are in practice much more complex, and beyond the scope of this book.

THE SEMI-CONDUCTOR DIODE

Resistors, capacitors, and inductors can usually be connected either way round, as current will pass equally well in both directions. The diode is, however, a uni-

directional device, since it will pass current in one direction, but not the other. Figure 3.14 shows two diodes connected in a resistive circuit. The 'point' in the diode symbol indicates the direction in which

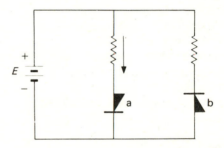

Fig. 3.14. Diode (a) allows current to flow, but diode (b) does not.

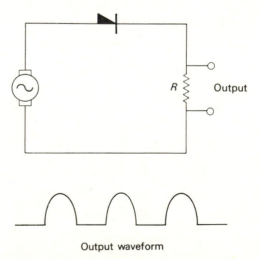

Output waveform

Fig. 3.15. The diode rectifies the generated sinewave.

conventional current (+ to −) will flow; so that diode (a) conducts but diode (b) does not. Diodes are frequently used as 'rectifiers', which allow signals of one polarity to flow, but reject signals of the opposite polarity. In Fig. 3.15 the diode rectifies the a.c. signal, so that positive half-cycles appear at the output, but negative half-cycles are blocked, and so do not.

AMPLIFIERS

The passive components considered so far are of limited use, since their function is always to reduce the size of the signal. In order to detect and 'condition' biological signals, some means of amplification must be available. Thermionic valves have, to a great extent been replaced by transistors as the fundamental constituents of amplifiers, and are often combined together in great number to perform but a single function. It is therefore unnecessary to have more than a superficial understanding of the mode of action of the single transistor.

Transistor action

The transistor is a 3-terminal device, in which a very small change of current into one terminal may induce a large change of current at another. Transistors come in two basic varieties: 'npn' and 'pnp'. Figure 3.16 shows an npn transistor operating as a

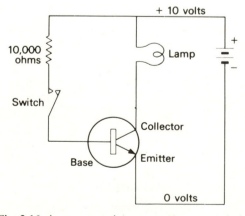

Fig. 3.16. An npn transistor operating as a switch.

current switch. When the switch in the base lead is open, no current flows from collector to emitter, the transistor is said to be 'off', and so is the light bulb. When the base switch is closed, a small current flows through the 10 kΩ resistor to the base, and through the transistor to the emitter. This has the effect of 'turning on' the transistor, so that current now flows from collector to emitter, and the bulb lights. The important point to appreciate is that the lamp current, which might be 80 mA, has been controlled by the base current of less than 1 mA. A pnp transistor could have been used, but since this passes current in the opposite direction, the power supply would have required reversal.

We have so far considered the transistor to be either 'off' or 'on'. It is possible to choose a base current which causes the transistor to be turned partly on. Any further change in base current will now be reflected by a much larger change in collector current.

Figure 3.17 shows a very simple amplifier. The collector is now connected to the positive power supply by a 2000 Ω resistor, and the emitter to the negative by a 500 Ω resistor. The base is 'biased' by current through the 100 kΩ resistor, which is chosen so as to turn the transistor partly on. The input signal is applied through a capacitor, which allows the a.c. signal to pass without upsetting the delicate d.c. bias on the base. When the input signal goes positive, the base current increases slightly, turning the transistor further 'on'. The voltage at the collector is pulled down towards that of the emitter, so that the output voltage moves in a negative direction. The nett effect is that a very small sine wave at the input appears as a much larger sine wave at the output, but 'upside down' (i.e. 180° out of phase). This is, therefore, the simplest possible *inverting amplifier*.

There are all manner of problems with this very crude amplifier, so that it is very rarely used in practice. The modern amplifier designer uses circuits in which large

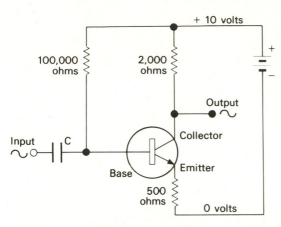

Fig. 3.17. A very simple a.c. amplifier.

numbers of transistors are combined in a single package to yield a device which is virtually devoid of non-linearity, temperature instability, frequency restriction, etc. (all features of the simple transistor). This multi-transistor device is known as an *operational amplifier*, and can be used as a 'black box' amplifier with no knowledge whatever of its internal structure.

THE OPERATIONAL AMPLIFIER

The operational amplifier can for the moment be considered to be an 'ideal' device, which is represented by the symbols in Fig. 3.18, and has the following characteristics:

1   The amplification of input signals is infinite. This implies that to produce a full-scale positive output, an infinitesimally small positive signal is required at the non-inverting input, or an infinitesimally small negative signal is required at the inverting input.

2   Neither input takes current from its

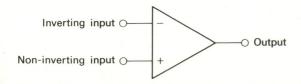

Fig. 3.18. The operational amplifier.

source. Both inputs therefore have an infinitely high input resistance.

3   The output can drive any load, irrespective of the current required. The output therefore has an infinitely low output resistance.

4   If the same input signal is applied to both inputs simultaneously, the positive and negative amplifications cancel out, so that no output appears. The ability to reject such signals is called the 'common mode rejection ratio', (CMRR) and is infinite for an ideal device.

5   All frequencies (including d.c.) will be amplified to exactly the same degree. It therefore has an infinitely wide band-width.

All practical amplifiers fail to reach these ideals, in some or all respects. Generally speaking, the more expensive the amplifier, the nearer to 'ideal' it will be. Operational amplifiers have increased in performance and decreased in cost in recent years (i.e. 50p will now buy a better amplifier than would £25 in 1965.)

The reader might at this point wonder as to the usefulness of an amplifier having infinite gain. The answer lies in the term *negative feedback*.

Consider Fig. 3.19 where two resistors are added to the basic amplifier. R_2, connecting the 'inverting' input to the output is called the 'feedback' resistor, and going to the negative input, carries a negative feedback current. If no input signal is applied (i.e. input terminals joined together), the output will settle at 0 volts. (If the output went positive, it would make the inverting input go positive, which would make the output go negative! The effect of this is a balance at which both the non-inverting and inverting inputs are at the same voltage (0 volts), so that the output does not swing in either direction.) If now, a voltage of $+1$ volt is applied to the input, the output will swing negative until the feedback current exactly balances the input current. Since by definition no current enters the amplifier itself, it will be evident that when the inverting input is at 0 volts, 1 mA must be flowing along R_1, and then

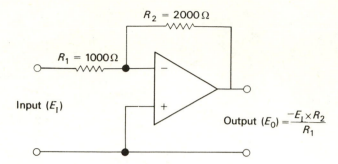

Fig. 3.19. An inverting amplifier, with a gain of 2.

along R_2. The output will therefore settle at that voltage which takes precisely 1 mA from R_2. By Ohm's law $E = IR$, $E = 0.001 \times 2000 = 2$ volts. The output therefore settles at -2 volts; precisely double the input voltage. It should now be clear why the *gain* (amplification factor) is the ratio of $R_2 : R_1$, with the amplifier itself simply acting as a sort of electronic lever. Thus the output voltage $E_0 = -E_1 \times R_2/R_1$. By choosing appropriate values for R_1 and R_2, any desired gain can be achieved, to an accuracy limited only by errors in the resistor values. Figure 3.20 shows how the same basic principle is applied to the design of a non-inverting amplifier. The input is applied to the positive, but the 'electronic lever' to the negative input. Note that the expression for the gain factor is slightly different.

In Fig. 3.21 the two basic amplifier types are combined to produce a *differential amplifier*, which amplifies the difference between the two inputs, but rejects any signal which is common to both of them. This type of circuit is widely used in amplifiers of biological signals, where considerable

interference by common mode signals may be encountered (see Chapter 4).

Figure 3.22 shows an additional refinement. This circuit is a straightforward inverting amplifier, but has a capacitor providing additional negative feedback. Since a capacitor passes more current at high than at low frequency there will be more feedback at high frequency. This means that the gain will be reduced at high frequencies, but will, under d.c. conditions, adhere to the simple $R_2 : R_1$ ratio. The circuit is, in effect a simple 'low pass' filter and the range of frequencies rejected can be selected by the choice of capacitor.

Capacitors can be used in operational amplifier circuits to perform special functions such as differentiation and integration.

Figure 3.23 shows how, by placing a capacitor in the feedback pathway, an integrator can be constructed. In this configuration, all the current passed down R_1 is stored by C, the output voltage showing the charge potential. The effect is to integrate the input voltage with respect to time. Such a device may be used, for example, to convert the flow signal from a pneumo-

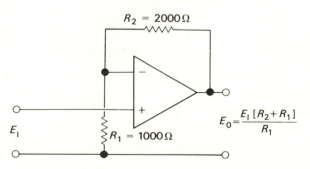

Fig. 3.20. A noninverting amplifier, with a gain of 3.

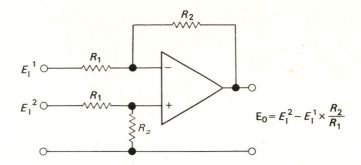

Fig. 3.21. A differential amplifier.

$$E_0 = E_I^2 - E_I^1 \times \frac{R_2}{R_1}$$

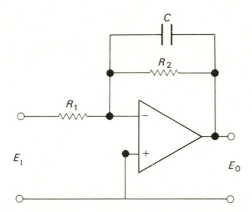

Fig. 3.22. An inverting amplifier with 'low pass' filter characteristics.

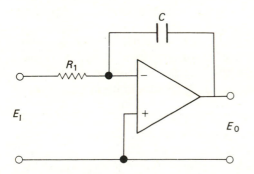

Fig. 3.23. Replacing R_2 with a capacitor creates an integrator.

derivative of the input. The values of R and C are chosen so as to provide a rate-constant of $R \times C$ (seconds) which will give a suitable output range for the range of 'rate of change' signals likely to be experienced at the input. The differentiator so produced may be used to derive the rate of change of left ventricular pressure which is used as an index of contractility (see Chapter 5).

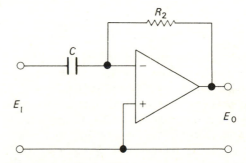

Fig. 3.24. Replacing R_1 with a capacitor creates a differentiator.

It should not have escaped the reader that this circuit is also a high-pass filter. Figure 3.25 shows the functions of integration and differentiation on various input signals.

Operational amplifier circuits are ubiquitous in modern instrumentation and may be very complex, as the designer's ingenuity may enable him to perform several functions simultaneously. Most circuits are, however based on those described here, so that by application of first principles the function of most operational amplifier circuits may be defined.

tachograph to volume. In Fig. 3.24 the converse arrangement is seen, with a capacitor in the input pathway. In this case, the current passing through the capacitor is amplified and appears at the output. Since the current through the capacitor is proportional to the rate of change of voltage (Fig. 3.7b), the output will also have this function. The output is therefore the first

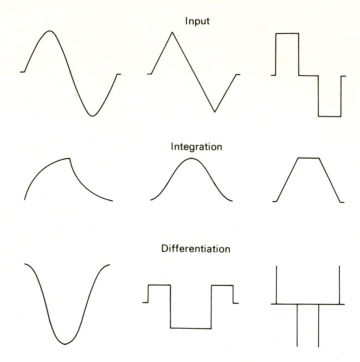

Fig. 3.25. Integration and differentiation of sine, triangular and square wave-forms.

IMPEDANCE MATCHING

We have so far assumed that amplifiers have infinitely high input impedance (Z_{in}) and infinitely low output impedance (Z_{out}). In practice, this is not quite true, but more to the point, the input and output impedances of complete circuits involving many other components are frequently far from ideal. We cannot therefore connect circuits (or even instruments) together with impunity without consideration of their impedances. Figure 3.26 illustrates the concept of input and output impedance. Z_{in} can be

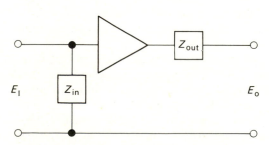

Fig. 3.26. The effects of input and output impedance can be calculated by imagining them to be included in the circuit, as shown above.

considered to be an imaginary impedance shunting the device input to ground (or more correctly, circuit 'common'), while Z_{out} can be imagined to be an impedance in series with the output. These impedances represent the nett effect of all the components involved in giving a circuit its input or output characteristics. The effect of input and output impedances upon circuit interconnection is shown in Fig. 3.27. In this case two devices A and B, having input and output impedances of 5000 ohms (5 kΩ) are interconnected. Z_{out} of A and Z_{in} of B form a voltage divider to ground, so that the potential 'seen' by B is

$$\frac{E_I \times Z_{in}}{Z_{out} + Z_{in}},$$

i.e. $0.5E_I$. This is a rather gross example of impedance mismatch, but it is very easy, when connecting devices whose impedances are unknown, to do much worse. It should be clear that wherever possible, output impedances should be low and input impedances high. It is perfectly correct to connect low output impedances to high

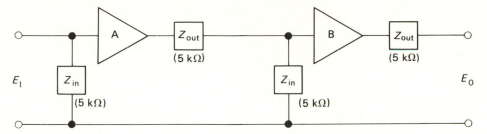

Fig. 3.27. The effect of impedance mismatch. If circuits A and B are both unity-gain amplifiers, with input and output impedance of 5 kΩ, then E_0 will only be $0.5E_1$. The attenuation error is due to Z_{out} (A) and Z_{in} (B) forming a potential divider.

input impedances, but *never* to connect a device with low input impedance to another with high output impedance. At best, the signal will be attenuated and perhaps distorted; at worst the output device may be damaged.

GAIN MEASUREMENT

In specifying the performance of a practical circuit, the amplification of the signal at different frequencies must be considered. The unit by which the *ratio* of output to input can be directly stated is the *decibel*, which is probably the least understood and most misused term in electronics. For this reason, some space will be given to its explanation. If the power dissipated in a resistor is increased from P_1 Watts to P_2 Watts, then the common logarithm of the ratio P_2/P_1 expresses the power gain in bels. 1 bel therefore represents a power gain of $\times 10$, 2 bels a gain of $\times 100$, and so on. Since the bel is rather a large unit, it is more conveniently expressed as 10 decibels. Thus $10 \operatorname{Log} P_2/P_1$ = gain in decibels. Thus a gain of $\times 10$ is $10\,\text{dB}$; $\times 100$, $20\,\text{dB}$; $\times 1000$, $30\,\text{dB}$; etc.

The expression $\text{dB} = 10\log P_2/P_1$ applies strictly to power, and cannot be indiscriminately applied to voltages. To express the voltage gain of an amplifier (i.e. Fig. 3.28) in decibel terms, it is first necessary to determine the power gain. For example, if the voltage gain is $\times 10$:

the power dissipation in $R_1 = E^2/R_1$
$$= 1/1000 = 1\,\text{mW}$$
the power dissipation in $R_2 = E^2/R_2$
$$= 100/1000 = 100\,\text{mW}.$$

Therefore, the power gain $= 10\log 100$
$$= 20\,\text{dB}.$$

It can now be seen that the power gain is in fact $20\log E_2/E_1$, so long as the resistances at the input and output are the same. If not, the power dissipation must be calculated for each as above. (If current gain is considered, the formula $\text{dB} = 20\log I_2/I_1$ is used, since $P = I^2R$.)

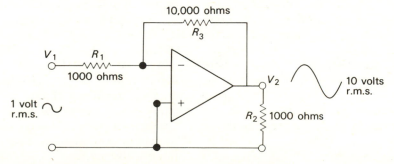

Fig. 3.28. $\times 10$ amplification of an a.c. signal. The power gain is 20 dB.

BRIDGE CIRCUITS

Circuits based on the *Wheatstone bridge* are to be found throughout medical electronics, but may be disguised by a number of other components. The principles of the bridge circuit are, however, universally applicable, so that time taken in their study is amply rewarded.

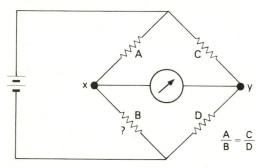

Fig. 3.29. The Wheatstone bridge.

Consider the circuit in Fig. 3.29. The object is to measure resistance B. The circuit consists of two resistive limbs, A–B and C–D, and current passes through both. Some current will also flow through the galvanometer (X → Y or X ← Y) unless points X and Y are exactly equipotential. A state of balance, indicated by a 'null' indication on the galvanometer, will exist when the ratio of resistors A : B is the same as the ratio of C : D, since the supply voltage will in each case be divided by the same fraction. Thus if C = D, and B is the unknown, we can substitute known resistances into position A until balance occurs. At that point, A = B.

If we put a known voltage across resistor B, and measured the current with an ammeter, we could, knowing Ohm's law, compute the resistance rather more simply than using the Wheatstone bridge. Consider, then, the effect of increasing resistor B by 1%. This will reduce the current by 1% and the meter deflection by 1%— a barely discernible decrement. In the bridge circuit, however, a 1% increase in B will raise the potential at 'X' by 1% while 'Y' remains constant. Since the galvanometer current reflects the potential difference be-

tween X and Y, it will rise from 'null' to a small indicated current which is in percentage terms, an infinitely large increase! The sensitivity of the bridge is therefore limited only by that of the galvanometer itself. Since the galvanometer does not have to carry the energising current (as in the simple Ohm's law circuit) it can be made very sensitive, and therefore able to detect very small changes in resistance. It should now be clear that the bridge has effectively isolated the change in resistance (ΔB) from the original value (B). Many transducers are resistive elements which change by a small fraction, so that, by using a bridge circuit which is initially set at balance, only ΔB is indicated. There is however, a complication. The current through the galvanometer is not linearly related to ΔB, so that it would appear that a bridge is only accurate at balance.

The output from a bridge circuit will however be linear if points X and Y in Fig. 3.29 are led to a differential amplifier whose input resistance is very high compared with the resistances in the bridge. Under these conditions, ΔB does not result in current flowing from X to Y, so that the output is directly proportional to ΔB.

Bridge circuits may feature reactive elements as well as, or instead of, resistors. Some pressure transducers, for instance, are variable capacitors, so that an a.c.-energized bridge is used to measure the very small change in capacitance (see p. 155).

MIXING AND MODULATION

Signals of different frequencies can be combined together to form complex waveforms. If signal B (high frequency) is simply added to signal A (low frequency), they are said to be *mixed* (Fig. 3.30). Passing the signal through a low-pass filter will block the high frequency 'B' component, so that signal A will appear alone at the output. Similarly, a high pass filter will block the 'A' component, so that signal B appears alone at the output.

If signal B (carrier frequency) is made to

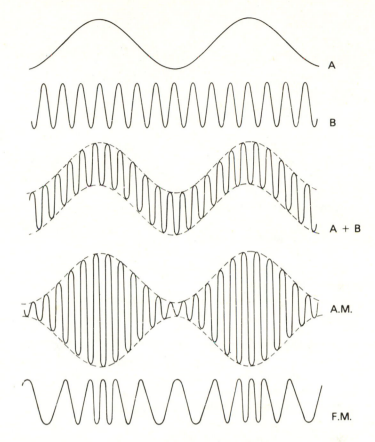

Fig. 3.30. Mixing and modulation. Signals A and B are simply added together to form the mixture A + B. In amplitude modulation, the carrier signal (B) is modulated by A. In frequency modulation the carrier (B) remains constant in amplitude, but fluctuates in frequency according the modulating signal A.

fluctuate in amplitude according to the waveform of signal A, it is said to be *amplitude modulated* (A.M.). The modulated signal consists of three signals mixed together; the carrier (signal B) and upper and lower side-band frequencies. (Upper side band frequency = frequency B + frequency A; lower side-band frequency = frequency B − frequency A). Since frequency A is not present in the mixture of carrier and side-band signals, the modulated signal cannot be separated into signals A and B by filtering. Separation can only be achieved by *demodulation*. If the modulated signal is fed to the circuit of Fig. 3.15 it will be rectified. The amplitude of the half-cycles will fluctuate at frequency A. Since the fluctuations of the upper side-band are no longer balanced by those of the lower side-band, a capacitor placed across resistor R will act as a low pass filter and remove the carrier frequency. The output will be

signal A added to a d.c. voltage corresponding to the rectified carrier signal.

If signal B (carrier) is made to fluctuate in frequency according to the wave form of signal A, it is said to be *frequency modulated* (F.M.). Signal B is said to be the 'centre frequency' and the degree of frequency shift depends upon the amplitude of signal A. (In amplitude modulation the range of frequencies depends upon the frequency of A.) An F.M. signal can be separated into its original components only by frequency demodulation. In its simplest possible form a demodulator is a rate meter (see Fig. 4.7). Practical demodulators are usually constructed using devices known as 'phase-locked loops', which are complex integrated circuits beyond the scope of this text.

Modulators and demodulators are ubiquitous in modern instrumentation and will be discussed further in later chapters.

Chapter 4
Biological Potentials

Activity in a nerve or muscle cell is accompanied by depolarization of the cell membrane. This temporarily reduces the potential difference which normally exists between the inside and the outside of the cell, and creates a potential difference between the active cell and its surroundings. The activity can thus be sensed with either an intracellular or extracellular electrode. Synchronous depolarization of a large number of cells results in more widespread changes of potential which often involve the skin. Such changes can be recorded by needle electrodes inserted into the subcutaneous tissue, or by surface electrodes which are electrically connected to the skin by a layer of conductive jelly.

Intracellular recording is usually carried out by inserting an extremely fine glass pipette filled with saline directly into the cell. The technique requires a high degree of technical skill and is only used in physiological research. Extracellular recording is effected with needle or wire electrodes and is again most commonly used in research applications. However, extracellular recording is being increasingly used in clinical measurement. For example, needle electrodes are inserted into muscles to record muscle action potentials (the electromyogram or EMG) and may be used to record conduction velocities in nerves. Electrodes are also placed directly onto the heart surface at operation so that complicated conduction patterns may be defined by epicardial mapping of the electrocardiogram (ECG or EKG). Surface electrodes are most frequently used for monitoring the ECG or the electroencephalogram (EEG), though they are also used in some situations for recording the EMG or the electrooculogram (EOG).

It may also be necessary to record changes in electrical potential or current when electrical impulses are passed through tissues for measurement purposes. For example, measurements of skin resistance may be used to assess autonomic activity whilst changes in impedance can be used to measure ventilation, lung water, cardiac output or limb blood flow.

All these applications have certain instrumental problems in common, although the relative importance of each problem varies with the application (Geddes 1972). Before considering the applications separately it will be convenient to discuss the general problems associated with the recording of biological potentials.

Interference

As was pointed out in Chapter 1, the first essential in any instrumentation system is that the signal : noise ratio should be high. Noise may originate in the patient or his surroundings and in the instruments used for recording, amplification and display. Instrumental noise can be reduced by careful design, the use of high grade components and adequate screening. However, noise arising from the patient or his surroundings is often more difficult to eradicate.

NOISE ORIGINATING FROM THE PATIENT

The electrical changes associated with the heart beat produce potential differences of about 0.5–2 mV on the surface of the body, whilst the EEG signal on the scalp has a magnitude of about 50 μV. The ECG signal may thus distort the EEG signal, whilst both these signals may be submerged by the much larger potentials produced by muscular movement. The choice of electrode and electrode site is important, and the use of amplifiers with high powers of discrimination may prove invaluable. For example, although the ECG signal is much larger than the EEG it is rarely a troublesome source of interference, since the ECG potentials are substantially in phase at all points on the head and can therefore be eliminated by using an amplifier which is able to attenuate the in-phase signals and amplify those which are out of phase. Muscle interference has a much higher frequency than the components of an EEG and can often be eliminated by cutting the high-frequency response of the amplifier to a level which does not interfere greatly with the characteristics of the EEG.

NOISE ORIGINATING FROM THE PATIENT-ELECTRODE INTERFACE

Unfortunately, recording electrodes do not behave as passive contact devices.

When a metal surface is brought into contact with an electrolyte solution, as occurs with a plain metal skin electrode, an electrochemical half-cell is produced. This will generate an e.m.f. If a differential amplifier is connected to a pair of such electrodes, a circuit will be completed, with the two half-cells in opposition. If they are identical, the potentials will cancel each other, but if not, they will produce an offset d.c. potential which will be 'seen' by the amplifier. Furthermore, the small current produced by the offset potential may change the characteristics of the electrodes themselves by electrolytic action, producing the phenomenon of *polarization*. A polarized electrode (such as platinum/ saline) will seriously distort any signal passing through it, since the cell potential varies with the direction and magnitude of the current. Electrodes which utilize a metal in contact with one of its own salts (e.g. silver/silver chloride) do not behave in this way and are described as *reversible* (i.e.

current can pass in either direction without altering the cell potential).

If materials such as iron were used for skin electrodes, corrosion would occur, developing a highly irregular electro-chemical potential. The corrosion potentials would superimpose on any recorded biological potential and, having a wide range of frequency components, would seriously reduce the signal : noise ratio.

Modern recording electrodes are almost invariably provided with Ag : AgCl surfaces, so that polarization and corrosion potentials should never be a practical problem.

Mechanical movement of recording electrodes may also result in large potential changes. These are due to an alteration of the physicochemical nature of the electrode half-cell, which changes the cell potential, and to an alteration of the skin-electrode impedance, which may impair the common-mode rejection ratio of the recording amplifier (see p. 41).

NOISE ORIGINATING FROM SOURCES OUTSIDE THE PATIENT

Interference from outside sources is due principally to electrostatic or electromagnetic induction from mains or radio-frequency sources.

Electrostatic induction

When a charged body is brought close to an uncharged one it will induce an equal and opposite charge on the uncharged body. If a patient is close to any object such as a cable or lamp element which is connected to the mains supply, he will develop a surface charge of equal and opposite potential *even though no current is actually flowing through the object*. Since the mains potential is a sinusoidal function, fluctuating between ± 339 V at a frequency of 50 Hz, the induced potential will have the same characteristics. The effect is the same as if the patient were actually connected to the source potential by a very small capacitor (stray capacitance). If the patient could be

electrically isolated from all his other surroundings, then his surface potential would
be the same at all points but fluctuating
at 50 Hz. However, in practice, there are
always other stray capacitances between
the patient and such objects as the bed
or operating table, the floor, nearby staff,
and electronic instruments. Many of these
bodies will be earthed, so that the patient
becomes part of a potential gradient between the source and ground, along which
a small a.c. current is flowing. It follows
therefore that his surface is no longer at a
single potential, but shows considerable
differences in a.c. potential, depending upon
the relative positions of all the bodies to
which he is electrostatically coupled. This is
illustrated by considering the surface
potentials detected by a simple noninverting
amplifier whose common right leg connection is grounded (Fig. 4.1). The patient is
subjected to stray capacitance from an a.c.

source close to his head. Electrode B is at
ground potential, so that an a.c. potential
gradient is established along the patient.
Electrode A is at a point along the gradient
and, so will detect and amplify the a.c.
potential at that point. Since the surface a.c.
potential may be as large as 1 V (rms), the
amplifier would be swamped with 50 Hz
interference. Moreover, the electrode lead
itself is also likely to have stray capacitance
to the source and this will add to the 50 Hz
signal which is detected. This effect will be
intensified if there is a high electrode contact
resistance.

Electromagnetic induction

This form of interference occurs in the
vicinity of wires carrying alternating
currents and is also illustrated in Fig. 4.1.
When a current flows it generates a
magnetic field: in the case of an alternating

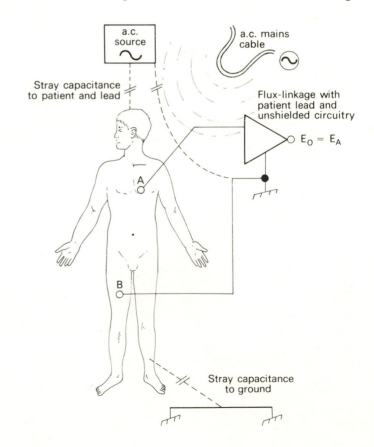

Fig. 4.1. A simple 'single input'
amplifier is subject to gross
interference from electrostatic
induction (left—a.c. source)
and electromagnetic induction
(right—a.c. mains).

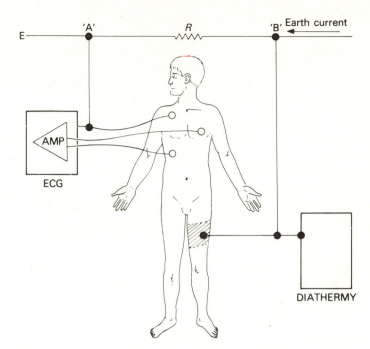

Fig. 4.2. Interference due to an earth loop. The earth current sets up a potential difference across a small resistance (R), and therefore between earth points 'A' and 'B'. This potential then appears across the patient, and causes 50 Hz interference. AMP = amplifier.

current the field is constantly growing and collapsing with successive half-cycles, so that any wire within the field will have a constantly changing flux linkage, and therefore an electromagnetically-induced current at the same frequency as the source. All cables carrying mains currents are surrounded by electromagnetic fields, the intensity depending upon the current flowing in the cable.

Since the simple electrostatic cable screens are readily penetrated by electromagnetic fields, electromagnetic interference would appear to be a major problem. Fortunately, the mains supply is usually arranged so that for every live cable carrying current to a device, there is a neutral cable carrying an exactly equal current away from it, these two wires lying either immediately adjacent to each other, or even better, twisted around one another. The electromagnetic effects are thus to a large extent self-cancelling. If at some point in the building, the neutral ˙cable is accidentally connected to ground, the supply will work perfectly well, but a large magnetic field will be generated, due to the

live : neutral mismatch. Similarly, when a machine or instrument develops a high leakage current, live and neutral currents are no longer equal and self-cancelling, so that an electromagnetic field is generated. Such a field induces an e.m.f. in all the wires within its vicinity, the effect being multiplied if the wires are coiled. The patient lead is most frequently affected, but inadequate protection of amplifier circuitry from electromagnetic fields may also result in inductive interference.

Earth-loop interference

If a patient is connected to two electrical devices, each of which is separately earthed, interference may arise due to the earth-loop effect. The mechanism is very simple and depends upon the two earth points having slightly different potentials (Fig. 4.2). This usually occurs in old installations, where the earth connections have deteriorated, so that any leakage current flowing along the earth (often from some quite separate, and even distant device) will set up a potential difference between two earth points in the same room. If the patient is now connected to the earthed plate of a diathermy machine, and to the leads of a non-isolated electrocardiograph in which one lead is earthed, there will be an a.c. potential gradient across the patient. Unless the electrocardiograph has good common-mode rejection, and the electrodes are correctly orientated to the potential gradient, 50 Hz interference will result. In modern devices, all circuits making contact with the patient must be isolated from ground, so that earth loops are now uncommon.

Radiofrequency interference

Radiofrequency (RF) noise can enter a recording system by three possible routes. Firstly, it may enter through the mains distribution system, mixed with the 50 Hz current. (Sources are diathermy machines, and unsuppressed sparking contacts as may be found in switch-gear and electric motors.) Secondly, it may be directly injected, as when a patient is touched by the active electrode of a surgical diathermy and coagulation performed. (In this case the noise behaves as if it were coming from the patient, and is detected by the recording electrodes.) Thirdly, it may be transmitted by radio-propagation. If the diathermy probe is simply held in the air and the circuit activated a nearby ECG system will show gross interference. Here the active diathermy electrode and its lead acts as a radio-transmitting aerial, and the patient lead as a receiving aerial. Radiofrequency potentials detected by the recording electrodes and patient leads present the greatest problem, as they are likely to be rectified by the input stages of the amplifier, and any low frequency signal with which the RF carrier was modulated therefore demodulated, and then subjected to the same amplification as the ECG signal. If this demodulated signal is large, the amplifier may 'block', so that no signal appears at the output, but more often a large 50 Hz signal appears which obscures the ECG

mixed with it. Newer diathermy machines (whose output waveforms are modulated at higher frequencies) may produce somewhat less interference, due to the limited band width of the ECG amplifier.

ELIMINATION OF INTERFERENCE

Mains-frequency interference can, to a large extent, be prevented by good amplifier design, but the user must be aware that noise-free recording is unlikely to be achieved in an environment littered with potential sources of stray capacitance, electromagnetic induction and radio-frequency radiations, however well the amplifier is designed.

An electrocardiograph amplifier should be of the *differential* type and should have both high input impedance and high 'common mode rejection ratio' (Fig. 4.3). The high impedance minimises the current taken from the electrodes. This is important because the electrodes also have a high impedance and this tends to vary with time. If the amplifier had a low impedance and drew an appreciable current from the electrodes the recorded potential would be very sensitive to small changes in electrode impedance. Furthermore the recorded potential would be less than the true potential at the electrodes. The high common mode rejection ratio (CMRR) means that the amplifier strongly attenuates signals (such as those due to capacitance coupling or earth loops) which are common to both inputs, but amplifies the difference between the two signals.

The efficiency of common mode rejection is also related to the size of the common signal to be rejected. Earthing the patient with a right leg electrode is undesirable for safety reasons, but it also intensifies the potential gradients on the patient's surface. By allowing the whole amplifier to 'float' at the same potential as the patient, these gradients are minimized so that common mode voltages are reduced, and therefore less difficult to reject.

Electrostatic induction in the leads is

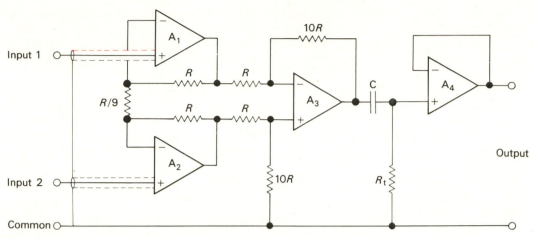

Fig. 4.3. A high-impedance, d.c. differential amplifier, with a gain of × 100, using 3 operational amplifiers. (A_1 and A_2 act as noninverting amplifiers, and A_3 as a differential stage.) Using suitable components, a CMRR of 10 000 : 1 can be achieved, with an input impedance exceeding 50 MΩ. Each lead is surrounded by an electrostatic screen which is connected to circuit 'common'. The final amplifier (A_4) is an a.c. voltage follower with a gain of 1, and a time constant of ($R_t \times C$) seconds.

prevented by surrounding each lead with a braided copper screen (connected with circuit 'common') so that the stray capacitances couple with the screen instead of the lead.

When EEG monitoring is disturbed by electromagnetic fields, a cure can be very elusive, since ordinary electrostatic screens are not effective. The circuitry itself can be protected by surrounding it with a copper enclosure, in which eddy currents are induced which produce opposing fields tending to cancel the effect of the original field. Materials with high magnetic permeability, such as mu-metal or iron, which concentrate the field within themselves can also be used for electromagnetic screens. Unfortunately, it is the patient leads which are most susceptible to this form of interference, and screening with sheets of iron is just not practicable! The only effective screening solution is to enclose the entire patient within an iron box (or room), together with the low-level stages of signal detection and amplification. Although this approach is widely used for low-level measurements (such as the EEG) it is not really suitable for clinical monitoring.

The effects of electromagnetic fields can

be mitigated by ensuring that all the patient leads are the same length, and are closely bound together, or even better, twisted together, until very close to the electrodes. This ensures that as far as possible, the induced signals are identical and therefore susceptible to common mode rejection. The only real cure is to eliminate the sources of the unwanted electromagnetic fields.

Radiofrequency interference (RF) from surgical diathermy has until recently presented insuperable problems, especially with spark-gap and valve-modulated generators. The solution is not in fact difficult, but requires an understanding of the problem. The RF signal is brought into the amplifier as both common-mode and differential signals which tend to saturate the input stages. Furthermore, the whole 'floating' input circuit, following the surface potential of the patient, 'floats' at a radiofrequency potential. This input circuit then radiates RF to all parts of the amplifier. Even worse, the sensitive input stages, floating at radiofrequency 'see' nearby earthed metalwork as a source of RF interference. The total effect is catastrophic, and all these sources of interference must be eradicated before a clean signal can be obtained.

Figure 4.4 shows the basic structure of a diathermy-immune ECG amplifier. The ECG signal passes through a filter before entering the floating input circuit, which is surrounded by a double screen. When combined with a simple filter in the power supply to block mains-borne radio-frequencies, these simple measures can result in total freedom from diathermy interference.

value in modern electrocardiographs). If small, high-impedance electrodes are to be used (as in the EEG), a high input impedance amplifier is especially important.

The band-width of the amplifier must cover the range of frequencies that are of importance in the signal. The American Heart Association (1967) standard for ECG machines specifies a flat response from

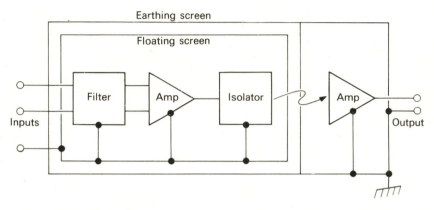

Fig. 4.4. The basic principles of a diathermy-immune ECG amplifier. AMP = amplifier.

Requirements of biological amplifiers

It has already been established that amplifiers for biological signals require high common-mode rejection and high input impedance. If the input impedance is too low it may cause both distortion and attenuation of the output signal. This is especially important where the augmented leads are concerned, since here the signals from two limb leads are averaged, and compared with the third. If one of the two signals to be averaged is attenuated due to high electrode impedance, the mean signal will be biased towards the other, with a resulting error in the geometry of the lead. To a much lesser extent, the bipolar leads are subject to the same type of distortion.

The CMRR for biological amplifiers should always exceed 1000:1, and is generally much higher. Input impedance must exceed 5 MΩ if the above problems are to be avoided. (10 MΩ is a common

0.14 Hz up to 50 Hz and allows up to 30 dB attenuation at 0.05 Hz and 100 Hz (30 dB is a 1000-fold loss). EEG's can be recorded satisfactorily using an amplifier with a similar band width but more voltage amplification, although purpose built machines usually have a band-width that extends from 0.5 Hz up to nearly 100 Hz. EMG's or nerve action potential recordings, require a flat response from about 20 Hz up to at least 1 kHz and preferably up to 10 kHz, to record the high frequencies contained in the signal.

Biological amplifiers are usually a.c. amplifiers with relatively short time-constants. D.c. amplifiers have a bandwidth down to 0 Hz and are unsuitable for ECG recording because the electrode resistance may vary considerably, and because the electrodes may develop slowly-changing potentials which, if amplified, would drive the trace right off the screen or recording paper.

These problems may be overcome by using an amplifier with an a.c.-coupled output stage (see Fig. 4.3). The RC network leading to amplifier A_4 will block any static or slowly-changing potentials present at the output of amplifier A_3, so that the circuit output shows only the a.c. components of the input signal. The network thus operates as a simple high-pass filter. If a step-change in input voltage occurs, this will appear at the output, but the resistor R_t will dissipate the charge exponentially, the process having a time-constant of $R_t \times C$ seconds. The step change at the output will therefore be followed immediately by an exponential restoration of the original baseline. Amplifiers designed for diagnostic ECG machines may have a time constant as long as 3 s, but those designed for monitoring applications (when trace continuity is more important than minor distortions) often have time constants of 1.5 s or even less. It is important to realize that while this circuit is a high-pass filter, it is also a low-frequency differentiator (see Fig. 3.24), so that if the time-constant is short, P and T waves will be both attenuated and biphasic and the $S-T$ segment distorted.

In commercial amplifiers trace restoration following an artefact is frequently much faster than could be achieved by this simple circuit. High speed restoration is achieved by connecting a transistor across R_t. This is turned on under overload conditions, thus reducing the effective resistance of R_t and thereby shortening the time constant. When the output returns to a value corresponding to the edge of the screen or paper, the transistor turns off, and the time constant resumes its normal value.

EEG machines provide a selection of time constants of 0.03, 0.1, 0.3 and 1 s. Since the selection of a very short time-constant effectively creates a high-pass filter it will result in the attenuation of the low frequency components of the recording. Special filters are usually incorporated to introduce additional attenuation at one or other end of the frequency range. For example, a high-frequency filter may be necessary to eliminate muscle artefacts from an EEG trace.

Calibration voltages may be incorporated so that the gain of the amplifiers can be correctly adjusted. It is customary to calibrate the ECG so that a 1 mV input will produce a 1-cm deflection of the trace, and the EEG so that $100 \,\mu V$ (0.1 mV) produces this deflection.

Electrodes

The importance of having an amplifier input impedance significantly greater than the electrode skin resistance has already been mentioned. At one time, biological signals could only be displayed using string galvanometers, and since these inevitably had a low input impedance, it was vital to lower the electrode-skin resistance as much as possible. This was achieved by using an electrode with a large area, applying electrically-conductive jelly, and abrading away the cornified layer of the skin in which the major part of the skin resistance resides. With the introduction of the valve amplifier, very high input impedances were easily obtained, rendering much electrode mystique pointless. With amplifiers having input impedances of over 2 MΩ it has been shown that perfectly satisfactory traces can be obtained using K-Y jelly, mustard, tomato ketchup, handcream, toothpaste, or even with no jelly at all (Lewes 1965). A further advantage is that electrodes with much smaller areas of contact can be used, although there has perhaps been a tendency to move too far in this direction without appreciating the consequences. For instance, subcutaneous needles have an appreciable impedance which, being largely capacitative, is marked at low frequencies. This gives rise to spurious features in the ECG, particularly diphasic T-waves and increased S-waves. It may also give the appearance of $S-T$ depression.

High electrode impedances are also undesirable (as mentioned previously) because a.c. interference may be accentuated, and differences between electrode impedances may lead to geometric errors. Signal distortion is also produced by polarized electrodes, and can be a major problem when the measured potentials are small, as in electroencephalography. Low-noise, reversible electrodes are best constructed of silver, coated electrolytically with silver chloride (Wiggins & Meldrum 1977).

The silver-chloride layer is very thin, and after a few uses becomes imperfect, so that re-chloriding or disposal is necessary. The best modern disposable electrodes have silver–silver chloride surfaces.

It has been found that movement artefacts are greatly reduced if the electrode surface is separated from the skin by a relatively thick layer of electrolyte. This ensures that mechanical distortion of the skin under the electrode does not significantly alter the electrode potential or resistance. This characteristic is often achieved by separating the electrode surface from the skin by a foam pad impregnated with electrolyte gel (Fig. 4.5). As stated previously, the electrolyte gel does not require specially conductive properties, but should be nonabrasive, non-allergenic, soap-free, and, ideally, sterile if the skin is not to be damaged during long-term use. Although it is not necessary to abrade the skin to achieve ultra-low impedances, it is a good idea to de-grease it with ether before applying an electrode. This reduces the resistance and ensures satisfactory adhesion. Needle electrodes are to be avoided unless strictly necessary, in which case special care must be taken to ensure that the signal is not distorted.

ELECTRODES FOR FETAL ELECTROCARDIOGRAPHY

Fetal electrocardiography has an established role in perinatal care. The fetal ECG can be recorded from abdominal skin electrodes on the mother, but the signal will be mixed with a much larger maternal ECG signal. If the maternal ECG is also recorded from chest leads, it will contain no fetal signals, so that with careful waveform matching, the maternal signal can be subtracted from the mixed one, leaving the fetal signal alone at the output. In the clinical environment, this is not a practical proposition, as the equipment is complex and requires very careful setting-up procedures. The fetal ECG can be more readily obtained by means of a scalp electrode. This may be a simple 'crocodile' type clip, or more recently, a stainless steel spiral, rather like a very small double corkscrew, which can be attached to the scalp through the cervix using a special applicator. A second electrode is attached to the mother's skin (usually on the inside surface of the thigh) and acts as a common connection to the fetus through the uterus and liquor. Using this technique, a good quality fetal ECG which is free from maternal artefacts, can be obtained early in labour. A high impedance amplifier is needed to avoid distortion (Finster & Petrie 1976; Steer 1977).

SIGNAL DISPLAY

All physiological signals are best seen on an oscilloscope screen, where distortions are at a minimum. Clinical ECG monitoring is now greatly facilitated by the digital storage oscilloscope, the use of which has become almost universal (see p. 74). Permanent records of ECG and EEG signals can be made using galvanometer pens, using either hot-stylus or ink-jet techniques. EMG signals cannot be reliably recorded using

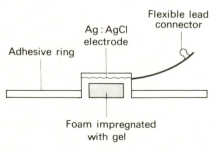

Fig. 4.5. A disposable ECG electrode, with Ag:AgCl electrode and foam pad.

these methods, due to their inadequate frequency response, so that it is conventional to either 'freeze' the oscilloscope trace and photograph it, or to use a paper recorder using an optically-coupled galvanometer and ultraviolet-sensitive paper.

Special applications involving measurements of induced potentials

TISSUE IMPEDANCE MEASUREMENT

The impedance of tissues depends on their constitution. When a small alternating current is applied across a portion of tissue, changes in its impedance can be detected as a change of a.c. voltage between the electrodes. Changes in impedance occur when the average composition of the tissue between the electrodes changes. This can occur, for example, in a limb which, because of vasodilatation, contains a greater amount of blood, or across the thorax when the intake of air causes a change in thoracic geometry.

Absolute calibration, based on the actual values of impedance, is virtually impossible, for so much depends on the position of the electrodes, the frequency of current employed, and the tissue structure of the individual. However, changes in impedance can often be shown to have a reasonably linear approximation to the function under examination, and the voltage changes can thus be calibrated empirically in an individual case (Geddes & Baker 1975).

The frequencies employed in impedance measurements are high enough to prevent polarization of the electrodes; for impedance spirometry frequencies of tens to hundreds of kHz are employed. At these frequencies, the threshold for sensation is appreciably higher than at 50 Hz so that currents of 1–2 mA can be used.

For impedance spirometry the electrodes are placed on either side of the chest in the mid-axillary line, and the gain is adjusted to give an adequate change of signal during the respiratory cycle. If a semiquantitative display is the only requirement, this is sufficient. If an accurate calibration is required, the actual impedance of the patient at end-expiration is determined by substituting a variable known resistance between the electrodes. Since the changes in impedance are mainly resistive, a noninductive resistance is used. The calibrating resistance is then altered in known steps, and the change in signal noted. This gives ΔZ, the change in impedance, and this must now be related to ΔV, the change in volume which produces the same voltage change when the patient is connected. This can be done by allowing the patient to breath in and out of a spirometer, or if paralysed, by inflating the lungs with a known volume of gas. If $\Delta Z/\Delta V$ is approximately linear, any change in impedance can then be directly calibrated in terms of volume (Baker & Hill 1969). These authors have also published a circuit diagram of a suitable apparatus (Hill & Baker 1969).

There is no inherent reason why the same technique, with differently placed electrodes should not be able to demonstrate the change in size of the heart with each heart beat (see Chapter 16). Impedance techniques have also been used to monitor changes in lung water (Severinghaus 1971).

In impedance plethysmography of a limb it is possible to calibrate roughly by the use of simultaneous venous occlusion or strain gauge plethysmography. However, if such a method is readily available, there is no need for the less accurate impedance measurements. Consequently, impedance measurements are employed when the actual values are not of interest and only changes in a state of varying magnitude are required. Thus the technique has been used as an objective indication of anxiety, since anxiety affects limb blood flow.

THE EEG AND THE CEREBRAL FUNCTION MONITOR

The diagnostic EEG is usually recorded from a number of electrodes which are placed in designated positions. Each channel records the difference in potential between a pair of electrodes and so permits functional abnormalities to be accurately localized. However, the EEG waveform represents the integrated activity of a large number of neurones so that the resultant signal is complex and relatively nonspecific. Although the signals can be displayed on an oscilloscope it is difficult to analyse such a complex signal during a brief display. On the other hand recording at normal paper speeds generates so much paper that it is quite unsuitable for clinical monitoring. Attempts have therefore been made to process the output so that the maximum amount of useful data is compressed into a small space on the record.

One of the earliest systems used was a frequency analyser which used a number of narrow band-pass filters, each of which accepted waves of a limited range of frequencies. The input to each frequency band was then averaged over a period of one minute and displayed as a histogram with intensity on the y-axis and frequency on the x-axis. This type of analysis has been further modified so that the histogram is smoothed into the form of a curve with intensity and frequency on the same axes, but successive sweeps across the frequency spectrum are plotted at progressively lower points on the y-axis.

The resultant image looks rather like a range of mountains, those in the foreground (i.e. at the bottom of the y-axis) showing the distribution of frequencies present in the EEG in the preceding few minutes whilst those higher up on the y-axis (which appear to lie in the background) display the previous information (Fig. 4.6). It is thus possible to display patterns of change in the frequency components of the EEG over any desired period of time.

These, and other techniques of analysis, involve expensive instrumentation and have not found wide favour (Smith 1978). However, an instrument which has been shown to be of practical value is the cerebral function monitor (Prior 1980). This instrument utilizes two silver/silver chloride

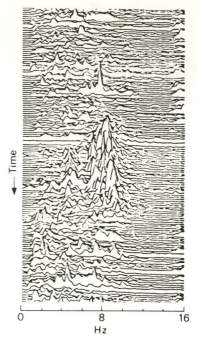

Fig. 4.6. Computer print out of sequential frequency analysis of the EEG.

recording electrodes (one on each parietal region) and a third guard electrode which is situated in the midline anterior to the vertex. The output produces two traces which are displayed on a slow speed, hot-wire recorder. The upper trace displays the mean amplitude and variation of cerebral activity on a semi-logarithmic scale. Increases or decreases in cerebral activity are shown by upward or downward movement of the trace whilst the amplitude of the trace displays the variability of the recorded signal. The instrument incorporates filters to restrict the activity displayed to the 2–15 Hz range, thus eliminating low frequency artefacts due to sweating and high frequency artefacts to RF or mains interference. The instrument is also designed to minimize capacitive interference due to lead movement or to the presence of static charges on clothing.

The lower trace presents a continuous measurement of the impedance between the electrodes. It thus provides a continuous monitor of the validity of the signal and indicates when the top trace is unreliable due to artefacts such as diathermy, mains interference or movement of the electrodes. The recording can be run at speeds of 2.5–9 cm/hr for ITU work or 36 cm/hr for monitoring more acute changes, for example in the operating theatre. The instrument is not designed to detect focal activity but has proved useful in monitoring cerebral function in situations in which cerebral perfusion may be impaired (Prior *et al.* 1971; Prior 1979). It has also proved useful in monitoring the response to anaesthetic drugs (Dubois *et al.* 1978).

Rate meters and warning systems

When a satisfactory signal has been isolated from the other electrical activity present in the body it may be processed in a number of different ways. Impulses arising from muscle or nerve are often displayed on an oscilloscope: the trace can then be photographed if a permanent record is required. The correct location of the tip of the electrodes used for this kind of work is often greatly facilitated if the impulses are channelled to a loudspeaker, since this allows the pattern of discharge to be easily recognized by ear. Another way of recording the frequency with which impulses are occurring is to display the count in the form of a frequency histogram. This is accomplished by counting the number of

impulses in successive time intervals; each of these counts is then displayed sequentially on a recorder (Sheppard & Kouchoukos 1976).

If a signal is occurring at regular intervals, as in the ECG, it is possible to measure the rate, which can then be displayed in analogue or digital form. Ratemeters are of two basic types; integrating and instantaneous. An *integrating rate meter* determines the average rate over a period, whereas an *instantaneous rate meter* measures a single period between pulses and then takes the reciprocal to yield a value for rate (i.e. it measures in the time domain, and converts to the frequency domain afterwards).

Clinical rate meters are usually of the integrating type, since the information is more useful in determining trends, even over short periods. The instantaneous rate meter in fact gives more information about rhythm than it does about rate; thus an instantaneous rate record from a patient with atrial fibrillation will show a wide scatter of rates corresponding to the inherent irregularity of the pulse.

A simple rate-meter consists of no more than a capacitor discharging through a resistor (Fig. 4.7). A quantum of charge is added to the capacitor with each input pulse, and leaks away to the 'virtual earth' of the amplifier through the resistor. It can be shown that the charge on the capacitor, and therefore the current in the resistor is

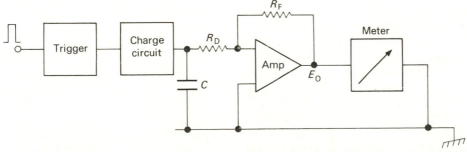

Fig. 4.7. A simple ratemeter. A quantum of charge is added to C each time the trigger is activated. C discharges through R_D to the virtual earth of the amplifier, so that the current through R_F must be equal and opposite. The output voltage E_O is therefore proportional to the current through R_D, which is determined by the charge on C, which is in turn proportional to the frequency at which quanta of charge are added.

directly proportional to the average frequency of the input pulse train, the averaging period depending upon the time constant ($R \times C$ seconds) of the circuit. Since the discharging resistor connects to the 'virtual earth' of the amplifier, the current in the feedback resistor is equal but opposite, so that the amplifier output voltage is proportional to the capacitor discharge current.

A display of this kind lends itself to further data processing, in which the signal is made to activate audible and visible warning devices when the rate transcends preset values (high and low) of rate. Needless to say the usefulness of such a warning system is dependent upon the quality of the signal whose rate is being measured. Early rate meters were notoriously unreliable, since the rate fell outside the limits whenever artefacts were present (due to the trigger circuit mistaking artefacts for QRS complexes, and failing to operate at all during recovery from large movement artefacts). Modern systems have largely overcome these shortcomings, as trigger circuits are commonly preceded by sophisticated filters which both remove noise and stabilize the trace. The reliability of alarms is also enhanced by the use of delay circuits, which prevent alarms sounding unless the alarm condition is sustained for a minimum period (usually approximately 10 s). A brief signal 'drop-out' due to movement is therefore not followed by an irritating false alarm.

Further developments in warning systems will undoubtedly accompany the present rapid spread of microprocessors through the field of clinical instrumentation. Already sophisticated computer-based systems have shown that certain types of irregularity are often seen to precede ventricular fibrillation, and may be useful as predictors. Certainly it is now clear that the careful monitoring and treatment of dysrhythmias greatly reduces the incidence of cardiac arrest in the management of acute myocardial infarction.

References

American Heart Association (1967) Report of a committee on electrocardiography. *Circulation* **35**, 583.

Baker L.E. & Hill D.W. (1969) The use of electrical impedance techniques for the monitoring of respiratory pattern during anaesthesia. *British Journal of Anaesthesia*, **41**, 2.

Dubois M., Savege T.M., O'Carroll T.M. & Frank M. (1978) General anaesthesia and changes on the cerebral function monitor. *Anaesthesia*, **33**, 157.

Finster M. & Petrie R.H. (1976) Monitoring of the fetus. *Anesthesiology*, **45**, 198.

Geddes L.A. (1972) *Electrodes and the measurement of bioelectric events.* London: Wiley—Interscience.

Geddes L.A. & Baker L.E. (1975) *Applied Biomedical Instrumentation. 2nd Ed.* New York: John Wiley & Sons.

Hill D.W. & Baker L.E. (1969) Impedance pneumograph. *British Journal of Anaesthesia*, **41**, 794.

Lewes D. (1965) Electrode jelly in electrocardiography. *British Heart Journal*, **27**, 105.

Prior P.F., Maynard D.E., Sheaff P.C., Simpson B.R., Strunin L., Weaver E.J.M. & Scott D.F. (1971) Monitoring cerebral function: clinical experience with a new device for continuous recording of electrical activity of brain. *British Medical Journal*, **2**, 736.

Prior P.F. (1979) *Monitoring cerebral function. Long-term recordings of cerebral electrical activity.* North Holland: Biomedical Press. Elsevier.

Prior P. (1980) Noninvasive monitoring of cerebral function. *British Journal of Clinical Equipment*, **2**, 54.

Severinghaus J.W. (1971) Electrical measurement of pulmonary oedema with a focusing conductivity bridge. *Journal of Physiology (London)*, **215**, 53.

Sheppard L.C. & Kouchoukos N.T. (1976) Computers as Monitors. *Anesthesiology*, **45**, 250.

Smith N.T. (1978) Computers in anesthesia, Chapter 13 in Saidman, L.J. & Smith N.T. *Monitoring in Anesthesia.* New York: John Wiley & Sons.

Steer P.J. (1977) Monitoring in labour. *British Journal of Hospital Medicine*, **17**, 219.

Wiggins K.E. & Meldrum (1977) ECG electrodes. *British Journal of Clinical Equipment*, **2**, 90.

Chapter 5
Data Processing and
Computation

It will be clear already that data acquisition is but the beginning of the process of measurement. In many instances we can simply feed the data into an oscilloscope or pen recorder and interpret it intuitively, as we are accustomed to do with the electrocardiogram. However, if the required information has to be derived from one or more data sources it is necessary to make a series of measurements from the recordings and then to compute the results. This process is often laborious and is always open to error. It is therefore obviously beneficial to have a system which performs the calculations by direct processing of the output data. Such a system is not only faster, and usually more reliable than manual computation, but is also independent of subjective influences.

Analogue processing

The process is best illustrated by a practical example. The function dP/dt (*max*), the maximum positive rate of change of pressure in the left ventricle, has been shown to be a useful index of cardiac contractility. By using a high fidelity pressure transducer a voltage may be obtained which is a faithful reproduction of the changing pressure in the left ventricle. This voltage could be recorded and the function dP/dt derived by measuring the slope of the pressure trace at the point where this was maximal. However, derivation of the slope by manual methods is very inaccurate and open to subjective error. By feeding the voltage representing the pressure into a suitable electronic circuit, differentiation can be performed continuously with a high degree of accuracy. The

record of the electrical output from such a circuit (Fig. 5.1) shows both positive and negative peaks because left ventricular pressure both increases and decreases

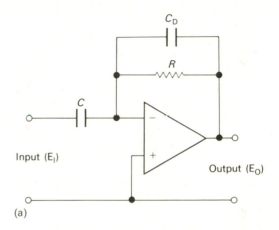

(a)

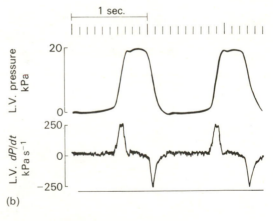

(b)

Fig. 5.1. Analogue differentiation of left ventricular pressure, to derive dP/dt (max). a. Circuit diagram of simple analogue differentiator. b. Record of left ventricular pressure and L.V. dP/dt showing that maximal deflections of dP/dt trace occur when L.V. pressure is rising or falling at maximal rate.

during the cardiac cycle, but it is a simple matter to read the peak value of dP/dt from the ordinate, providing this scale has been previously calibrated.

One way of calibrating this scale is to use a triangular waveform generator of known amplitude and frequency. The rate of rise of the voltage signal from the signal generator is governed by the amplitude and frequency of the waveform and can thus be adjusted to produce a signal which is comparable in magnitude with the observed dP/dt (max). Since this signal rises at a constant rate, the rate of change is constant. The triangular input waveform thus produces a square wave signal when differentiated (Fig. 5.2). As the voltage output of the pressure transducer can be measured, and the rate of rise of the voltage output from the generator is known, it is possible to calibrate the ordinate in terms of the rate of increase in pressure. It will be appreciated that the power of the analogue method lies in its ability to compute continuously from rapidly changing input functions which are, in purely mathematical terms, very complex, but in electronic terms, very simple.

Digital processing

An alternative method of computing dP/dt is to use digital processing. The first step is to convert the electrical signal from the pressure transducer into digital form (analogue-to-digital conversion, or ADC). This is done by measuring the pressure signal at regular intervals with an electronic voltmeter which then expresses the results in digital form.

Most electronic devices used in processors are capable of assuming one of two stable and unique states. Thus a switch can be on or off, a transistor can be conducting or nonconducting, a magnetic field can be orientated clockwise or anticlockwise. For this reason, computers use binary arithmetic rather than the more familiar decimal notation which would require devices that could assume ten unique, stable states. To illustrate the use of this system let us take the binary number 10011001. It is 8 digits or *bits* long, and the value of each bit is always either '1' or '0'. The least significant 'bit' is on the right (as in a decimal number), and represents either 1 or 0. The next bit is twice as significant again, so that a '1' represents 2, and a '0' nothing. The next bit is twice as significant again, so that a '1' represents 4. Successively significant bits therefore double in value, so that the '1' in the most significant bit (far left), represents 128. The decimal equivalent of the number 10011001 is the sum of the values of the four 1's in the binary number, i.e. $128 + 16 + 8 + 1 = 153$. An 8-bit number (properly called a

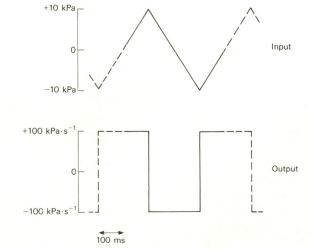

Fig. 5.2. Calibration of an analogue differentiator. A 'triangular' input waveform produces a 'squarewave' first derivative. Since the rate of rise is 10 kPa in 100 ms the calibration is 100 kPa s^{-1}.

byte) can resolve a given analogue signal with an accuracy of 1 part in $1 + 2 + 4 + 8 + 16 + 32 + 64 + 128 = 255$ parts. This is an accuracy of 0.4% of full scale. For more accurate applications a 12-bit byte resolving to 1 part in 4095 or 0.02% of full scale may be required. However, this is not the only factor governing the accuracy of analogue to digital conversion, for sampling frequency must also be considered. Whilst a relatively low sampling frequency may provide a representative sample of values for a slowly-changing waveform it may prove quite inadequate for one containing higher frequency components (Fig. 5.3). The detail with which the input voltage is digitised thus depends upon the length of the data byte and the sampling frequency, a frequency of 100 bytes per second (or correctly 100 bauds) being adequate to

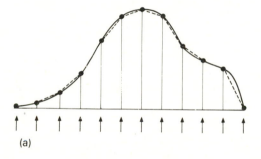

(a)

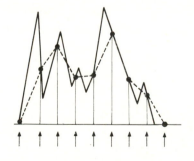

(b)

Fig. 5.3. Analogue-to-digital conversion. The sampling rate indicated by the arrows would provide a reasonably accurate reproduction of the slow variations in waveform a, but would not provide an accurate representation of waveform b. The waveform which would be reconstructed from digital data is shown as a dotted line.

capture the fastest likely rate of change of pressure in digital form.

After analogue-to-digital conversion each 12-bit byte can be led in parallel to a microprocessor. (Parallel connection means that 12 wires connect the two devices, each carrying a yes/no bit of information corresponding to one of the 12 bits in the byte.) The processor consists of three essential parts:

1   An arithmetic logic unit (ALU) which can perform simple arithmetic operations, and has several temporary storage locations for single bytes. These are usually referred to as registers or accumulators.

2   A fixed memory (program).

3   A larger, addressable memory, which can be used by the processor for both storage and recall of data bytes during the computation.

The whole process is under the control of the programme memory, which has been programmed to acquire bytes from the ADC, store them in the addressable memory, perform the necessary arithmetic manipulations in the logic unit, scale the answer to that required by the user, and send the information to an output device.

The output device takes the byte representing the answer to the problem and converts it back into a form intelligible to the user. In this very simple application, all these functions can be performed by a single microprocessor chip on a circuit card, which is programmed by devices known as *read only memories* (ROM's). These are memory circuits which are programmed during construction, so that when inserted into a microprocessor system, they will correctly instruct it to perform the required function.

The use of a microprocessor to solve this simple problem may seem to be excessively complex. It is, however, very simple from the designer's point of view, since all the component parts are readily available as 'large scale' integrated circuits (LSI) and are relatively inexpensive. Patient monitoring instruments whose data are processed by built-in microcomputers are now becoming commonplace. The overwhelming advantage of the method is that the processor can easily be programmed to perform much more sophisticated tasks at no extra cost. For example, the processor might take dP/dt (*max*) for successive cardiac cycles and after each cycle, print out the running mean of the last ten values, so as to minimize beat-to-beat variations and show underlying trends. Whilst this task is technically possible in an analogue computer, it would be extremely complicated.

MINI-COMPUTERS

Bigger problems require bigger processors, which can be programmed to perform many functions. The mini-computer, which might have a storage capacity of between 8000 (8K) and 64 000 (64K) bytes, finds widespread applications in medical instrumentation. Some instrumentation systems (such as that required for a cardiac catheterization laboratory), are available complete with a mini-computer which is ready programmed for specific tasks which are appropriate to its specifications.

The basic architecture of such a minicomputer system is shown in Fig. 5.4. The system consists of the computer itself, and a number of peripheral units such as papertape punch and paper-tape reader, keyboard, magnetic tape recorder, disc store, and visual display unit (VDU).

The heart of the computer is the central processing unit (CPU) which does all the calculating. It is connected to all the other parts of the computer by the 'data bus' which often consists of 16 parallel data lines, which can transmit data wherever required at very high speed. The CPU operates under the control of the instructions sent out by the program memory, but for relatively simple and specific tasks it might be programmed by a 'read only' memory (ROM).

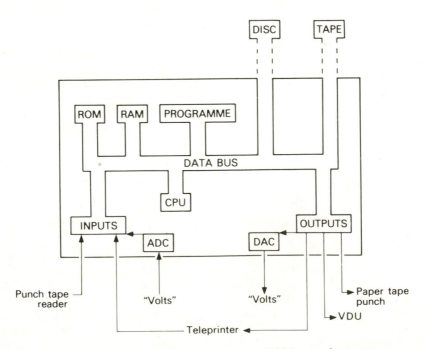

Fig. 5.4. The essential architecture of a minicomputer system. RAM = random access memory. ROM = read only memory. CPU = central processing unit. ADC = analogue-to-digital conversion. DAC = digital-to-analogue conversion. VDU = visual display unit.

The CPU may be supported by a number of back-up data stores. The random access memory (RAM) is rapidly accessible but of limited size and is used to store the binary numbers during processing. Information which does not need to be retrieved quite so quickly can be stored in a magnetic disc system. The disc rotates rapidly and may contain up to 100 000 bytes of information any of which can be retrieved within a few milliseconds. Less urgent data is recorded on magnetic tape where millions of bytes can be recorded on a single spool. These tapes may have to be searched by the computer to pick out the relevant information (e.g. the references on a particular topic in a library retrieval system) and this may take a period of minutes.

Some peripheral devices (e.g. a disc store) may be connected directly to the data bus. More often, peripheral units are not fully compatible with the data bus, and so must be connected to it via an *interface* circuit. This is simply a circuit which converts data bus signals into a form intelligible to the peripheral, and *vice versa*. It frequently has to synchronize the two devices, since the peripheral unit will usually operate at a much slower rate than the CPU. If, for instance, a paper-tape punch is instructed to punch a character, the interface circuit shows a 'flag' signal which stays until the punch cycle is complete. The CPU 'watches' the flag and does not send a second punch command until it is clear.

The input to the computer may be typed in directly from a teleprinter. However, the computer can receive data at a rate which is many times greater than normal typing speeds, so it may be more efficient to transfer the data to punched tape at a remote terminal and then to feed the tape into a tape reader connected directly to the computer. The computer teletype is thus reserved for simple instructions such as 'input tape', 'print out', etc. The output from the computer may be printed out directly by the teleprinter or may be transferred to punched-paper tape for subsequent typing, or graphical plotting. Alternatively it may be displayed visually on a cathode ray screen as an analogue or digital display.

PROGRAMMING

The microinstructions, in the form of binary numbers tell the CPU how to perform each basic task. (Thus the instructions 'take a number from location A, multiply it by 2, and put the answer in location B' might well require more than 10 microinstructions). Since programming in microinstructions would be very tedious, most minicomputers have a much higher level set of built-in instructions, called machine code, each of which executes a number of microinstructions. These instructions are very powerful, but are still in the form of binary numbers. To facilitate programming, a number of 'languages' have been developed, which substitute nmemonics (key-words) for binary numbers, and perform the necessary translation. In addition to simple nmemonics, high level languages have many powerful instructions of their own, each of which can execute many machine code instructions in sequence to perform a particular function. For example, a language suitable for the physiologist might have available the instruction 'LN'. When executed, this will perform all the manipulations necessary to compute the natural logarithm of a number. This would involve many machine code instructions, and literally thousands of microinstructions, but would occupy but a single step of the program written by the user.

The program is first written in the form of a flow-diagram, and then in the selected user language. It is then placed in the program store where it sequentially instructs the computer in its task. Big computers are often able to use any of several languages, but the mini-computer must first be 'loaded' with the required language. It is, of course, possible to have a fixed language in the form of a read-only memory, which makes the system very easy to use, but somewhat less flexible. In this form, the mini-computer is really a programmable calculator. The distinction between these two devices, which was once clear, is now rather blurred.

Let us take a very simple example of how a programme flow diagram might be constructed to solve part of the physiological problem of dP/dt (*max*) discussed earlier. Rate of change is determined by comparing successive differences between digital samples of the voltage waveform. dP/dt (*max*) will therefore be represented by the biggest positive successive difference, and knowing the binary number equivalent to say 10 kPa, and the time period between samples, the actual rate of change can be calculated easily. If three addressable storage locations are labelled A, B, C and the instruction ADC → A means 'do one analogue-to-digital conversion, and put the answer in store A', a very simplified flow diagram might appear as shown in Fig. 5.5.

In instruction (1), all the stores are set to zero. In (2) the first sample is digitized and put in Store A, then in (3) shifted to Store B. In (4), a further value is sampled and stored in A. In (5) the difference (B − A) is computed. Step (6) is a 'conditional branch'. If (B − A) is positive, the program goes to step (7) where a second conditional branch is found. Here the programme asks whether (B − A) is less than the previously stored value in C (which is of course zero in this first 'circuit' of the program). Step (8) shifts (B − A) into C, as it is, as yet, the biggest positive difference, and in step (9) loops back to step (3), where the value of A is shifted into B, and in (4), a new value put in A. The program can be seen to circulate, so long as the value (B − A) remains positive. If (B − A) is bigger than any previous value, it is stored in C (step 8), otherwise the program simply returns to (3). When a *negative* difference is detected in (6), the

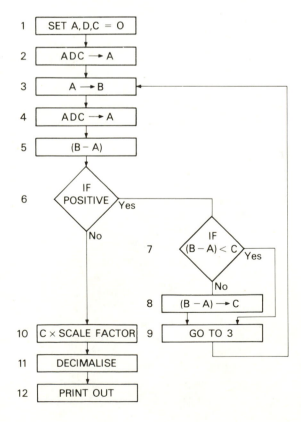

Fig. 5.5. A simple flow diagram to find the largest positive successive differences between serial analogue-to-digital conversions.

peak of the pressure waveform has been passed, so that it is now time to take the latest value of C, multiply it by a scaling factor (11), and print out (12). This very simple program must be instructed to start again at step (1) for a new cardiac cycle.

A practical program would be much more complex, as it must take into account all possible eventualities. The computer will only do exactly as it is told however ridiculous the instruction may prove to be in that particular circumstance, hence the saying 'garbage in–garbage out'.

So far, it has been assumed that the computer is linked directly to the data source. This is said to be *on-line*. This is not always possible, as computers often have several users. One could, instead, have tape-recorded the voltage waveform and replayed the data into the computer at a more convenient time. This is called 'off-line, real-time' processing, as everything is still being done at the same speed as before. A great deal of computer time can, however, be saved by using time-contraction techniques. The tape recorder is replayed at exactly 4, 8 or 16 times the speed at which it was recorded so that processing takes proportionately less time. This poses few technical problems, since ADC can be performed thousands of times per second if required, each computation literally taking microseconds. It is, of course, necessary to tell the program how fast the tape is going, or dP/dt (*max*) will be interpreted as being in the 'bionic' range!

LARGE COMPUTERS

Large computers, such as those to be found in university computing departments, are almost invariably unsuitable for the kind of task we have so far considered, since it is uneconomic for a single user to have uninterrupted access to the CPU. These large machines generally operate on a 'time-sharing' basis, so that a large number of operators, using teleprinter terminals, can be served almost at once, the amount of

central processor time actually used by each operator being very small.

The time-sharing computer can be likened to a chess player playing numerous exhibition matches simultaneously. He is in fact sharing his time between opponents, giving each his undivided attention for a brief period, making a move, and then going on to the next opponent who is ready for him. Because he analyses problems so quickly and has a large memory, he can effectively oppose each player almost as if the others were not present.

The time-sharing computer, with its extensive programme library and vast storage capability is of great use to a worker who needs to handle very large quantities of data (such as population statistics), but is of relatively little value to the physiologist who requires on-line data computation. In this application, the microprocessor and the ROM-programmed minicomputer are likely to reign supreme for many years to come.

COMPARISON OF ANALOGUE AND DIGITAL COMPUTERS

Although digital methods of computation are tending to replace analogue computers there are certain applications for ,which analogue methods are ideally suited. Although analogue computers can perform the four arithmetic functions of addition, subtraction, multiplication and division, it is their ability to perform continuous differentiation or integration with respect to time which makes them unique. Thus they can be used to provide a continuous indication of the volume entering or leaving the lung by integration of the flow signal; body displacement can be differentiated to give velocity and then differentiated again to give acceleration in the ballistocardiogram; or the area under a dye-dilution curve can be obtained by integrating the area under the curve after establishing the pattern of exponential decay (Chapter 16). The larger analogue computers usually have 50 or more operational amplifiers which can be connected in an appropriate manner to solve complex equations so that a large number of calculations may be performed simultaneously. For example, it is possible to study the uptake and distribution of drugs by modelling a series of body compartments with different blood flows and different capacities for the drug, and then to study how regional variations in blood flow might affect drug distribution. Since each constant in each equation is controlled by one knob on the control panel it is a simple matter to produce a perturbation in one part of the system and to observe its effect on the remainder of the system. In all these applications the amplitude of the input voltage is scaled to match the variable under observation while the time scale is adjusted to provide a reasonable duration for the computation. Amplitude and time scaling add greatly to the versatility of the instrument for they enable processes with very long or very short time scales to be simulated at a rate which can be adjusted to provide the most information in the available time. For examples illustrating the use of analogue computers see Fletcher & Bellville (1966), Bellville and Hara (1966), Wald, Murphy and Mazzia (1968) and Hull and McLeod (1976).

Digital computation has made enormous strides since the advent of the microprocessor, for this discovery has enabled both the cost and size of the installations to be reduced by staggering amounts. Indeed its importance has been compared to the advent of the wheel. The new technology started with the invention of the transistor in 1948. Subsequently a small piece of semiconductor material was processed to perform as a group of transistors or other components of a circuit. The complexity of the microcircuits increased rapidly as the production technology advanced. By 1960 there were about 10 components on each small silicon 'chip'. By 1970 there were several hundred and by 1976 large scale integration (LSI) resulted in over 10 000 components per chip. Very large scale integration (VLSI) will bring 100 000 components per chip in 1980 and over 1 million components are expected to be incorporated in a $6\,mm^2$ chip by the mid-1980's. Microcircuits can now be programmed to perform various functions and thus form the basis of the digital computers of today. Microprocessors are very reliable and since each element functions in an on/off mode they are not subject to problems of electronic drift. Even complex calculations can be performed very rapidly and the input and output can be in analogue or digital form. The ability to pre-program the microprocessor now simplifies the programming of large computers but also greatly widens the usefulness of microprocessors in other fields. Thus they are being increasingly utilized in specialized computing applications such as control systems.

In medicine small dedicated digital computers are used to calculate acid base variables from the outputs from P_{O_2}, P_{CO_2} and pH electrodes (Chapter 18), to calculate cardiac output from indicator dilution curves (Chapter 16) or from the arterial pressure trace (Wesseling *et al.* 1974). Digital processing has also been used in the analysis of the ECG. For example digital storage is used to permit the ECG waveform to be 'frozen' for closer scrutiny, whilst programs have been devised to provide a detailed analysis of the ECG complex or to detect differences in the R-R interval as an indication of the presence of dysrhythmias (Glaser & Thomas 1975). Many computer-assisted studies of the EEG have also been carried out (Smith 1978). On-line computation of pulmonary function is now standard in many pulmonary function laboratories and has also been used to monitor patients on mechanical ventilators. An entirely new field is that of computed trend analysis in which the analysis of monitored data is used to predict the likelihood of an impending complication. This, together with medical record or literature retrieval demands a huge storage capacity which can only be accommodated in the digital computer.

Glossary of computer terms

Algorithm A fixed step-by-step procedure for accomplishing a given task. It is often defined in algebraic terms.

Alphanumeric characters Alphabetical and numerical symbols.

Analogue signal A continuously varying signal representing the instantaneous magnitude of a variable.

Arithmetic section of central processing unit (ALU) The section of the computer in which the logic and arithmetical operations are carried out.

Assembly language Program instructions in the form of symbols or mnemonics which are converted into machine code by the computer.

Backing store Magnetic tape or disc units.

Baud One byte per second.

Bit A contraction of *binary digit*.

Byte A sequence of bits processed as a unit.

Character A digit, letter or symbol.

Compiler A program which converts high level language statements into machine code.

Computer A device for processing information received in a prescribed and acceptable form according to a set of instructions.

Control section The section of a computer which controls the operations of the other parts.

Direct access store Store in which data are not accessed in a serial manner and in which the time taken to access a location does not depend on the position of that location in the store.

Disc store A backing store in which data are stored on a number of concentric circular tracks on magnetic discs. These rotate at high speed and give direct access.

Hardware The physical components of a computer system such as the central processing unit, the memory and the peripheral devices.

High level language A programming language orientated to the natural language of the programmer. Each instruction generates a number of machine code instructions.

Hybrid computer A computer which solves problems using both analogue and digital hardware.

Interface The common boundary between two computers or between a computer and an external device. Interface circuits ensure compatibility between the devices.

Machine language (code) The basic computer language, each instruction having a numerical code to describe the operation or the location of data.

Memory The part of the computer which stores information in bytes for use by the central processing unit. The memory may consist of magnetic cores (permanent magnets) or may be a solid-state memory. A solid-state memory is smaller and faster than core memory, but the information may be lost when the supply voltage is removed. (Often referred to as a volatile store.)

Off-line Not directly connected to the computer, not operating simultaneously with the computer.

On-line Equipment or function in the system connected to the computer.

Programme A set of instructions which tells the computer how to handle a specific problem. They may be direct instructions in machine code or higher level mnemonic instructions which themselves control a series of direct machine code instructions. Such mnemonics form the basis of a high-level computer language, such as BASIC, FORTRAN, ALGOL, etc.

Real-time Processing of data by a computer sufficiently rapidly for events to be detected or influenced as they occur.

Routine Part of a programme.

Software The programs associated with a computer system. Some of these are provided by the manufacturer and may be integrated into the computer design but others are written by the programmer to deal with specific problems.

Store The computer memory.

References

BELLVILLE J.W. & HARA H.H. (1966) Use of analog computers in anesthetic research. *Anesthesiology*, **27**, 70.

FLETCHER G. & BELLVILLE J.W. (1966) On-line computation of pulmonary compliance and work of breathing. *Journal of Applied Physiology*, **2**, 1321.

GLASER D.H. & THOMAS L.J. (1975) Computer monitoring in patient care. *Annual Reviews of Biomedical Engineering*, **4**, 677.

HULL C.J. & McLEOD K. (1976) Pharmacokinetic analysis using an electrical analogue. *British Journal of Anaesthesia*, **48**, 677.

SMITH J.T. (1978) Computers in anesthesia, Chapter 13 in *Monitoring in Anesthesia*, Eds. L.J. Saidman and N.T. Smith. New York: John Wiley & Sons.

WALD A.A., MURPHY T.W. & MAZZIA V.D.B. (1968) A theoretical study of controlled ventilation. *Biomedical Engineering*, **15**, 237.

WESSELING K.H., SMITH N.T., NICHOLS W.W., WEBER H., DEWIT B. & BENEKIN J.E.W. (1974) Beat to beat cardiac output from the arterial pressure contour. *Measurement in Anaesthesia*. Eds S.A. Feldman, J.M. Leigh & J. Spierdijk. Leiden: University Press.

Chapter 6
Displaying the Signal

In the past most biological signals were processed by analogue methods and displayed as an analogue signal on a scale or cathode-ray tube. However the advent of the microprocessor has revolutionized digital processing so that digital processing methods are now rapidly replacing those based on analogue principles. Digital processing units require much less maintenance, retain their accuracy longer and have greater inherent flexibility than analogue units. As a result of this processing revolution signals which were commonly displayed in analogue form are now often displayed digitally.

Analogue displays

An analogue signal is one in which the variable biological signal is represented by a physical quantity whose amplitude continuously represents the magnitude of the input variable. The signal may be displayed in many ways. For example the intensity of the signal may be represented by the intensity of a light bulb, by the number of lights in an array which are illuminated, or by the intensity of sound from a loudspeaker (as in instruments using Doppler ultrasound p. 115). More commonly the signal is displayed by the movement of an indicator over a scale. Such *scalar* displays enable information to be assimilated rapidly and are of particular use when it is desirable to indicate whether the signal is in the normal range, or above or below this range. By choosing the appropriate scale length for each variable and colour coding the scale in segments for the high, normal and low ranges, it is possible for an observer

to monitor many displays simultaneously and yet to be able to identify an aberrant reading immediately. Analogue displays on a cathode-ray oscilloscope have the advantage that they provide a continuous indication of the variable and can thus reveal trends, whilst they are often more easily visible from a distance or in poor lighting conditions than some other forms of display. In certain circumstances, for example ECG monitoring, the information can be displayed in no other way.

SCALAR DISPLAY

The scale may be linear or curvilinear, and the signal may be displayed directly or by electronic means. The simplest example of a direct linear display is that produced by the mercury column in a mercury-in-glass thermometer or in a sphygmomanometer, or by the bobbin in a rotameter. Electronic forms of display are utilized when the signal is processed before being displayed. For example a blood pressure signal may be processed to yield systolic and diastolic pressures and heart rate and this may then be displayed by producing an illuminated column beside a linear scale. This form of display was adopted because this type of image is familiar to doctors and nurses and it is easy to display high/low limits or alarm states.

More commonly the magnitude of the signal is displayed on a meter which is based on the moving-coil or moving-iron galvanometer. The former consists of a coil of wire suspended in a magnetic field (Fig. 6.1). When a current is passed through the coil a magnetic field is generated which interacts with that of the magnet to create a force which rotates the coil against the torsion of the suspension. The degree of rotation of the coil is then displayed by the movement of a needle attached to the coil.

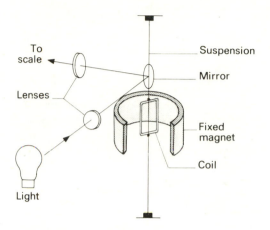

Fig. 6.1. Moving coil galvanometer using light source and mirror to display the signal on a translucent scale.

Since meters are usually used for the display of slowly-changing signals, the mass of the moving parts is not critical and a large coil can be used to increase sensitivity. The other system commonly used for driving the meter is the moving-iron system, in which a permanent magnet (attached to the pointer) is mounted inside a fixed coil. A variation in signal strength in the fixed coil varies the strength of the electromagnetic field and so alters the position of the permanent magnet and the pointer.

The movement of a coil may also be displayed by shining a narrow beam of light onto a small mirror attached to the coil. The reflected beam is then directed onto a translucent scale. The use of a mirror allows the mass of the moving parts of the instrument to be greatly reduced and so increases the frequency response (p. 78). Furthermore by increasing the length of the light path, usually by reflecting the light back and forth between a system of fixed mirrors, it is possible to produce a great increase in the sensitivity of the system. Mirror galvanometers are therefore commonly used when it is desired to obtain maximum sensitivity and speed of response. The movement of the light beam can also be recorded by directing it onto moving photographic film or onto special paper which is sensitive to ultraviolet light (see Chapter 7).

CATHODE-RAY TUBES

This form of display is utilized when diagnostic information is contained in the shape of the analogue signal or when it is important to display trends. It is the only form of display unit which can produce an image of very high frequency signals.

Usually the variable is displayed on the y-axis with time on the x-axis but for some purposes (for example pressure–volume curves of the lung or vectorcardiography) a second variable is applied to the x-axis so that a two-dimensional shape is described on the display screen.

There are two types of cathode-ray tube, *electrostatic* and *electromagnetic*. The electrostatic type of tube is the standard laboratory instrument which is used to display high frequency analogue signals on a relatively small screen, whilst the electromagnetic tube is employed when a high velocity electron beam is required to produce a bright display over a large area, for example in television and radar receivers. Both types of tube consist of a glass cylinder with a conical or tetrahedral expansion at one end. The narrow part of the glass tube contains the electron 'gun'. This consists of a heated cathode which generates a stream of electrons, a cylindrical grid which controls the intensity of the electron beam (and hence the brightness of the display) and a series of positively-charged anodes which accelerate the beam and focus it onto the fluorescent screen lining the flat surface at the expanded end of the tube, thus rendering it visible (Fig. 6.2a). Between the anodes and the screen there is a mechanism which deflects the electron beam in the x and y axes.

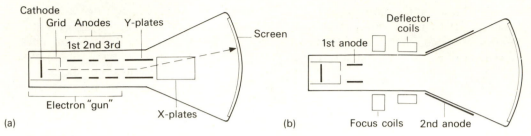

Fig. 6.2. Cathode-ray tubes a. electrostatic, b. electromagnetic.

In the electrostatic tube the deflection is produced by applying potentials to two pairs of deflection plates situated within the tube. One pair of plates is mounted horizontally and deflects the beam in a vertical direction (y-plates) whilst the other pair is mounted vertically and deflects the spot horizontally (x-plates). Normally a potential from a special time-base circuit is applied to the x-plates. This potential resembles a saw-tooth waveform for it increases gradually and at a constant rate and then suddenly drops to zero. Thus the spot is drawn at a constant rate from left to right across the screen and then suddenly returned to the left side again before commencing another sweep. If a potential proportional to the input signal is now applied to the y-plates, an image representing signal amplitude versus time will be produced, thus re-creating the original analogue input signal. When desired the time-base can be switched off and a second input signal applied to the x-plates; a graphical plot then results.

In the electromagnetic tube large deflections of the electron beam are required and electrostatic deflection becomes impracticable. Deflection is therefore accomplished by electromagnetic deflector coils situated outside the tube between the focus coils and the second anode (Fig. 6.2b). The speed of deflection in an electromagnetic tube is slower than in an electrostatic tube. This affects the way in which multiple signals are displayed.

Multiple signal inputs to an electrostatic scope can be displayed by utilizing several separate beams of electrons and deflecting each beam independently. However, this makes the equipment bulky and expensive. More commonly a single electron gun is used in association with a beam-switching technique which causes each input to be sampled in turn. Each input channel is associated with a certain value of 'y-shift' so that the time-base deflection corresponding to it is located at a certain height on the tube face, the rate of switching between channels being designed to maintain an adequate quality of signal on each trace. Thus a switching rate of 10 kHz would be adequate to display concurrently four signals each having a frequency of 1 kHz. (This beam-switching can often be identified on the trace when the writing speed is high, for the trace then appears as a series of dots.)

The 'fly-back' of the time-base tends to interfere with the display of multiple analogue signals so that it is customary to diminish the intensity of the electron beam whilst it is travelling back to commence another sweep or switching between channels. This intensity, or z-modulation, is synchronized with both beam switching and the resetting of the time-base and is known as 'fly-back blanking'.

The relatively slow deflection of the spot in electromagnetic CRT's precludes high-speed beam-switching so that a *raster* display is used instead. In this form of display the electron beam is repeatedly moved in a very fine zig-zag pattern over the whole screen, the actual display being generated by altering the brightness of the spot as it moves across the screen. The raster pattern may be horizontal, in which the spot moves progressively down the screen in a series of horizontal passes, or vertical, in which it moves across the screen in a series of vertical passes. The technique thus permits complex displays to be generated (including alphanumeric characters) and the frequency of signal that can be handled is a function of the number of times that the spot can cover the screen each second.

In the simplest application (for example the display of an ECG signal) a vertical raster is moved across the screen at such a speed that the horizontal movement is equivalent to the paper speed of a direct recorder. As the beam moves up the screen on each raster line the intensity is kept switched off until the raster voltage equals that of the signal. It is then briefly turned on and off so that the screen glows at that point. Successive raster sweeps thus gradually build up a waveform. In this type of display a long persistence phosphor is essential: this is usually chosen so that the beginning of the trace has disappeared by the time the raster returns to the left-hand side of the screen. In more advanced systems, such as the visual display unit (VDU) of a computer, the whole raster pattern fills the screen many times a second, the spot modulation being controlled by the computer. As a result flicker-free displays of great complexity and uniform brightness can be generated. Since the entire display is refreshed many times a second a short persistence phosphor is used.

The display on an oscilloscope screen can be photographed with a Polaroid or standard camera or the time-base can be switched off and the vertical deflection of the spot recorded on a film moving in the horizontal plane. CRT's with a fibre-optic face plate produce an image which is bright enough to record directly onto ordinary photographic paper. However, for some applications it is desirable to be able to hold the image until it has been examined more closely and then to banish the image and restore the usual display. This has now been made possible by the development of storage oscilloscopes.

Storage oscilloscopes

Several different principles are employed to permit retention of the image. One type is known as a *direct-view bistable storage tube*. This is illustrated in Fig. 6.3. This tube contains two electron guns. In the narrow part of the tube there is a *writing gun* which can be focussed and deflected as in a conventional electrostatic or electromagnetic cathode-ray tube. The second cathode which generates the electrons for the *flood gun* is usually annular in shape and situated at the narrow end of the conical part of the tube. Electrons emanating from this source are collimated by an electrode in the conical part of the tube (often a carbon coating in the inside of the tube itself) so that they form a wide parallel beam of equal density which floods the screen with electrons. Parallel to the screen and close to it are two fine wire meshes, the *storage mesh* and the *collector mesh*. The side of the storage mesh remote from the screen is coated with an insulating material which has good secondary emission charac-

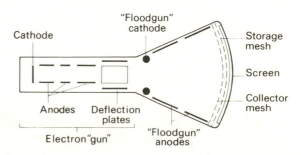

Fig. 6.3. Bistable storage cathode-ray tube.

teristics. When this material is bombarded with fast-moving electrons it emits more electrons than it receives and so becomes positively charged.

The image on the 'screen' is created by the stream of fast-moving electrons from the writing gun. These electrons impinge on the storage mesh and displace electrons so that the written area is positively charged with respect to the rest of the mesh. Meanwhile the flood gun showers the whole area of the screen with low velocity electrons which have inadequate energy to cause secondary emission. These areas therefore become negatively charged and cease to attract further electrons from the flood gun, the electrons being accelerated instead to the positively-charged, 'written' areas. Their velocity is high enough for them to penetrate the storage mesh and so to cause persistence of the image on the screen. This image tends to fade if storage periods are more than about 10 min because the rest of the screen tends to brighten with time. The brightening is caused by leakage of electrons across the insulator surface and by bombardment with positively-charged ions formed within the tube. However, this can be prevented by switching off the flood gun when the display does not have to be viewed. The image can be erased completely by applying a single positive pulse to the storage mesh. It is also possible to carry out a 'continuous erase' by applying a succession of smaller pulses so that the image fades at a controlled rate ('variable persistence'). This type of display is much used in the radar field, for moving objects then show up as a trail with a bright head and fading tail, whilst stationary objects remain uniformly bright as their image is up-dated by each sweep of the writing gun. In the medical field storage tubes are used for the display of images built up from the output of a gamma camera or ultrasonic imaging device.

An alternative method of storing an image is exemplified by the *digital storage oscilloscope*: this is now commonly used in the display of the electrocardiograph signal.

The ECG signal is first fed into a analogue-to-digital converter (Chapter 5) and the data then stored in a computer type of memory. This contains data from the preceeding few seconds and is continually up-dated by data from the incoming signal. The memory is constantly scanned by a digital-to-analogue converter at much higher speed (above the flicker-fusion frequency) and the output displayed on the screen. The screen thus continuously displays the ECG recorded during the preceeding few seconds, whilst the use of a short persistence phosphor and repeated refreshing of the image produces a high quality image which does not fade. As the memory is up-dated, the data shifts so that the trace appears to move across the screen. If the memory is not up-dated its contents are unchanged, so that a static image appears on the screen. The display can thus be frozen at any desired moment to facilitate recognition of individual ECG complexes. This type of apparatus can be connected to a conventional direct writing recorder or to a digital computer for further analysis of the signal. It can also be programmed to record traces at given intervals of time. It therefore provides a most useful facility in the ECG monitoring field.

Recorder displays

For much slower analogue signals it is possible to use any of the recorder systems outlined in Chapter 7 as display units. Again, the most common display is one in which the variable is expressed on the y-axis with time (paper speed) on the x-axis. Certain flat-bed recorders have an additional facility which permits separate signals to be recorded on the x and y axes, the paper being kept stationary. These are useful for recording shapes like pressure–flow or pressure–volume loops. By an extension of this principle it is possible to display results in graphical form, each point being printed at the appropriate intersection of the x and y axis.

Digital display

This form of display is most suitable when the information is required in the form of figures, e.g. counts of nerve impulses, radioactivity, temperature etc.

The figures may be generated by gas-filled tubes, light emitting diodes or liquid crystal display units, displayed on an oscilloscope screen or printed on paper. Obviously, the number of digits available must cover the range and accuracy required. Digital displays can convey more information in a given area than many other forms of display but are often difficult to read when viewing conditions are poor and are not suitable for rapidly-changing signals. This type of display eliminates errors due to faulty scale reading, but may introduce others, for example, in correctly identifying the position of the decimal point.

CHOICE AND POSITION OF DISPLAY UNITS

The selection of the form of display is crucial. Choice of the wrong form of display leads to the presentation of inadequate data, increases the likelihood of errors from misinterpretation of the data and increases the strain on the observer. Although manufacturers are now greatly improving the design of display systems, it is rare to see them used to maximal advantage in hospitals. Display units should be placed in situations where they are easily visible to the appropriate observer, but not visible to the patient, and the lighting conditions should be adjusted so that the display stands out clearly from the background. It is often difficult to achieve such conditions in the hospital environment but strenuous efforts should be made to do so, for the patient's life may depend on the accurate relay of information to the observer.

Chapter 7
Recorders

Recording and display are usually carried out by separate instruments. However, in some systems it is easy to visualize the signals as they are being written on the paper, thereby eliminating the need for a separate display unit, whilst in others the display itself is photographed for record purposes.

Choice of recorder

There are three main types of recorder: direct writers in which a writing arm or ink jet makes a direct imprint on the paper (Figs 7.1 and 7.2); photographic or ultraviolet, in which the impression is made by a beam of white or ultraviolet light (Fig. 7.3); and magnetic, in which the data is stored on magnetic tape, or in a computer 'store'.

The choice of recorder is determined primarily by the frequency of the signal which is to be recorded. The frequency components of some typical biological signals are shown in Table 7.1. It may be seen that they vary from a steady current or voltage (d.c.) to a frequency of up to 5000 Hz. Potentiometric recorders can only deal with d.c. or low frequency signals. Few recorders with a long writing arm are capable of accurately recording frequencies above 75–100 Hz. Ink-jet recorders can handle frequencies up to 500 Hz whilst photographic or ultraviolet recorders are capable of reproducing frequencies up to 2000 or even 8000 Hz provided that the galvanometers are specially chosen for this purpose. Higher frequencies can be recorded by photographing the movements of an electron beam on the fluorescent screen of a cathode-ray tube, by recording on to magnetic tape, or by temporary storage in a computer store followed by 'read out'

Table 7.1. Frequency and amplitude of some typical biological signals.

Signal	Approximate frequency range (Hz)	Approximate magnitude
ECG	0.1–100	1 mV
EEG	0.5–70	50 μV
EMG	10–70	100 μV (skin electrode)
	3–5000	1 mV (needle electrode)
EOG	d.c.–120	0.5 mV
Arterial pressure	d.c.–20	
Left ventricular		
dP/dt (*max*)	d.c.–100	
Phonocardiogram	20–2000	
Respiratory		
airflow	d.c.–30	

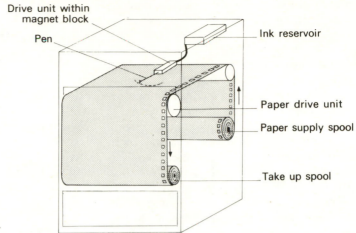

Fig. 7.1. A simple pen recorder.

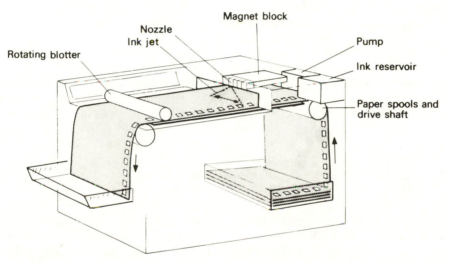

Fig. 7.2. An ink-jet recorder.

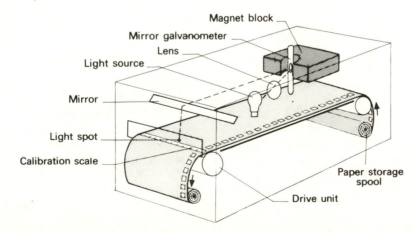

Fig. 7.3. An ultraviolet galvanometer recorder.

into a conventional recorder at a much lower data rate.

The second factor to be considered is the accuracy required from the recording. For example, when recording arterial blood pressure it is usually adequate to display the trace on a channel which is 50 mm wide. When the gain of the recording system is adjusted to produce a full-scale deflection of 250 mmHg, each millimetre on the record then represents 5 mmHg. This accuracy is quite satisfactory for most clinical purposes. On the other hand, a dye dilution curve must be recorded with an amplitude of 10–20 cm so that the logarithmic replotting of the exponential part of the curve can be accomplished with sufficient accuracy (p. 211). Since the dye curve has only low frequency components and since most galvanometric pen recorders become non-linear when the deflection is large, it is better to choose a potentiometric recorder for this application.

The third factor determining the choice of recorder is the environment in which the recorder is to be used. For example, heated stylus recorders are usually more reliable and cleaner in use than ink-pen recorders and are ideal for the clinical situation. Photographic or ultraviolet recorders do not produce an immediate image and are more difficult to adjust, but may have to be used if high frequency recordings are required or if more than 4–6 channels are to be recorded simultaneously. Tape recorders are clean, compact and can incorporate a voice channel thus obviating the need to write down details of events, but they must usually be combined with a display unit so that the recording can be monitored.

The fourth factor is cost. Pen recorders are relatively cheap to buy and to run. Heated stylus recorders are more expensive and require special recording paper, as do ultraviolet and photographic recorders. Paper costs must be considered in relation to the quantity likely to be used. For example EEG recordings are always made with pen recorders on plain paper because the cost of photographic or heated stylus papers would be prohibitive when recordings may extend to half an hour or more.

Recorder performance

When analysing the performance of a recorder it is necessary to consider the frequency response, linearity and the possibility of timing errors.

FREQUENCY RESPONSE: AMPLITUDE AND PHASE DISTORTION

If a writing arm is oscillated at gradually increasing frequency by a sine wave signal of constant amplitude it responds in a characteristic fashion (Fig. 7.4a). At low frequencies it faithfully follows the sine wave input but as the frequency is increased a point is reached at which the excursion of the pen arm begins to increase. As frequency is further increased the excursion of the arm reaches a peak and then declines, the amplitude of the recording at the highest frequencies being scarcely discernible. The increase in amplitude is due to resonance, and the frequency at the peak deflection represents the resonant frequency of the vibrating system. At higher frequencies the movement of the pen fails to follow the applied waveform and finally settles in a mean position. This is a characteristic response of all vibrating systems and is discussed further in Chapter 13; however, some basic considerations must be appreciated at this stage.

First, the response illustrated in Fig. 7.4a is the response of a freely oscillating system. This has its own natural frequency of oscillation determined by the effective mass of the writing arm and the tension of the spring tending to return the writing arm to its zero position. The resonant frequency can be increased by reducing the effective mass of the arm (by decreasing its weight or its length) or by increasing the stiffness of the spring. This will permit higher frequencies to be recorded without encroaching on the resonant frequency but will still leave much of the potential of the system untapped.

As well as needing an adequate frequency response, an efficient and accurate system needs to be appropriately damped. This may be done hydraulically (for example by suspending the driving galvanometer in a viscous fluid) or electronically (by incorporating an inductance in the system). A system is said to be critically damped when the damping is adjusted to such a level that it follows a step change at the input with maximum velocity but does not overshoot (Fig. 7.4b). However, this degree of damping markedly slows the response to a square wave input signal. The optimal rate of response with minimal overshoot (approximately 6–7%) occurs when the damping is adjusted to be about 64–66% of critical.

A system which is damped in this manner has a 'flat' response (i.e. the amplitude distortion is less than ±2%) up to frequencies which are two-thirds of the un-

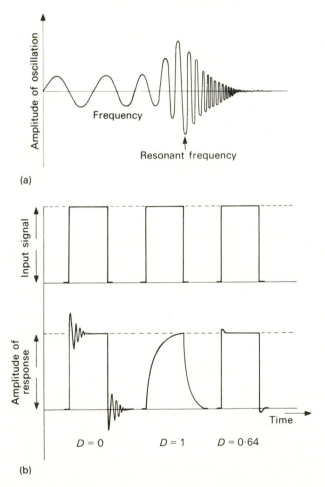

(a)

(b)

Fig. 7.4. a. Effect of increasing frequency on amplitude of recorded signal with constant amplitude sine wave input. b. Response to square wave input. Left: minimal damping showing overshoot and oscillation. Centre: critically damped (overshoot just abolished). Right: damping 64% of critical showing maximum speed of response with minimal overshoot. D, damping factor.

damped natural frequency of the system. Thus to record the higher harmonics of an arterial pressure waveform (usually considered to be about 20 Hz) it is necessary to use a recorder with an undamped natural frequency of 30 Hz and then to apply damping until this is 64% of critical. Optimal damping therefore minimizes amplitude distortion and enables a much greater proportion of the undamped natural frequency to be used for recording (Fig. 7.5).

When considering frequency response it is important to take note of phase delay as well as amplitude distortion, for both of these factors will distort the output signal (p. 167). Phase delay occurs because the inertia of the vibrating system causes it to lag behind the applied waveform. The phase lag varies with both the frequency and with the degree of damping (Fig. 7.6). Phase lag is small at low frequencies but increases to one quarter of a cycle (90°) at the resonant frequency of the system. To secure an accurate registration of all the harmonics of a complex wave it is essential that the time delay imparted to all harmonics should be the same so that their time relationships

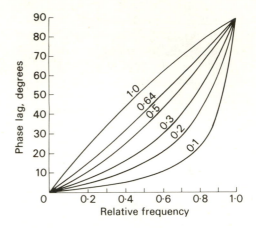

Fig. 7.6. Phase lag with increasing frequency. $D = 1.0$ represents critical damping. $D = 0$ is undamped. Phase lag is proportional to frequency when $D = 0.64$.

with each other are undisturbed. Now a phase lag of 90° with a wave having a frequency of 1 Hz represents a delay of 1/4 second, whereas a similar phase lag with a 2 Hz wave would be 1/8 second. To secure the same *time* delay it is therefore essential that the phase lag should increase in proportion to the frequency. As shown in Fig. 7.6 this condition is satisfied when the damping is adjusted to be 64% of critical. Thus optimal damping secures the optimal frequency response and minimizes both amplitude and phase distortion.

LINEARITY AND TIMING ERRORS

Ideally a recorder should respond to a square wave input signal by producing an identical square wave on the recording paper. Unfortunately such an ideal is difficult to achieve. Let us first consider a pen recorder in which the angular displacement of the pen is linearly related to the input signal. Such a pen will describe an arc across the paper, thus distorting the recorded signal. Since we are concerned with both the amplitude of the signal (i.e. vertical displacement) and the timing of the signal (horizontal displacement) we must assess the magnitude of the errors introduced by this method of recording. Since the

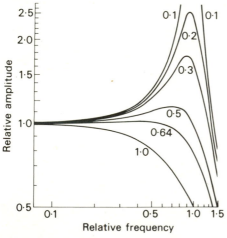

Fig. 7.5. Amplitude distortion with increasing frequency $D =$ damping factor. $D = 1.0$ represents critical damping. $D = 0$ is undamped. When $D = 0.64$ the recorded amplitude is accurate to within 2% up to about two thirds of the undamped natural frequency. (Relative frequency = fraction of undamped natural frequency).

length of the arc is directly related to the length of the writing arm (R) and the angular displacement (θ radians) the length of the arc must be directly related to the input signal (Fig. 7.7). However the vertical displacement of the writing point from the zero position is given by $R \sin \theta$, where θ is expressed in degrees. Each successive increment of angular displacement will therefore produce a smaller vertical displacement than the previous one, so that the recorded amplitude is not linearly related to the input signal. This *sine* error is minimized by using small angular displacements and is not significant with a pen arm (10 cm long) moving through an angular displacement of $\pm 20°$.

A larger error is produced on the time axis (Fig. 7.7). This timing error (t) can be calculated from the expression $t = R - R \cos \theta$. As may be seen from Table 7.2 and Fig. 7.8 this error can create major

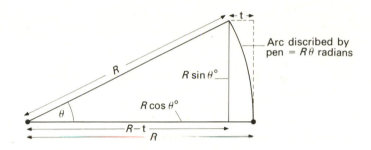

Fig. 7.7. Sources of distortion in a pen recorder. The pen (of length R) describes an arc whose length is $R\theta$ radians. The vertical displacement of the pen tip is $R \sin \theta°$ and the timing error is $t = R - R \cos \theta°$. The sine error causes the vertical displacement to be less than it should be at large angular displacements.

Table 7.2. Effect of angular displacement of writing arm on sine, timing and tangent errors

| Angular displacement (degrees) | Length of arc (cm) | Linear displacement (cm) | | |
		vertical	horizontal	vertical
	$(= R \theta \text{ radians})$	$(= R \sin \theta°)$	$(= t)$	$(= R \tan \theta°)$
0	0.00	0.00	0.00	0.00
10	1.75	1.74	0.15	1.76
20	3.49	3.42	0.60	3.64
30	5.23	5.00	1.34	5.77
40	6.98	6.43	2.34	8.39

Displacement along the arc, vertical and horizontal axes calculated for a writing arm 10 cm long. Since a tangent error arises from an effective lengthening of the writing arm it is assumed that the arm is 10 cm long at zero displacement (see Figs. 7.7, 7.8 and 7.12).

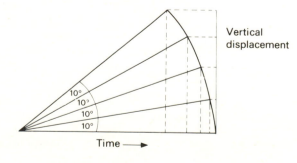

Fig. 7.8. Angular displacements of writing arm of 10°, 20°, 30° and 40° to show relative magnitudes of sine error and timing error with 10 cm long arm.

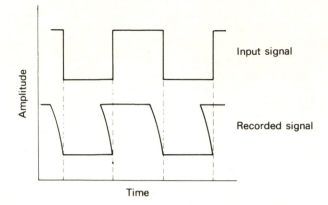

Fig. 7.9. Use of curvilinear co-ordinates to eliminate pen distortion. Although the time and amplitude of the event are now correctly recorded the shape of the waveform is distorted.

inaccuracies in timing even with relatively small angular displacements of the pen.

The simplest method of overcoming these problems is to mark the recording paper with curvilinear co-ordinates which parallel the arc inscribed by the pen. This eliminates both sources of error but the shape of the trace is distorted (Fig. 7.9). A second method is to mount the writing arm vertically and to shape the paper into a corresponding arc by pulling it along a curved trough (Fig. 7.10). This is a simple solution in single-channel recorders but creates technical problems when a number of signals must be recorded on the same roll of paper.

A more satisfactory alternative is to draw the paper over a knife-edge and to use a heated stylus to mark heat-sensitive paper.*

* This type of paper has a coloured base and is covered with a thin layer of white cellulose. When the cellulose is melted the coloured base shows through.

The heated stylus is usually about 1–2 cm long and is mounted at the tip of the writing arm in its long axis. The knife-edge is mounted at right angles to the direction of travel of the paper (Fig. 7.11). When the writing arm is deflected laterally the point of contact of the heated stylus with the knife-edge moves towards the tip of the writing arm. This effectively lengthens the arm as it moves laterally and so ensures that the time co-ordinate is unaffected by lateral displacement of the writing arm. A similar effect is achieved in the ink-jet recorder where the jet is mounted above the paper and the angular displacement of the jet results in a vertical displacement of the trace (Fig. 7.2).

Unfortunately both these methods introduce yet another problem, that of tangent distortion (Fig. 7.12). In this case the deflection along the vertical axis is $R \tan \theta$

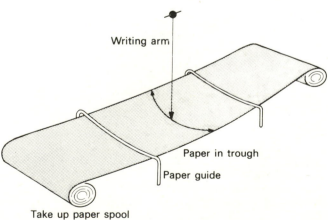

Fig. 7.10. Use of curved trough and vertical writing arm to overcome sine distortion.

and at large deflections is greater than it should be. Again the error is not significant at small angles of deflection (Table 7.2) but if larger deflections are used (as in the ink-jet and galvanometer recorders) the error must be corrected electronically.

In a few recorders sine distortion is overcome by lengthening the arm mechanically. To accomplish this without decreasing frequency response requires engineering of high precision: such recorders are therefore very expensive (Fig. 7.13).

Types of recorder

DIRECT-WRITING RECORDERS

The disadvantages of pen recorders have already been outlined. Nevertheless their relative simplicity, the immediacy of the image and the cheapness of the recording paper make them a popular choice for many types of recording where linearity and time distortion are not of paramount

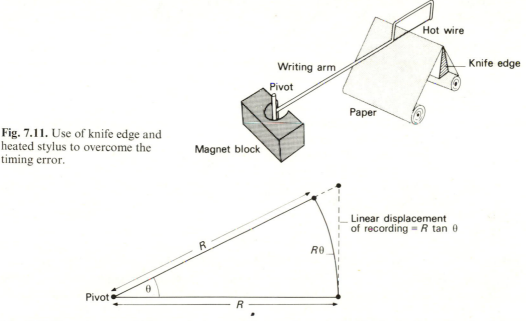

Fig. 7.11. Use of knife edge and heated stylus to overcome the timing error.

Fig. 7.12. Tangent error which must be corrected in recorders using knife edge and heated stylus, ink jet or mirror galvanometers. The error in vertical displacement gets larger as the angular displacement increases.

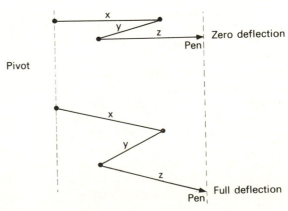

Fig. 7.13. Use of mechanical linkage to lengthen the writing arm and so obviate time distortion.

importance (e.g. EEG, ECG). By suitable modification many of the disadvantages can be minimized. Heat-sensitive paper is much more expensive than ordinary recording paper, but the use of a heated stylus recording over a knife-edge is one of the easiest ways of overcoming sine distortion. Other methods of producing an image are a cold stylus writing on pressure-sensitive paper and the use of electrolytic paper. The latter conducts electricity and an imprint is produced where a current flows from the pen onto the paper.

All direct recorders display hysteresis, i.e. the pen does not return exactly to zero after it has been deflected by the current. By correct design of the spring which returns the pen to zero, hysteresis can be reduced to less than 2% of the maximum deflection.

The flat frequency response of most pen recorders is limited to 75–100 Hz. Some recorders contain very simple amplifiers, which may require an input signal of 0–1V fsd, but many have sophisticated pre-amplifiers which will accept signals in the microvolt range with input impedances of $> 1\,M\Omega$.

PHOTOGRAPHIC RECORDERS

Cathode-ray oscilloscope

When this instrument is used for display the trace can be photographed directly with a time exposure. It is often difficult to adjust the trace to the correct brightness at the first attempt, but the use of a Polaroid camera enables a print to be obtained immediately so that the appropriate adjustments may be made.

When prolonged periods of recording are required the time base on the oscilloscope may be switched off and the film moved continuously through the camera. The oscillations of the light spots in the y-axis then produce continuous traces on the film. This form of recording greatly enhances the versatility of the instrument but some care is necessary to ensure correct exposure.

Although a fairly high voltage must be applied to the plates to produce a deflection (e.g. 10 volts/cm deflection) high gain amplifiers are usually incorporated in the chassis so that input signals as small as $100\,\mu V$ can produce a 1-cm deflection. Although a certain amount of experience with the technique is necessary to produce good records, there is no alternative to the oscilloscope when one wishes to record components of a waveform having a frequency greater than about 8 kHz.

Recent developments in design have widened the application of oscilloscopes in the recording field. For example the storage oscilloscope permits the image to be selected and then 'frozen' whilst it is photographed. Furthermore oscilloscopes with fibre-optic face plates produce such bright images that traces can be recorded directly onto photographic paper without the necessity for interposing a negative film (see p. 112).

Mirror galvanometers

Photographic recorders utilizing the mirror galvanometer (Fig. 7.3) have been used for many years, but they have suffered from the disadvantage that the trace had to be developed and fixed before the image could be inspected. However, the introduction of ultraviolet sensitive paper, on which an image appears after a delay of about 15 s, has once again brought the mirror galvanometer recorder back into popularity, though the image lacks the contrast which is obtainable with most other kinds of recording. The image is semipermanent, but the paper blackens if it is exposed for prolonged periods to bright light. The image can be preserved by chemical treatment or by spraying the paper with a protective yellow varnish.

The use of galvanometers has a number of advantages. Many channels (sometimes up to 50 or 100) can be recorded on the same strip of paper and the traces can be overlapped so that each trace can sweep the full width of the paper. Identification marks can be superimposed on each trace and a time scale and calibration grid can be printed onto the paper as it passes through the recorder. The light spots can also be projected onto a ground-glass screen so that the zero and calibration points can be adjusted and the recording monitored visually. Perhaps the greatest advantage is the wide choice of galvanometers which permits each galvanometer to be matched exactly to the character of the input signal. Since each galvanometer is carried as a complete unit in a cylinder about 6 cm × 0.5 cm, it is a simple matter to change galvanometers when required.

Choice of a galvanometer. The sensitivity of a mirror galvanometer depends on the length of the optical writing arm (mirror to paper distance) and on the deflection of the mirror produced by a given current or voltage. The deflection can be increased by increasing the density of the magnetic field or by increasing the size of the coil. There is a limit to the density of the magnetic field which can be achieved and the larger the coil the greater is the mass and therefore the lower is the undamped natural frequency. Although the sensitivity is also affected by the internal resistance of the galvanometer, sensitivity is approximately inversely proportional to the square of the natural frequency. There is therefore no advantage to be gained from using a galvanometer with a higher frequency response than that required for the purpose in hand. For this reason the first step in choosing a galvanometer is to decide on the maximum frequency which it will be called upon to handle. The undamped natural frequency is then calculated by multiplying this by a factor of 1.6 since, if it is correctly damped, the frequency response should be flat to 60–65% of its natural frequency.

In addition to undamped natural frequency and sensitivity it is necessary to ensure that damping is optimal. In galvanometers with undamped natural frequencies up to 300–400 Hz damping is applied electromagnetically, but with galvanometers with undamped natural frequencies above about 1 kHz fluid damping is used. Electromagnetic damping is achieved by inserting a known resistance into the galvanometer circuit so that the reverse current which is induced in the coil by the deflection of the coil produces the required degree of damping. The magnitude of this resistance can only be calculated if the resistance of the current source is known, for optimal conditions exist when the resistance of the source equals the resistance of the damping resistance. When these resistances are not equal, a series or parallel resistance may need to be incorporated in the circuit. Details are given in the manufacturers' literature.

Some typical values for galvanometer characteristics are given in Table 7.3. This illustrates how sensitivity decreases as frequency response increases.

Table 7.3.

Natural frequency (Hz)	Flat frequency response (± 5 per cent) (Hz)	Galvanometer sensitivity	
		(mA/cm)	(mV/cm)
35	20	0.0008	0.038
450	300	0.05	6.0
1000	600	0.34	25
5000	3000	25	1050

POTENTIOMETRIC RECORDERS

This type of recorder is used when it is desired to write across a wide strip of recording paper (e.g. 15–25 cm) with high accuracy. Sensitivity can be made very high (e.g. 1 mV for full-scale deflection) but the response is slow compared with galvanometric recorders. In standard instruments the pen may take up to 2 s to traverse the full width of the paper although it is possible to obtain slewing speeds of $75 \, cm \cdot s^{-1}$ in sophisticated models.

This type of recorder is based on the potentiometer circuit (Fig. 7.14). A battery or power supply supplies a constant current to a slide wire A, B. The slide wire has a uniform cross-section throughout its length so that the resistance per unit length is constant. The input voltage is applied between one end of the slide wire and the moving contact, C. When the position of the contact is such that the voltage drop between B and C is the same as the input voltage there will be no current flow through the galvanometer, G. In the potentiometric recorder the galvanometer

is replaced by a servo-amplifier which feeds a servo-motor and which, in turn, moves the sliding contact through a cable linkage. Thus if the input voltage to the recorder exceeds that across B–C the bridge will be out of balance and the motor will be activated to move the sliding contact in the direction which tends to minimize the difference in potential between the input and B–C. If the input voltage is less than B–C it will move the contact in the opposite direction. Thus the position of the sliding contact is continually adjusted to match the input voltage. Since the pen is directly linked to the sliding contact a continuous record of the input voltage is obtained.

Potentiometric recorders are used in many monitoring applications and for such relatively slow signals as indicator dilution curves or gas chromatograms. Sampling recorders, printing out distinctive marks for a number of different variables in rotation, are used for such applications as the monitoring of temperature from a number of different probes. Another variation is the x–y recorder, in which two potentiometer movements drive the pen along axes at right-angles to each other. This may be used for plotting two simultaneously changing variables, such as pressure and volume in lung mechanics measurements. They may also be used as curve plotters on the outlet terminals of computers. The best modern recorders can follow signals up to about 10 Hz.

MAGNETIC RECORDERS

Magnetic recording is used for both analogue and digital data. Analogue data are stored on magnetic tape but digital data can be stored either on magnetic tape or in some form of computer store.

Tape recorders for analogue data

There are basically two types of analogue tape recorder. The first utilizes a *direct-recording* system in which the magnitude of

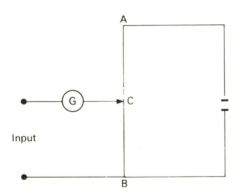

Fig. 7.14. Principle of a potentiometric recorder. A constant current is passed along the slide wire A, B. A sliding contact C is moved along the wire by a servo-amplifier and servo-motor which is activated when a potential difference is detected at G. The motor thus moves the sliding contact in such a way that the potential difference across B–C always matches the input voltage. Since the pen is linked to the sliding contact it produces a record of the input voltage.

the signal is recorded by altering the magnetic flux on the tape. This is the method used in *audio* recorders. The highest frequency which can be recorded depends on how small an area of the tape may be independently magnetized, and on the tape speed. In general direct recording systems provide a relatively wide frequency bandwidth even with low tape speeds. However, they have several disadvantages: the handling of signals below 100 Hz is poor, the amplitude response varies markedly with frequency and the signal:noise ratio is relatively low.

The second type of recorder uses *a frequency-modulation* (FM) system. In this machine the input voltage is represented on the tape by an audio tone whose pitch is directly related to the input voltage (p. 46). For example, the modulator might produce a note with a frequency of 1000 Hz when there is zero input to the recorder. This is known as the *carrier frequency*. Input voltages of $+10V$ or $-10V$ might then be represented by notes of 1300 Hz and 700 Hz respectively so that the full range of input voltages would be covered by a bandwidth of 600 Hz. The reproduction of the recorded signal is then achieved by passing the output signal through a demodulator which translates the variation in frequency into an output voltage.

Frequency modulation systems have the advantage that the amplitude response is relatively flat from d.c. to the upper frequency limit of the recorder and that the signal:noise ratio is relatively high. However their upper frequency limit is generally less than that obtained in direct recording systems. The multichannel FM recorders used for physiological work are generally known as 'instrumentation' tape recorders.

One of the main problems in tape recording is the maintenance of a constant tape speed. Because of the variations in tone noted in audio recorders low frequency variations were known as 'wow' and high frequency variations as 'flutter'. In instrumentation recorders these variations in speed lead to timing errors, signal distortion and a decrease in the signal:noise ratio. There are two methods of reducing the FM recorder's sensitivity to variations in tape speed, both methods requiring the sacrifice of a tape channel. In one method an unmodulated steady note is recorded. Variations in the pitch of this note are sensed on replay and used to correct the pitch of the frequency-modulated signals on all the other channels. In the second method a stable, high repetition rate pulse train is recorded and used to control the speed of the tape motor on replay.

Analogue recorders are most commonly used for temporary storage of data or for prolonged monitoring. Recorders using 0.6 cm ($\frac{1}{4}$ inch) tape can provide up to four parallel data channels whilst 1.25 cm ($\frac{1}{2}$ inch) tape can carry up to eight channels. It is often advantageous to use one of these channels to record a spoken commentary and the remainder for recording the physiological signals.

One example of the use of tape for temporary storage of data is the tape-loop. This consists of a complete loop of tape which can be varied in length to provide a period of recording which suits the chosen application. As the tape passes through the recording head the previous signal is erased and the new signal is recorded. This system can be used for monitoring patients who are likely to develop a cardiac arrhythmia or arrest. If the nurse stops the machine when such an arrest occurs, the ECG for the previous 5 or 10 min will be retained on the tape and can be played back to reveal the pattern of events leading up to the arrest. Magnetic tape may also be employed when it is desired to select small periods of a long recording for detailed analysis, for example when analysing the incidence of arrhythmias over a 24-hr period. The tape can be scanned at high speed and relevant portions of the record played back into a direct-writing or photographic recorder at the original speed to obtain a permanent visual record. The tape can then be re-used. Compact cassette tape recorders running at a slow speed have also proved useful in monitoring the response to drugs used in the treatment of hypertension (Stott 1977).

Tape recorders for digital data

The ability to apply a positive or negative pulse to the tape makes it very suitable as a medium for storing digital data in binary form. Whilst many analogue machines could be used for this purpose it is now usual to use a specially designed machine. Digital machines use 1.25-cm ($\frac{1}{2}$-inch) tape with seven or nine tracks. Digital tape is specially inspected for defects before use and one track is usually used for error-detecting or error-correcting procedures. The remaining 6 or 8 tracks are used to store the binary information in parallel, i.e. each byte is stored as a column running across the tape.

Digital tape recorders are mostly used to record data for subsequent computer processing. The original data may be in digital or analogue form; in the latter case it is subjected to analogue-to-digital conversion before recording.

Computer store

There are now several types of computer store which are used for temporary storage of small quantities of digital data. One type of store consists of an array of ferrite rings each of which can be magnetized in a specific direction to record the 0 or 1 of the binary information. Since the ferrite rings are permanent magnets the information is retained when the power supply is cut off. Another type of store is the solid state memory in which the bits of information are stored as one of two states of integrated circuit bistable multivibrators. This type of store is smaller and faster than core memory but the information is usually lost when the supply voltage is removed.

With the advent of microprocessors digital stores are now being increasingly used in small items of equipment such as oscilloscopes, monitoring systems and analytical apparatus. For example digital electrocardiographs contain an analogue-to-digital converter which continuously samples the ECG waveform and updates a digital memory. The latter is continuously scanned and the resulting analogue signal displayed on the screen. By using digital techniques it is possible to make the trace move across the screen so that the image appears to have been written by an invisible pen behind one edge of the screen. Alternatively the trace can be 'frozen' at any time for closer inspection. Digital storage also forms the basis of one type of storage oscilloscope (p. 73).

PAPER TAPE

In applications where the data are subsequently to be fed into a computer it is often convenient to record the data in digital form on paper tape. Each digit or letter is represented in binary code by a row of holes (usually eight) punched across the tape, and the tape is then fed directly into the tape reader attached to the computer. Additional information may be typed onto the end of the tape by a teletype machine which automatically punches a series of holes in the tape corresponding to the keys on the keyboard. Paper tape can be read visually, is cheap and there is a very low incidence of reading errors. However a given amount of data occupy a relatively large storage space so that paper tape is really only suitable for storing relatively small amounts of data. For large-scale storage magnetic tape is invariably used.

References

STOTT F.D. (1977) Ambulatory monitoring. *British Journal of Clinical Equipment*, **2**, 61.

CASHMAN P.M.M. (1980) Foundations of medical technology. Recording methods. *British Journal of Clinical Equipment*, **5**, 172.

Chapter 8
Electromagnetic Radiation and Optical Measurement

The various forms of electromagnetic radiations are usually given distinct titles such as *ultraviolet*, *infrared*, *radiowaves*, etc., although it should be remembered that they all form part of a continuous spectrum and are qualitatively identical. The spectrum of electromagnetic radiations which is shown in Fig. 8.1 stretches from the very short wavelength and highly energetic cosmic and gamma rays through to the relatively low energy radiowaves. Out of the whole range of these electromagnetic radiations only a small segment of wavelengths is capable of stimulating the eye. This is the visible region. The limits of this band are ill-defined but may be regarded as terminating at a wavelength of about 390 nm at the ultraviolet end and at 750 nm towards the infrared zone.

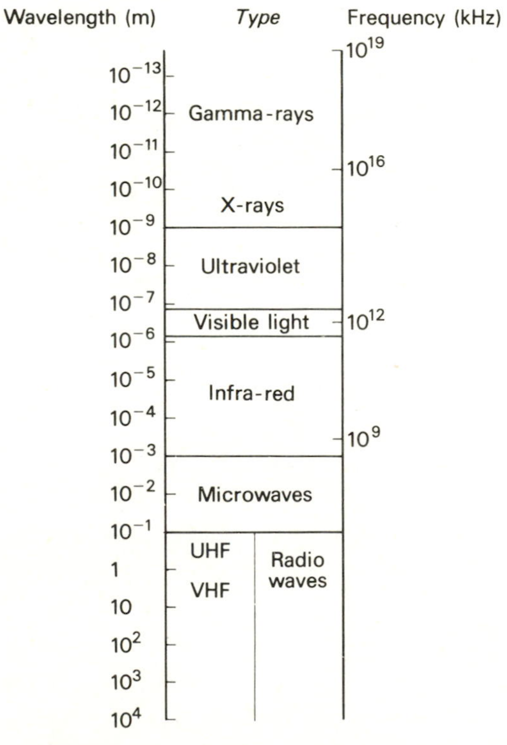

These radiations are all examples of energy being transmitted in a waveform in accordance with the laws:

$$\lambda f = c$$

and

$$E = hf$$

where λ = wavelength in metres

f = frequency in Hz (cycles per second)

c = velocity of light = 3×10^8 m·s^{-1} (in a vacuum)

h = Planck's constant (Joules·s)

E = energy in Joules.

These relationships apply when radiation is propagated as if it were a wave motion. However, it should be appreciated that when electromagnetic radiation interacts with matter, it exhibits both wave and particle properties. Some of the interactions can best be described by considering the wave-like properties while other phenomena suggest particle behaviour.

For the purpose of this chapter a detailed understanding of electromagnetic radiation is not required and no further distinction between the two characteristics will be drawn. As can be seen from the expressions above, frequency and wavelength are inversely related, while energy is proportional to frequency. Thus the radiowaves with their long wavelengths have low frequencies with little energy whilst the gamma rays at the opposite end of the spectrum have short wavelengths, high frequencies and considerable energy. Although it is possible

Fig. 8.1. The electromagnetic spectrum.

90

to define any particular point within the spectrum by referring to its wavelength, frequency or energy, the wavelength is the usual term (except in scientific circles where frequency or wave number—the reciprocal of wavelength in cm—is often used). The units of wavelength in use nowadays are the nano-, micro- and centimetre, but the terms millimicron ($m\mu$) and Angström (Å), now becoming obsolete, are still encountered.*

The tremendous importance of electromagnetic radiations to the scientist resides in their interactions with matter. From the standpoint of the biological and medical sciences, most of the interest concerns the narrow part of the spectrum with wavelengths from 200 nm to 10 μm—the near ultraviolet to the far infrared. Within this range many organic molecules absorb radiation, a process which can be exploited in two ways. Firstly, when dealing with an unknown compound, it can be used for identification or the interpretation of particular structural features. Secondly, the concentration of the absorbing component can be calculated by measuring the amount of energy that is absorbed. Thus the techniques that have grown up based on these interactions have several attractions; analyses can be performed more rapidly and specifically than with chemical procedures, information is gained about molecular structure that is inaccessible by other means and the radiation rarely destroys the material under investigation.

All molecules have natural vibration frequencies which correspond to the molecule oscillating between two states. Most have many such natural vibration frequencies. These states may be electronic transitions where an orbital electron passes from a low energy (ground) state to a higher energy (excited) state or positional movements of atoms with respect to each other, for example, the stretching, flexing or rotation of bonds. Atoms or molecules

can only absorb or emit energy in discrete quantities, in fact integral multiples of *hf*. These packets of energy are referred to as quanta. If the molecule receives electromagnetic radiation of a frequency corresponding to one of its natural vibrations, the radiation will be absorbed. Generally speaking more energy is required for an electronic transition than a vibrational oscillation, which, in turn, is at a higher level than rotational movement. The electronic transitions are found in the ultraviolet and visible regions, vibrational in the infrared and rotational in the microwave. It is perhaps easier to consider the process involved by concentrating the discussion on the absorption of visible light.

Within a molecule, certain groupings, termed chromophores, absorb light of particular wavelengths. These chromophores have structural features such that the energy of the light quanta at that wavelength coincides with the energy required for a particular energy transition. The molecule absorbs the energy and passes into an excited state. Having moved to the higher energy state the excess energy is dissipated via one of several routes:

1 to neighbouring molecules as heat,

2 the energy may be sufficient to rupture a bond so causing the molecule to dissociate, or

3 after certain internal rearrangements the molecule may re-emit the excess energy as electromagnetic radiation—a process termed fluorescence.

Different molecules exhibit these three modes of energy dissipation to varying degrees although in the vast majority of cases loss of energy as heat predominates. Light of other wavelengths possesses incorrect energy to cause the transition to the excited state; it is not absorbed and passes unhindered through the sample. Thus, within a molecule each grouping absorbs selectively certain components of the spectrum. When the substance is viewed in white light only the remaining parts of the spectrum are transmitted or reflected so that the substance appears to

---

* $1\,m\mu = 1nm = 10^{-9}\,m$ or $10^{-7}\,cm$
  $1\,\text{Å} = 0.1\,nm = 10^{-10}\,m$ or $10^{-8}\,cm.$

be coloured. When the substance is placed between a source of white light and the prism system of a spectroscope, the spectrum obtained is not continuous but has dark bands corresponding to those wavelengths which are removed. If the sample absorbs all the incident light, it will appear black. By measuring the extent of the light absorption as a function of wavelength, an absorption spectrum is obtained which, because of its dependence on chemical structure, is a diagnostic characteristic of the compound.

By considering the absorption process that takes place when a quantum of light interacts with a chromophore, certain laws may be derived. If a beam of monochromatic light (light of a single wavelength) passes through a solution of a chromophore, the extent of the absorption depends upon three factors: (a) the thickness of the absorbing material through which the radiation passes, (b) the concentration of the chromophore, and (c) the efficiency of the chromophore at absorbing light at that wavelength.

As the quanta pass through a thin layer of the solution, the interactions between quanta and absorbing chromophores can be expressed in terms of probabilities of collision. Thus the probability that within a given time interval a particular chromophore will absorb a quantum of light is proportional to the number of quanta passing through the solution, i.e. the quantum flux, which is itself proportional to light intensity. Therefore, the thin layer of solution will absorb a certain proportion of the light which falls on it regardless of the intensity of that incident light. For example, if the incident light intensity is 10 arbitrary units and 10% is absorbed by the layer of solution, the emergent light intensity will be 9 arbitrary units, while an increase in incident intensity to 100 units will result in an emergent intensity of 90 units, namely still 10% absorption. The total absorption cell containing the solution can be considered to comprise a large number of these very thin layers of chromophore and each of these layers absorbs the same proportion of the light which falls upon it (Fig. 8.2a). If the light intensity is 100 arbitrary units and each section removes 10%, then 90 units emerge from the first

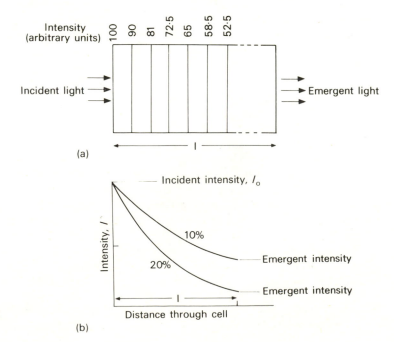

Fig. 8.2. Absorption of light passing through a solution.

layer and enter the second. Thus, $90 \times 90\%$ emerge from the second; $(90 \times 90\%) \times 90\%$ emerge from the third, etc. This type of decrease in light intensity across the cell is termed an exponential decay (Fig. 8.2b), which mathematically can be expressed:

$$I = I_0 e^{-kl} \qquad \text{(i)}$$

where k is a constant, l is the length of lightpath through the solution, I_0 is the incident light intensity, and I is the emergent light intensity. Taking logarithms and re-arranging:

$$\log_{10} \frac{I_0}{I} = \frac{k}{2.303} l. \qquad \text{(ii)}$$

The entity $\log_{10} I_0/I$, which is the logarithm of the ratio of incident to emergent light intensities, is referred to variously as the absorbance, extinction or optical density. The first term, absorbance, is preferred. Thus the expression (ii) states that the absorbance is proportional to the thickness of the absorbing layer. This is Lambert's Law.

The probability that a particular quantum will interact rather than travel unimpeded through the solution is dependent upon the density of the chromophores, i.e. the concentration. By doubling the chromophore concentration, the probability of a quantum being absorbed is doubled. Taking the example quoted above, the thin layer of chromophore absorbed 10% of the incident light. If the concentration is doubled, then 20% of the light is absorbed. This is repeated through the series of layers of which the total thickness of solution is composed. The variation in the light intensity across the solution for the two situations is shown in Fig. 8.2b. Note that doubling the concentration does not halve the emergent intensity.

Mathematically, it is found that the concentration term is present in the constant, k, of equation (i) thus:

$$I = I_0 e^{-k'cl}$$

where k' is a constant and c is the concentration of chromophore. Taking logarithms:

$$\log_{10} \frac{I_0}{I} = \varepsilon.c.l.$$

where ε is the absorption coefficient. However, since $\log_{10} I_0/I$ is the absorbance (A) this equation can be written:

$$A = \varepsilon.c.l. \qquad \text{(iii)}$$

In words, expression (iii) states that the absorbance is proportional to the chromophore concentration. This is Beer's Law.

If concentration (c) is measured in moles per litre and length (l) in cm, ε has units of litre moles^{-1} cm^{-1} and is referred to as the *molar absorption coefficient*. It is the absorption which would be recorded at that wavelength of a 1M solution in a 1 cm lightpath cell. The magnitude of the molar absorption coefficient reflects the probability that radiation at that wavelength will cause an electron to be excited. If the probability is high that the structure of a molecule will result in absorption, then the absorption coefficient is large. If the coefficient is small, it signifies that the efficiency of absorbing radiation is poor. Thus the positions of the absorption maxima and their intensities provide information on the structure of the molecule in question and constitute a fingerprint for identifying it. Because the efficiency of light absorption varies with wavelength, the molar absorption coefficient will likewise be dependent upon the wavelength.

Although these laws have been discussed from the standpoint of the absorption of visible light, the concepts are just as valid for the non-visible parts of the electromagnetic spectrum. The absorption of ultraviolet, infrared, and other forms of radiation obeys exactly the same principles. It is in spectrophotometry, the application of these concepts, that the relationships between absorbance, concentration and wavelength are exploited as an analytical technique. The importance of spectrophotometry in the analytical laboratory resides in its reliability in terms of accuracy and reproducibility and also because it is possible to detect and measure many materials at low concentrations. Usually these measurements are unaffected by the presence of other compounds. The technique may be extended to chemicals which do not themselves absorb. Often such compounds which are transparent to visible light can be easily converted into a coloured, and therefore absorbing species, through a simple chemical procedure.

To take advantage of the potential of spectrophotometry it is essential to be able to measure light intensities accurately at defined regions of the spectrum. The photometric instruments which achieve this all contain the same four basic units, namely, (a) an energy source generating radiation in the appropriate region of the spectrum, (b) a system for selecting particular limited parts of this spectral region, (c) a sample chamber, and (d) a means of detecting the intensity of the radiation in use. On the second part of the instrument, wavelength selection, it should be remembered that the Beer and Lambert Laws are based on the assumption that the incident radiation is all of one wavelength. This is difficult to achieve without incurring a high cost penalty, for example, by using lasers. In practice, the instruments have either monochromators which will produce light that has a very narrow bandwidth of wavelengths or filters which transmit a broader spread of radiation. The former type of instrument is termed a spectrophotometer while the latter is a colorimeter. Since the filters in colorimeters transmit light of non-absorptive as well as absorptive wavelengths through the sample, deviations from the Beer and Lambert Laws are more likely with this type of instrument.

COLORIMETERS

The original analytical technique of colorimetry was performed by eye. In the early instruments colours were matched visually in white light against either a selection of permanent coloured-glass standards or a series of solutions prepared from known concentrations of the substance under assay. The analyst used his own judgement in estimating which of the standards most closely matched the unknown. This subjective approach has disappeared and has been replaced with a photoelectric device that converts the residual or unabsorbed radiation emerging from the sample into an electric current. The magnitude of the signal is related in a defined way to the intensity of the light. Two further advantages were gained by the use of such photoelectric devices: determinations could be performed in the presence of interfering colours and the technique could be applied to the analysis of pale colours or absorptions outside the visible range.

The present-day colorimeter is a fairly simple instrument in which the light detector is either a selenium photocell which generates a current proportional to the light intensity or a cadmium sulphide resistor whose resistance varies with light intensity, so changing the current flowing in the circuit. The current is measured by a galvanometer which is calibrated logarithmically in absorbance units. The light source is an incandescent tungsten filament lamp and the required region of the spectrum is selected by filters. A diagramatic representation is given in Fig. 8.3.

As mentioned above, it is the filter system

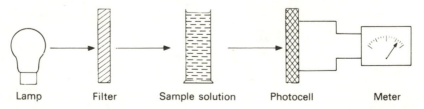

Lamp   Filter   Sample solution   Photocell   Meter

Fig. 8.3. Diagram of a colorimeter.

of wavelength selection which creates the primary limitation and source of inaccuracy in using a colorimeter. Some wavelengths transmitted by the filter (those close to the wavelength of maximum absorption) are absorbed by the chromophore, while the remainder are less efficiently removed. Thus even when the concentration of the chromophore is very high and absorbing all the light at the wavelength of maximum absorption, light of other wavelengths will be unabsorbed and be converted into an electric current by the photocell, so giving a false reading.

SPECTROPHOTOMETERS

In a spectrophotometer a monochromator placed between the light source and the sample replaces the filter system of the colorimeter. The light entering the monochromator is dispersed by either a prism or a combination of a prism with a diffraction grating into a continuous spectrum. Since a very narrow part of this spectrum is selected the sample is illuminated by light that is almost monochromatic and

the Beer–Lambert Laws are more closely obeyed.

For operation in the visible region the radiation source is a tungsten filament lamp, although recently quartz-halogen bulbs have been used by some manufacturers. The voltage applied to the lamp is stabilized to prevent variations in filament temperature which would create fluctuations in the intensity of the emitted light. The light detection system of a spectrophotometer is likewise more elaborate than that of a colorimeter, the two devices in most common usage being the phototube and photomultiplier. A phototube is a vacuum tube whose cathode emits electrons in proportion to the light intensity. These electrons are collected by the anode and the resultant small signal amplified before display. Instruments designed for operation at low light intensities usually have photomultipliers as their detectors. These devices are effectively photocells which have several stages of internal amplification but they have the disadvantage of requiring a stabilized high voltage supply. The resultant signal is dis-

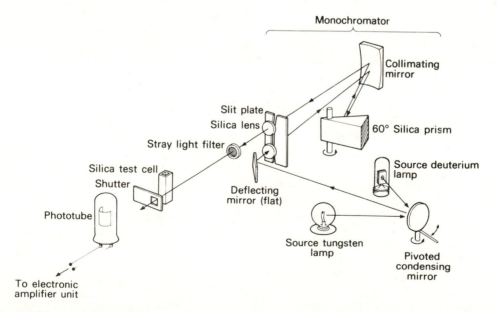

Fig. 8.4. Diagram of a spectrophotometer.

played either in analogue form, for example as a deflection of a meter needle, or in a digital form. Most spectrophotometers have provision for the external recording of the readings on a chart recorder or an automatic printout unit. The layout of a spectrophotometer in diagrammatic form is given in Fig. 8.4. The collimated beam of white light is dispersed by the prism (or diffraction grating) so generating a spectrum which falls on the slit plate. The sample is illuminated only by the portion of the spectrum which passes through the narrow slit aperture. By rotating the prism the spectrum is caused to move along the slit plate, past the aperture, so changing the wavelength of the light emerging from the slit. The wavelength of the selected narrow band may be read off a graduated scale that is related through a suitable gearing system to the angular position of the prism.

Most laboratory spectrophotometers are also capable of operating in the ultraviolet region although certain design modifications are required. A second radiation source is needed, and this is a deuterium arc lamp. The glass prisms and lenses are replaced with quartz equivalents because glass is an efficient absorber at wavelengths shorter than 330 nm.

A feature often encountered in spectrophotometers is a double beam capability. With this type of instrument the light from the monochromator is split into two beams —one of which passes through the test sample and the other through a reference sample. The detection system, usually a photomultiplier in this type of instrument, generates two signals corresponding to the sample and reference light intensities by sampling each in turn. The electronic system compares the two signals and generates an output proportional to the difference. This gives greater stability because fluctuations due to the instrument will affect both reference and sample beams equally and thus the difference remains constant. Furthermore, when scanning the absorption spectrum with the double-beam spectrophotometer it is unnecessary to 'zero'

the instrument each time the wavelength is changed: the reference beam automatically compensates for the source emitting different intensities of radiation at different wavelengths and the detector having a sensitivity that is wavelength dependent. In view of the greater complexity of spectrophotometers they are larger and considerably more expensive than colorimeters.

When making a measurement the first criterion is selection of the appropriate wavelength. Normally this should be the wavelength that gives maximum absorption, for at this wavelength the sensitivity is the greatest and thus the error on the reading will be the least. Sometimes this rule does not hold. For example, many biological oxidation-reduction processes involve the redox pair NAD^+ and NADH. These two compounds have different and characteristic absorption spectra (Fig. 8.5). The best wavelength to employ in monitoring the interconversion is not at the absorption maxima but at 340 nm, the point of maximum difference between the two forms. At 340 nm NADH has a molar absorption coefficient of 6.2×10^3 while NAD^+ is transparent. This change in absorption as NAD^+ is reduced or NADH oxidized is the basis of many biochemical assays. Similar considerations apply if two or more

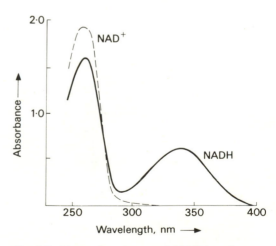

Fig. 8.5. Absorption spectra of NAD^+ and $NADH^-$ both solutions in 0.1 mM.

components are present and their absorption spectra overlap. Usually by judicious wavelength selection a point can be chosen where the interfering components contribute little absorption compared with the substance of interest. Quite gross variations in the concentration of interfering components will then have little effect on the total absorption, although small changes in concentration of the test substance are easily detected.

The same basic principles are employed in oximetry. Here we may regard the two mutually interfering substances as the oxygenated and unoxygenated forms of haemoglobin. Their relative spectra are illustrated in Fig. 8.6 and it can be seen that the maximum difference in the absorption of the two forms of haemoglobin occurs at a wavelength around 650 nm, while at 800 nm the *absorption coefficient* is the same in both forms. In any mixture of two components, a point at which the absorption coefficients are identical is referred to as an *isobestic* point. Applying Beer's Law the concentration of oxyhaemoglobin is proportional to the absorption difference of the two forms at 650 nm. Unfortunately by making a measurement at a single wavelength of 650 nm the oxyhaemoglobin content cannot be calculated

because both forms are contributing to the absorption and the total amount of haemoglobin present in the sample is unknown. However, a measurement of the light absorbed at the isobestic point is independent of the degree of oxygenation and standardizes the system in terms of the quantity of haemoglobin. It also serves as a reference point for the adjustment of the oximeter to compensate for variations in sample size and fluctuations in light intensity. Having created a reference point, the difference between the absorption value at 800 nm and that at 650 nm is proportional to the degree of oxygenation. A full discussion of the design and operation of various types of oximeters has been given by Reichert (1966).

In a colorimeter or spectrophotometer the length of the lightpath is fixed usually by the availability of cuvettes with defined dimensions. Commonly these range from 0.2 to 4 cm with the 1-cm light path cuvette being by far the most widely used. In the case of liquids, having decided on the wavelength and light path, the absorbance is proportional to concentration. However, where gases are concerned, changes in pressure affect the quantity of substance in the light path and thus the determination is performed at a defined pressure.

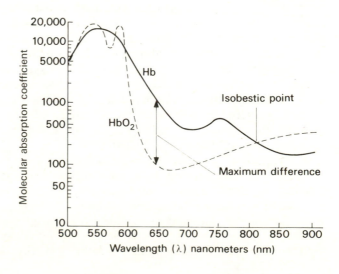

Fig. 8.6. Absorption spectra of reduced (Hb) and oxygenated haemoglobin (HbO_2).

The concentration of a chromophore may be calculated by comparing its absorbance with that given by a solution of known concentration. However, rather than rely on the accuracy of one standard, it is better to plot a calibration curve using a series of standards of known concentrations. This also serves to verify that the Beer–Lambert relationship holds for the particular system being studied. If the Beer–Lambert laws are known to be valid for the system and if the molar absorption coefficient is known for the particular wavelength, an alternative procedure is to apply equation (iii) on page 93, directly.

The term absorbance, as defined in equation (iii), is a ratio—the logarithm of incident light intensity to emergent intensity. Thus effectively two readings are required. Firstly the instrument is set for zero absorbance by placing a cuvette containing water or other suitable reference solution in the light beam. This value is taken as equivalent to the incident light intensity. In addition this reference solution provides a correction for the small absorbance of the cuvette windows and a stable absorbance to refer to in case the energy emitted by the light source changes. Having obtained a 'zero' reference, the second reading, the unabsorbed light emerging from the sample, is taken and displayed as an absorbance value. Some assays depend on the generation of a coloured derivative via a sequence of chemical reactions in which the reagents themselves may contribute to the light absorption. By processing blanks through the entire procedure this error is minimized.

The optical clarity of solutions is essential. Light is scattered by particulate matter so creating the illusion that the solution is absorbing more light than is actually the case. Although normally such particles are removed before taking an absorbance reading, in certain specialized situations advantage is taken of the scattering effect. For example, a standard procedure for estimating the density of a bacterial suspension is to measure the amount of light able to penetrate the culture. As the bacterial density increases during growth the turbidity increases and less light reaches the photocell.

If the solution contains semi-absorbent particles, such as red blood corpuscles, some light is reflected back, and some is absorbed in passing through the corpuscles. Both components may then be reflected off other corpuscles and scattered in all directions, including the forward direction. The high degree of transmission through blood is due to the fact that a proportion of the light is subject to multiple reflection and is thus transmitted through the liquid without passing through the solid elements. A simple instrument which utilizes this property is the pulse detector, in which a light source and a photosensitive detector are positioned so that either reflected or transmitted light impinges on the detector. By using a detector which is only sensitive to red light, outside daylight interference is minimized. The rhythmic electrical output can be displayed either by a moving pointer, via a ratemeter or used to actuate an intermittent light or audible device.

The use of time-versus-concentration curves of dye dilution, sensed by an oximeter type of cuvette, has been a common method for measuring cardiac output. The dye, indocyanine green, was chosen because its peak absorption occurred at 800 nm, the isobestic point on the oxygenated and unoxygenated haemoglobin spectra (Fig. 8.6). Consequently, the sensing device was unaffected by any changes in the state of oxygenation of the haemoglobin in the sample during the course of sampling the dye curve. The determination of cardiac output is discussed in detail in Chapter 16.

INFRARED SPECTROSCOPY

Many molecules of biological interest absorb in the infrared region. The absorptions occurring at infrared wavelengths originate from the natural vibrations of the bonds between atomic nuclei. The bond linking two atoms behaves rather like an elastic force and thus will vibrate in much the same way as a spring with a weight at each end. For a diatomic molecule in which the masses and electric charges of the two atoms are different, for example CO or NO, the oscillation of the atoms creates a similar regular fluctuation in the magnetic dipole moment. This arises because as the atoms move apart the lighter atom moves further than the heavier one in order to keep the centre of the mass for the molecule stationary (Fig. 8.7). An analogy can be drawn to balancing two dissimilar weights on a beam across a fulcrum: to achieve equilibrium the heavier weight is the closer of the two to the fulcrum. Should the heavier weight be displaced away from the fulcrum, the lighter one must be moved a much greater distance in the opposite direction to restore the balance. To return to the oscillating diatomic molecule, the distance apart of the two charges carried by the atoms is varying and because the charges are dissimilar a fluctuating magnetic field or dipole moment is created. Such a system absorbs energy from an oscillating electromagnetic field, provided the field frequency and the vibration frequency of the dipole are identical. Radiation of this resonant frequency will be absorbed and removed from the spectrum. The frequency at which the absorption occurs is dependent on the bond strength and the masses of the atoms linked by the bond. The stronger the bond and the lighter the atoms, the faster is the vibration and the higher the absorption frequency. (For symmetrical diatomic molecules such as O_2 and N_2, in which the atoms have equal masses, the atoms move equal distances and since the charges are identical, no change in dipole moment occurs and hence there is no absorption.)

There are other influences which can lead to a fluctuation in the dipole moment of an asymmetric diatomic molecule, for instance, the rotation of the molecule around its axis. All such oscillations in the dipole moment lead to absorption of electromagnetic radiation in the infrared region, each absorption being characteristic of the type of bond.

In a polyatomic molecule the situation is considerably more complex and is beyond the scope of this chapter. Basically all absorptions originate from factors which cause dipole moments to oscillate, such as stretching and bending of bonds, but these frequencies may be modified by the environment in which the particular bond occurs. At first sight it would seem that with so many oscillations the absorption spectrum of a complex molecule would have too many absorption bands to be useful. In practice, compounds possessing particular functional groups do have absorption bands at

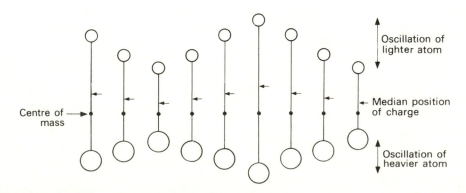

Fig. 8.7. Stretching vibration of an asymmetric diatomic molecule.

characteristic wavelengths. Examples of such groups are OH (stretching) at $2.8\,\mu m$, C=O (stretching) at $5.7\,\mu m$ and C—O—H (bending) at $8\,\mu m$. Thus with relatively simple molecules the infrared spectrum is characteristic of the molecule itself while for more complex compounds it aids the detection of specific features within the molecule.

The principles underlying the design of an infrared spectrophotometer are essentially the same as described above for ultraviolet/visible instruments. The differences are necessary to cope with the longer wavelengths being studied. Two common sources of infrared radiation are a heated nichrome wire and the Nernst filament (zirconium oxide together with other rare earth oxides). In the instruments that use prisms rather than diffraction gratings to disperse the radiation, the prism material is NaCl, KBr or a similar salt, glass not being transparent to infrared radiation. KBr, which exibits very little absorption throughout the infrared region, is used also as a supporting medium for studying solid samples. The material under investigation is ground into a fine powder with KBr and compressed to form a translucent disc. This form of sample presentation overcomes the problem of finding suitable solvents that do not absorb in the infrared region. Materials that are liquid or gaseous are analysed directly. The unabsorbed radiation is focussed on a thermal detector, the change in temperature of which is measured with a thermopile* or Golay cell. The Golay thermal detector is a pneumatic device which, although responding to a wide range of wavelengths from ultraviolet to microwave, is normally only encountered in infrared instruments. It is similar in principle to the Luft analyser (see p. 232). The radiation enters the detector through a window that forms one end of a closed, gas-filled chamber. In the middle of the

* A thermopile consists essentially of a number of thermocouples connected in series, one set of junctions being exposed to the heat source and the other set being shielded from the radiation.

chamber a membrane of very low thermal capacity absorbs the radiation, so warming up the gas, usually xenon. The other end of the chamber is sealed with a membrane that incorporates a mirror. When the gas expands, this mirror moves in sympathy. An optical system monitors the small movements of the mirror.

FLUORESCENCE

The spectroscopic techniques described so far have centred on the absorption of energy while the fate of this energy within the excited molecule has been ignored. As mentioned earlier in this chapter most molecules on absorbing energy dissipate it as heat. On the other hand, after excitation, the electrons in certain molecules instead of returning directly to the ground state pass to a metastable state intermediate in energy between the ground and excited states. The electrons return from this metastable state to the ground state with the emission of energy in the form of electromagnetic radiation. The process is termed fluorescence. Since the energy gap between metastable and ground states is less than the energy absorbed during excitation, the wavelength of the emitted radiation will be longer than that of the absorbed light. (If no loss in energy occurred during the process, the emitted and absorption wavelengths would be identical.) A characteristic of fluorescence is that the compound absorbs radiation, so exhibiting an excitation spectrum, and re-emits at longer wavelengths in the form of an emission spectrum (Fig. 8.8). Furthermore, the fluorescent radiation is emitted in all directions, not just following the path of the original beam.

Fluorescence is studied by modifying the arrangement of the sample chamber and detector of a spectrophotometer. The sample is illuminated with monochromatic light of a wavelength at which the molecule absorbs energy. Since the fluorescent emission has lost the directionality of the excitatory beam, it is measured usually at right angles to the incident light. This confers on fluorescence as a technique several advantages over absorption spectroscopy. The main benefit is much increased sensitivity for although the emitted light intensities are low, they are measured with reference to no light. This contrasts with absorption spectroscopy where the measurements depend on the difference in the intensities of the light entering and leaving the sample or comparing the light beams

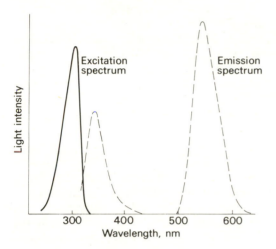

Fig. 8.8. Fluorescence spectrum of 5-hydroxytryptophan in acid solution:— excitation spectrum; — — emission spectrum.

emerging from the sample and reference cells. An analogy might be loosely drawn: the contrast is between comparing two light bulbs, one of 100 watts and the other of 99 watts, and viewing a 1-watt light bulb in an otherwise completely dark room. It is far easier to measure accurately the emission from a 1-watt bulb than to detect a 1% change in a 100-watt bulb.

Unfortunately, fluorometric measurements are susceptible to interference from a variety of factors. These originate partly from the sensitive nature of the technique. For example, trace impurities in reagents that would not have affected an assay based on absorption, can pose significant problems with fluorescence. Another technical difficulty concerns particulate matter such as dust which scatters the incident light into the detector. Interference from this effect is minimized by using two monochromators; one to select the excitatory radiation and another to analyse the emitted radiation—the scattered light being of the same wavelength as the incident beam is ignored by the emission monochromator. This arrangement involving two monochromators increases the cost of the instrument considerably. A compromise is to eliminate the scattered light with a filter. A further variable that must be controlled is temperature. In fluorescence, an excited molecule loses its energy via two routes—to other molecules by collision, or release as light. As the temperature increases, the kinetic energy of the molecule is raised, so making intermolecular collision more probable. With a greater proportion of the absorbed energy being dissipated in collisions less is emitted as fluorescence. Thus for accurate quantitative measurements, temperature control is vital.

ATOMIC ABSORPTION SPECTROPHOTO-METRY AND FLAME PHOTOMETRY

The technique of flame photometry was developed many decades ago and has become a standard procedure in clinical laboratories for it constitutes a rapid and accurate method for the determination of many inorganic ions. Many flame photometers are fully automated to dilute the sample into the correct concentration range, inject it into the flame and, by reference to the response given by standards, calculate and print out the concentration in the original sample.

With flame photometry the sample is dispersed into a flame from which the metal ions draw sufficient energy to become excited. On returning to the ground state, energy is emitted as electromagnetic radiation in the visible part of the spectrum, usually as a very narrow wavelength band. These coloured emissions—sodium (orange), potassium (lilac), calcium (red)—

have long been recognized as characteristic of many metals. The radiation is filtered to remove unwanted wavelengths and the resultant intensity measured.

The related technique of atomic absorption is more recent, but it has already developed into an extremely sensitive and specific technique, in routine use in most laboratories, for the analysis of metals and semi-metals.

In atomic absorption the sample is injected likewise into a flame which imparts sufficient energy to dissociate it into the constituent atoms but not enough to move the individual atoms out of their ground state. These atoms can absorb energy from a light beam passing through the flame if the wavelength of the radiation is correct for the promotion of an electronic transition. The Beer–Lambert Laws also apply to this system so the absorbance is proportional to the concentration of atoms in the flame. The absorption wavelengths are characteristic of the element in question and, unlike the spectrophotometric absorptions described previously, have very narrow bandwidths. As an analytical technique atomic absorption is far more sensitive than flame photometry. The detection limits for most metals using atomic absorption are in the ng/ml range. The reason for this difference in sensitivity is that in flame photometry only a small proportion of the atoms are excited and hence emitting radiation while with atomic absorption all the atoms present can contribute potentially

to the absorption, thus giving a much greater response. In addition to sensitivity, atomic absorption has the further advantages of simplicity and speed. Because interference from other materials in the sample very rarely causes problems, sample processing prior to analysis is usually very straightforward.

The organization of the components of an atomic absorption spectrophotometer is shown in Fig. 8.9. The instrument itself closely resembles a spectrophotometer. In place of the sample chamber there is a burner in which sample, fuel and oxidant are mixed. Typical fuel mixtures are air/acetylene and N_2O/acetylene. The burner is designed to generate a long flat flame aligned so that the light beam passes along the length of the flame. This arrangement ensures that the maximum number of atoms are in the beam.

The sample is illuminated with radiation created by a special type of source, termed a hollow cathode lamp, which emits radiation only of the wavelengths characteristic of the element under analysis. Thus the sample is illuminated only by the wavelengths that it is capable of absorbing. A different hollow cathode lamp is required for each element to be analysed.

MAGNETIC RESONANCE

Electron spin resonance (ESR) and nuclear magnetic resonance (NMR) are a pair of related techniques which, although still

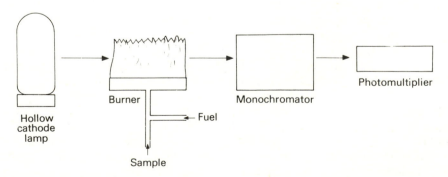

Fig. 8.9. Schematic representation of an atomic absorption spectrophotometer.

concerned with the absorption of electromagnetic radiation, differ considerably from
other spectroscopic procedures. Both phenomena arise from the magnetic property
possessed by certain atoms; this property
enables them to absorb electromagnetic
radiation. The difference between ESR and
NMR lies in the origin of these magnetic
properties: in ESR the electrons are
responsible while with NMR the composition of the subatomic particles in the nucleus
creates the magnetic field.

Nuclear magnetic resonance

Each of the protons within the nucleus
carries a single positive charge. The protons
usually form pairs; one proton having
opposite spin characteristics to the other so
that from a magnetic point of view they
cancel each other out. For an atom having
an odd number of protons one of the
protons remains unpaired and, because it
has both spin and charge, the nucleus will
behave like a small magnet. Normally, the
nuclei have no directional organization but
point randomly in all directions. However,
when they are placed in the field of another
magnet the two fields interact, leading the
nucleus to adopt one of two orientations;
the first being alignment with the external
field and the second against this field. These
orientations possess different energy levels,
the lower energy state being where the
alignment is with the field. Imparting energy
in the form of electromagnetic radiation
causes the nuclear magnets to jump from
the low to the high energy states, and the
absorption of this energy can be measured.
This is the basis of the technique of NMR.
The energy required to effect this transition
is quite small and therefore the radiations
absorbed are at the comparatively long
wavelengths in the radiowave part of the
spectrum.

The great advantage of NMR as a technique is in the ability to study a single type of
atom within a molecule to the exclusion of
all other nuclei. Only those atoms with
magnetic properties are accessible so within
organic molecules the isotopes ^1H, ^3H,
^{13}C, ^{17}O and ^{31}P, are potentially open to
study. Most investigations have centred on
^1H because it has a high natural abundance
and does not require the chemical synthesis
of the compound from suitably labelled
precursors. When studying a hydrogen atom
in a particular molecule the other atoms,
while not participating in the magnetic
resonance phenomenon themselves, are not
without influence for they create local environments that slightly disturb the natural
resonance of the hydrogen atom. For
instance, a hydrogen atom within a methyl
group has a different resonance to the same
atom in an hydroxyl group. In consequence,
the oscillation of the magnetic nucleus in
the external magnetic field yields considerable information on the structure of the
parent molecule.

One such hydrogen containing molecule
which is amenable to study is water. The
ability to investigate the state of hydration
within the soft tissues has recently been the
subject of interest since the freedom of
movement of water molecules in tumour
cells and normal tissue appears to differ.

Electron spin resonance

With ESR the magnetic properties arise
from the spin and charge possessed by
unpaired electrons. In much the same way
as described for NMR, if the molecule
containing such an atom is placed in a
magnetic field, it can adopt one of two
possible attitudes, each possessing different
energy levels. Absorption of electromagnetic
radiation will promote the transition to the
higher energy state although the frequencies
required to observe this resonance are in the
microwave region rather than the radiowave
range employed in NMR. ESR has proved
particularly useful for studying transition
metal ions and so has been employed in
investigating natural metalloproteins.

References and further reading

KNOWLES P.F., MARSH D. & RATTLES H.W.E. (1976) *Magnetic Resonance in Biomolecules.* New York: John Wiley.

METZLER D.E. (1977) *Biochemistry*, chapter 13. New York: Academic Press.

REICHERT W.J. (1966) The theory and construction of oximeters. In: *Oxygen Measurement in Blood and Tissues and Their Significance* Eds J.P. Payne and D.W. Hill. London: Churchill.

STERN E.S. & TIMMONS C.J. (1970) *Electronic Absorption Spectroscopy in Organic Chemistry.* London: Edward Arnold.

VAN DER MAAS J.H. (1969) *Basic Infrared Spectroscopy.* New York: Hayden Book Co.

Chapter 9
The Use of Ultrasound in Clinical Measurement

Ultrasound was first used in diagnostic medicine in about 1937 but it was not until 1945 that A-scanning techniques were introduced. B-scans first appeared in 1950 and instruments using the Doppler effect were introduced in 1958. Ultrasound techniques permit tissue interfaces to be detected and their shape and size described: they are of most use in situations where X-rays yield poor images, such as the definition of soft tissues, or are contraindicated, as in pregnancy. They have the additional advantage that movement of surfaces within the body can be detected and measured

with a useful degree of accuracy, whilst information about the nature of a tissue (e.g. solid or cystic) can often be obtained. The introduction of Doppler techniques has also provided a useful means of deriving qualitative information about blood flow. Since the energies used in diagnostic ultrasound techniques appear to be harmless, the measurement can be used repeatedly on the same patient. Similarly, there is no risk to the operator. However, there are still a number of problems. It is often difficult to locate the structures of interest and the interpretation of ultrasonic images can be

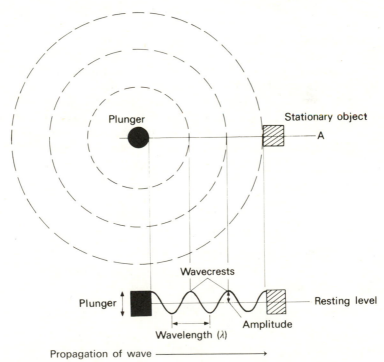

Fig. 9.1. Above: surface view of plunger creating ripples on surface of water. Below: section through water surface from plunger to A showing movement of water molecules at right angles to direction of propagation of wave.

difficult. Image detail is somewhat limited in many machines and instruments have a large number of controls. Successful ultrasonic diagnosis therefore depends on the appropriate choice of instrument and on the correct use of its facilities by a skilled operator.

Before dealing specifically with the generation and special properties of ultrasound it is necessary to consider some of the general properties of wave motion.

Sound energy

Sound energy is generated by an oscillating source and travels through a medium in the form of a wave. Planar wave motions can be fully defined by only three terms, namely their frequency, wavelength and amplitude. The simplest way to visualize wave motion is to consider the action of a plunger which is moved up and down in a regular manner on the surface of water (Fig. 9.1).

The plunger interacts with the water particles immediately surrounding it and causes them to oscillate in a similar manner. This oscillatory motion is transmitted in an outward direction from one group of particles to the next and so forms a series of ripples. The maximum displacement of the water surface from its resting level represents the *amplitude* of the wave, the distance

between the crests of the waves defines the *wavelength* (λ) whilst the number of ripples impinging on a stationary object in their path each second indicates the *frequency* of the oscillation (f). The *velocity* with which the wave front moves (c) is then given by the equation:

$$c = \lambda f.$$

When waves are formed on the surface of water the particles move at *right angles* to the direction of wave propagation, the transmission of the wave thus being similar to the transmission of an oscillation imparted to one end of a piece of rope. However, sound waves are transmitted by the movement of particles in the *same direction* as wave transmission. The movement is thus similar to the oscillation seen in a row of railway trucks when a shunted truck hits the end of the row. This is illustrated in Fig. 9.2. In this type of wave motion the distance between the successive peaks of high pressure defines the *wavelength*, and the amplitude (the difference in pressure between ambient and the peaks of the waveform) governs the loudness or *intensity* of the sound. The *pitch* of the sound is determined by the frequency, which is again defined by the number of high (or low) pressure pulses which can be detected per unit time by a pressure transducer placed in the path of the oncoming wave. At the present time it is possible to

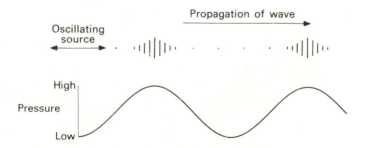

Fig. 9.2. Above: Longitudinal propagation of sound wave. The position of the oscillating source is shown on the left, the dense areas showing how the zone of high pressure is transmitted along the line of particles. The intermediate low pressure zones travel in a similar direction. Below: The pressures recorded in the transmitting medium.

generate sound waves with frequencies ranging from less than 1 cycle per second (1 hertz or 1 Hz) up to 10 000 000 000 cycles per second, i.e. 10 000 megahertz (MHz). However, the human ear can only detect frequencies within the range 20–20 000 Hz. In the elderly the upper limit of audibility is commonly reduced to 15 000 Hz or less. Sound waves generated at a frequency above that which can be distinguished by the human ear (i.e. $> 20 000$ Hz) are therefore termed ultrasound. In diagnostic ultrasonics the most commonly-used frequencies are in the range 1–10 MHz. Since the velocity of wave propagation (c) is fixed by the tissues at about $1500 \, \text{m} \cdot \text{s}^{-1}$ the resulting wavelengths can be calculated from the equation $c = \lambda f$ or $\lambda = c/f$. Thus for a frequency of 1 MHz the wavelength will be $1500 \div 1 000 000 = 1.5$ mm whilst for a frequency of 10 MHz the wavelength will be 0.15 mm ($150 \, \mu$m). Since the ability of the ultrasound apparatus to resolve small distances increases as wavelength is reduced the best resolution is achieved with the highest frequencies.

In practice the oscillating source is not restricted to a single line of particles but imparts its energy to particles in contact with the whole of its oscillating surface. This results in planes of high and low pressure which move at right angles from the oscillating surface of the generator and so create a beam of ultrasound (Fig. 9.3a). This beam normally tends to diverge but by making the shape of the oscillating surface concave it is possible to focus the beam so that the diameter of the beam becomes narrower before diverging again (Fig. 9.3b). Acoustic lenses and mirrors can also be used to control the width and direction of the beam. However, in ultrasound apparatus the lenses are commonly of opposite curvature to their optical equivalents (Fig. 9.3c). This is because in most materials ultrasound travels faster in the solid lens material than in the surrounding liquid or tissue, whereas light travels slower in glass than in air.

Natural sources of ultrasound are few.

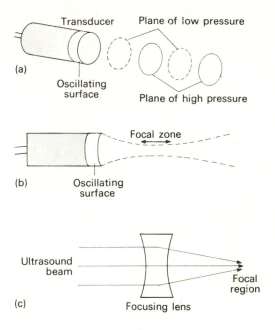

Fig. 9.3. a. Generation of a plane wave by a flat oscillating source. b. Generation of a focused beam using a concave oscillating source. c. Focusing by lens.

Bats and porpoises transmit and receive information at frequencies up to 100 kHz whilst grasshoppers can generate similar frequencies. The paucity of naturally-occurring sources of ultrasound has hampered investigations into the long-term effects of ultrasound on man. However, the evidence which is gradually accumulating suggests that the short-term diagnostic use of ultrasound is relatively free from hazard.

Generation of ultrasound

Most diagnostic apparatus produces a narrow beam of ultrasound which is highly directional and can thus be aimed at the target. In some instruments ultrasound is transmitted continuously along the beam but in others the ultrasound is emitted in a series of short bursts.

The resulting pulse travels through the medium at a velocity which is determined by the medium; but because the pulse duration is characteristically only two or three cycles in length the pulse only affects a limited region of tissue 2–3 mm thick at any particular instant. Unfortunately very short pulses of ultrasound contain oscillations of varying frequencies and amplitudes and this complicates the way in which they are affected by tissues. Nevertheless pulsed ultrasound has proved invaluable in many clinical applications for it forms the basis of the echo techniques for identifying tissue interfaces.

The generation and sensing of ultrasound is performed with transducers which are usually manufactured from crystals displaying the piezo-electric effect. When such crystals are subjected to pressure an electrical charge appears on their surfaces. The charges are positive on one side and negative on the other and are generated because the structure of the crystal is disturbed when pressure is applied. Such crystals are used both to sense the pressure waves produced by ultrasound and also to generate the ultrasound beam. The generation of ultrasound is accomplished by applying an alternating potential difference to the two sides of the crystal which then changes its thickness and so produces ultrasonic radiation of the same frequency as the applied voltage.

The piezo-electric effect is exhibited by naturally occurring crystals such as quartz or Rochelle salt (potassium sodium tartrate). Most ultrasonic transducers are now made from ceramic materials containing lead zirconate and lead titanate. These substances are cheap, easily shaped and very efficient in transforming mechanical to electrical energy. The crystal thickness determines the operating frequency of the transducer and must be matched to the alternating voltage which excites it. A 1 MHz transducer might have a diameter of 2 cm and a thickness of 1.8 mm whilst a 10 MHz device might have a diameter of 2 mm and a thickness of 0.18 mm. The front and back surfaces of the crystal are coated with metal and connected by wires to the electronic circuits which generate or detect the alternating voltage. The whole transducer is then surrounded with an accoustic insulator (Fig. 9.4). Pulsed ultrasound is produced by applying a step change of voltage which shocks the crystals into a brief burst of vibration.

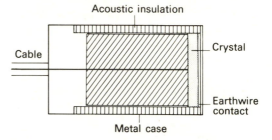

Fig. 9.4. Ultrasound transducer.

Although ultrasound can be produced by other types of transducers (e.g. the magnetostrictive transducers used in ultrasonic cleaning baths) most have not yet been used in diagnostic applications because they are much less efficient at the frequencies used in diagnosis.

Properties of ultrasound

The characteristics of a plane ultrasound beam are described by its frequency, wavelength and its amplitude. It has already been pointed out that wavelength is important in determining the possible resolution of an image. Amplitude is important because it determines the intensity of the ultrasound beam. The intensity, which would correspond to loudness in the audible range, is defined as the rate of flow of energy crossing a unit area held at a right angle to the beam at that point, the units being watts per square meter ($W \cdot m^{-2}$). The intensity of the beam is important because it determines the sensitivity of the instrument and thus governs the number and size of echoes recorded. The total power of the instrument is the product of the intensity and the cross-sectional area of the beam. Its dimensions are:

$$\frac{\text{watts}}{\text{m}^2} \times \text{m}^2 = \text{watts}.$$

Ultrasound is absorbed by tissues and reflected and refracted at tissue interfaces. The intensity of the beam decreases in an exponential fashion as it passes through tissue so it is convenient to express the intensity at any point with respect to an arbitrary reference level. For example, when the attenuation of ultrasound by a given medium is being measured the reference intensity and amplitude levels are normally taken to be those on the surface of the medium nearest the generator.

The intensity and amplitude levels within the medium are then said to be a given number of decibels down with respect to the initial levels, i.e.

relative level (dB)

$$= 10\log_{10}\frac{\text{power of observed wave}}{\text{power of reference wave}}$$

Attenuation is expressed in terms of decibel loss per cm or sometimes in terms of the $d\frac{1}{2}$—the distance at which the intensity is reduced to half (approximately 3 dB down) at a frequency of 1 MHz (Table 9.1). Attenuation is affected not only by the character of the tissue but also by temperature and, most importantly, by the frequency of ultrasound used, attenuation (in dB/cm) increasing linearly with frequency in many tissues. Thus the greatest penetration of the beam is generally achieved with the lowest fre-

quency. However, at low frequencies resolution is poor because wavelength is long. It is therefore common practice to utilize the highest frequency which will ensure adequate penetration of the tissues being investigated. For example frequencies of 2–3.5 MHz are used for abdominal scanning whereas frequencies in the 10 MHz range may be used in ophthalmological investigations.

The absorption of ultrasound by the tissues results in the generation of heat. This is the basis for its use in physiotherapy. However, the attenuation of an ultrasound beam is produced not only by absorption but also by reflection, scattering, refraction and wave divergence.

The reflection of the ultrasound beam from the junction between two tissues or from tissue-fluid or tissue-air interfaces forms the basis of the majority of diagnostic techniques. An echo is generated if the acoustic impedances of the two tissues are different, the magnitude of the echo depending on the difference between the two impedances. The characteristic impedance is the product of the density of the tissue and the velocity of sound in that tissue. Unfortunately, the differences between the characteristic impedances of most tissues are quite small whilst there are large differences between most soft tissues and the values for air (very low) and for bone (very high) (Table 9.2). Reflections at most soft tissue interfaces are therefore very weak

Table 9.1. Attenuation of ultrasound by tissues.

	Attenuation coefficient (dB/cm)	$d\frac{1}{2}$ at 1 MHz (cm)
Strong:		
air, bone, lung	>10	>0.1
Intermediate:		
fat, muscle	>1	~3
Weak:		
blood	0.2	~15
Very weak:		
water	0.00	~1500

Table 9.2. Velocity and characteristic impedance of ultrasound in some materials.

	Velocity of sound ($\text{m}\cdot\text{s}^{-1}$)	Characteristic impedance ($\text{g}\cdot\text{cm}^{-2}\cdot\text{s}$)
Air (NTP)	330	0.0004×10^5
Blood	1570	1.61×10^5
Bone	4080	7.80×10^5
Fat	1450	1.38×10^5
Kidney	1560	1.62×10^5
Liver	1550	$1\cdot65 \times 10^5$
Muscle	1580	1.70×10^5
Water 20°C	1480	1.48×10^5

(less than 1% of the energy being reflected) whilst a bone/fat interface may reflect 50%, and a soft tissue/air interface 99% of the incident energy. This renders detailed examination of structures through the lung and the skull almost impossible.

Although the angle of reflection from a tissue interface equals the angle of incidence (in just the same way as light is reflected from a mirror) some degree of scattering also occurs. The intensity of the reflection is very much affected by the angle of the incident beam, the reflection being strongest when the beam is at right angles to the tissue plane.

At poorly-reflecting interfaces a high proportion of the incident beam is transmitted. When such a beam strikes an interface at anything other than a right angle it is refracted in a manner analogous to light passing through a lens or prism. Although the deviation of the beam produced by this mechanism is usually relatively small it can lead to errors of location in some applications (Fig. 9.5).

Display of ultrasound information

Since the signals developed by most ultrasound apparatus have a short duration and high repetition rate the only practicable form of display for many applications is the cathode-ray oscilloscope (p. 71). However the choice of instrument is governed by the scanning technique and the type of information being sought. Further details of methods of displaying and recording the signal will therefore be given with the descriptions of scanning techniques.

A-scan (amplitude scan or A-mode)

This is the simplest technique. The crystal, acting as the transmitter and receiver of pulsed ultrasound, is coupled to the skin by a liquid coupling medium, such as oil or water, and pointed at the area of interest. The echoes which are reflected back to the crystal are delayed by time intervals which are governed by the distance of the interface from the transducer and the velocity of sound in the intervening tissues. In soft tissues a time delay of 1-μs corresponds to a tissue distance of about 1.5 mm (i.e. a tissue *thickness* of 0.75 mm). The scan is displayed by initiating the sweep of the time base on the oscilloscope at the moment that the pulse is transmitted. When an echo is received the spot is deflected vertically for the duration of the echo. It then returns to the baseline and continues its horizontal traverse until another echo is received or another sweep of the time base is initiated by another pulse of ultrasound. If the tissue planes are stationary the echo pattern will be repeated in exactly the same place at each sweep of the time base. Because of the persistence of vision the display will appear to remain static provided that the pulse repetition frequency is at least 20 Hz. The size of the vertical deflection represents the amplitude of the echo whilst the position of the deflection along the time base is a measure of the time taken for the echo to return to the receiver and hence is related to the distance of the tissue interface from the crystal (Fig. 9.6). Unfortunately it is rare to receive a single echo from biological

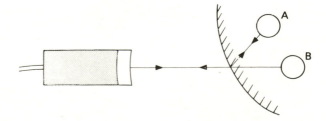

Fig. 9.5. Effect of refraction of ultrasound beam on apparent position of interface. Object A is interpreted as being at position B.

tissues for there are usually many interfaces and often multiple reflection artefacts. One source of interference is the artefact due to multiple reflection within the crystal itself. This can usually be minimized by careful design of the crystal. Another problem is that part of the echo that is received by the crystal is reflected and so initiates a second echo with double the time delay of the first. This process may lead to multiple echoes but these can usually be recognized by the regular spacing and decreasing amplitude of the signal.

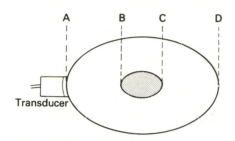

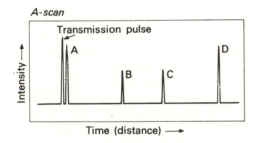

A-scan

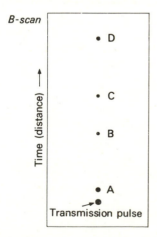

B-scan

Fig. 9.6. *A*-scans and *B*-scans showing reflections from surfaces A, B, C, and D.

Since echo signals from deep structures are attenuated more than those from superficial structures most machines incorporate a swept gain function generator which progressively increases the amplification of the echo signal as the time base moves from left to right. This provides a substantial improvement in the quality of the information provided.

The *A*-scan is relatively simple to understand and the equipment is fairly inexpensive. It is most useful where the anatomical structures are not complex and where accurate measurement of dimensions is required. Examples are the identification of the midline of the brain when space-occupying intracranial lesions are suspected and the measurement of the depth of the chambers of the eye. It is also useful for differentiating solid from cystic lesions (e.g. in the kidney) and can be used to facilitate further examination of an image identified on the *B*-scan.

B-scan (brightness scan or B-mode)

It often proves difficult to identify the source of all the echoes received during one-dimensional A-scanning and identification may become impossible if the structures are moving. Use of the *B*-scan obviates some of the difficulties by modifying the form of the display. The principle is illustrated in Fig. 9.6. The depth of the echo is still recorded by the sweep on one axis of the oscilloscope but the site of the echo is now recorded by a bright spot on the sweep line, the brightness of the spot being proportional to the intensity of the echo. In its simplest form the B-mode is usually displayed as shown in Fig. 9.7a. The vertical axis now displays the depth of the reflecting surfaces from the transducer. If any of the echoes are moving this will be shown by movement of the bright spots along the vertical axis. Since this scan is produced by rapid repetition of the ultrasonic pulses a graphical display of the movement can be obtained by adding a time

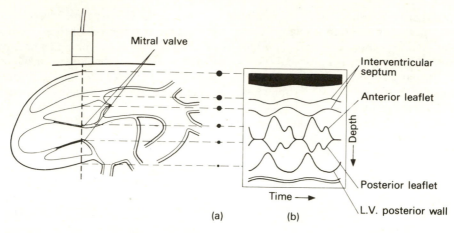

Fig. 9.7. B-scan: time-position recording on oscilloscope a. static B-scan b. with addition of time base.

base on the horizontal axis. This yields an M-scan. The time base may be relatively slow. For example, in studies of the movement of cardiac valves the traverse may take 3 seconds so that one or two cardiac cycles are displayed. The screen can then be photographed by a time exposure (Fig. 9.7b). Alternatively the signals may be displayed on a long-persistence screen or on a storage oscilloscope (p. 73). If more prolonged periods of recording are required the M-scan is displayed on a cathode-ray oscilloscope with a fibre-optic face plate. This produces an extremely bright image of the M-scan y-axis which can then be converted to a continuous record by driving ultraviolet recording paper across the face plate at right angles to the direction of the depth scan (Fig. 9.8). Such scans are also called time–motion scans (T–M scans), or

time–position scans (T–P scans). They are of most use in assessing the movement in heart valves or ventricular wall (Traill & Gibson 1977). Another use of the B-mode is illustrated in Fig. 9.9. In this type of scan the transducer is moved linearly across the object and the movement of the transducer is linked mechanically and electronically to the horizontal sweep of the cathode-ray oscilloscope. The depths of the reflecting surfaces are marked in the vertical direction by spots of varying brightness, and the shape of the underlying structure is then built up as the transducer is moved across the object. In order to record the scan as it is produced it is necessary either to display the scan on a storage oscilloscope or to use a time exposure photograph of a standard oscilloscope screen. B-scanning has now been developed to incorporate

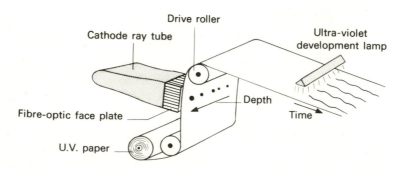

Fig. 9.8. M-scan: time-position recording on ultraviolet paper.

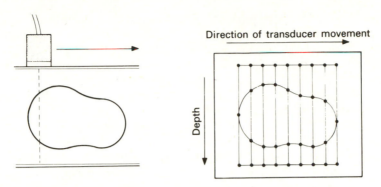

Fig. 9.9. M-scan: time-position recording of moving scanner.

more complex scanning patterns, for the image is greatly improved by increasing the number of interfaces struck at right angles by the ultrasound beam. The accurate registration of the movement of the transducer and its synchronization with the oscilloscope trace naturally add greatly to the complexity and cost of such apparatus. There are also problems associated with the coupling of the transducer to the skin. However, the tremendous improvement in the images obtained has greatly extended the scope of the method.

Two-dimensional scanning is used mostly in obstetrics. It is of value for measurement of fetal size, detection of multiple pregnancies, diagnosis of fetal abnormality and localization of the placenta. It is also used in the diagnosis of abnormalities of many other systems and has proved particularly useful in assessing the mobility of heart valves and the movement of cardiac muscle.

Real-time scanning

Until recently two-dimensional scanners were generally designed to produce sharp black and white images which emphasized the shape of organ boundaries. These could be displayed on the bistable direct view storage tube (p. 73). However, it has now been demonstrated that the echo amplitude also conveys useful diagnostic information and that grey-scale displays are valuable

supplements to black and white images. These are best displayed on a transmission control direct-view storage tube, which has a limited but useful grey-scale capability, or by the scan conversion memory (p. 114).

The maximum pulse repetition rate in B-scanners is limited by the time taken for the echoes and their reverberations to return to the transducer. For a penetration of, say 15 cm the sweep time of the time base is about $200\,\mu s$. This is followed by a dead period of about $500\,\mu s$ in order to allow the reverberations to die down. The resultant maximal pulse repetition rate is about 1500 per second. Since each pulse contributes a single line to the B-scan, the rapidity with which an object can be completely scanned will depend on the number of scan lines required to build up a satisfactory image. For a pulse repetition rate of 1500 per second an image built up from 100 scan lines can be scanned completely 15 times per second. It is thus possible to produce a series of moving images which are comparable to those recorded by the separate frames on a cine-film.

Instruments are now available which produce and display images at more than 20 frames per second. These are said to operate in 'real-time', and permit moving structures to be studied in great detail.

There are basically three types of real-time scanners. In one the probe contains an array of 20–64 separate transducer elements. These are operated either individually or in small groups to produce a rectangular image of the moving anatomy lying underneath the probe. A second type of machine incorporates a high speed mechanical scanner using one or more transducer probes. If this is in contact with the skin its movement is limited to rotation around the point of contact. The third type of apparatus uses a phased-transducer display. The probe consists of about 20 transducer elements mounted in parallel so that they would normally view a field in their long axis. However, by introducing time delay circuits in the signal paths associated with each transducer element it is possible to steer the beam through a sector and to record the image as the sector is scanned.

Real-time scanning has recently been used to study fetal heart movements and fetal respiratory patterns, the image closely resembling that obtained by fluoroscopy. Indeed this technique has recently led to the discovery that some babies suffer hiccups in utero. The scope for further developments is obviously boundless!

C-scanning

This resembles a tomograph in that a plane is scanned at right angles to the direction of the ultrasonic beam, the plane being situated at a defined distance from the plane of motion of the transducer. This method has not received much clinical application for the scanning system is complicated and it does not seem to have many advantages over other scanning techniques.

THE SCAN CONVERTER

Scan-converter systems can store and display large-area images which exhibit a range of grey shades. Since the image is presented on a television monitor, colour presentations of echo intensity can also be achieved. Furthermore, since the echo signals are stored electronically within the scan converter it is possible to process the signals after the scan has been performed or to record them on video tape. The scan-converter tube resembles a small cathode-ray tube in which the screen phosphor has been replaced by a target which is capable of retaining a pattern of electronic charge on its surface. The target consists of a wafer of electronically-conductive material backed by an array of several hundred thousand strips or squares of insulating material. The beam is deflected across the target by electrostatic or electromagnetic fields and passes through a field mesh which ensures that the beam hits the target at right angles to its surface. The velocity of the electrons is increased whenever an echo is received and the accelerated electrons then eject other electrons from the insulating strips on the target. Thus each echo is recorded as a positively-charged area on the target, the amount of charge being proportional to the intensity of the echo. However, the recording mechanism is so arranged that if a structure is detected from more than one direction of the ultrasound beam only the strongest echo is recorded.

To read the image a lower intensity electron beam is caused to scan the target in a series of parallel lines whilst a second electron beam in a television tube performs a similar scan. The brightness of the image on the television tube then reflects the pattern of charge on the target in the scan-converter tube. The image can be read repeatedly so that a steady image appears on the television tube and can be erased at will. The scan-converter system may also have facilities for magnifying sections of the image or for presenting a number of separate images on different parts of the screen. The resolution of the image is good and it can be recorded by photographing the image directly (usually from a second TV screen), by using electrostatic recorders, or by transferring the image to video tapes.

Analogue scan converters are subject to drift and ageing of the components so that their performance deteriorates with time. They are therefore now being replaced by digital processing and storage systems which are not subject to these disadvantages.

Detection of motion by the Doppler effect

PRINCIPLE

When an ultrasound beam is reflected from a stationary object the frequency of the reflected wave equals that of the transmitted wave. However, when the reflector is moved towards the transmitter it encounters more oscillations in a given time than a stationary reflector so that the frequency of the waves impinging on the reflector is apparently increased (Fig. 9.10). This is known as the Doppler effect. If the transmitted frequency is f_0, its wavelength λ, the velocity of sound in the medium c, and the velocity of the reflecting object moving towards the source is v, the frequency of the waves impinging on the reflector will be

$$\frac{c + v}{\lambda}.$$

Since the reflector then acts as a source which is moving towards the transmitter/receiver the actual frequency sensed by the receiver (f_r) must be

$$f_r = \frac{c + 2v}{\lambda}.$$

Thus, the apparent *increase* in frequency is given by:

$$f_r - f_0 = \frac{c + 2v}{\lambda} - \frac{c}{\lambda} = \frac{2v}{\lambda}$$

or since $\lambda = c/f$,

$$f_r - f_0 = \frac{2vf_0}{c}.$$

This equation assumes that the velocity of the reflector is small compared with the velocity of sound in the medium, a condition which exists in most clinical situations. Substituting some typical values in the equation, e.g. $c = 1500 \, \text{m} \cdot \text{s}^{-1}$, $f = 2 \, \text{MHz}$, $v = 0.1 \, \text{m} \cdot \text{s}^{-1}$ indicates that:

$$f_r - f_0 = \frac{2 \times 0.1 \times 2\,000\,000}{1500} = 266 \, \text{Hz}.$$

The Doppler signal can be detected using the *heterodyne principle*, which states that when signals of two similar frequencies f_1 and f_2 are mixed together, the resultant waveform will be 100% amplitude-modulated at the frequency $f_1 - f_2$ (see Chapter 3, p. 47). Simple demodulation and low pass filtering yields the side-band frequency, which is of course the Doppler signal.

Fig. 9.10. Doppler effect. An object moving towards the transmitter encounters more cycles per second than a stationary object so that the reflected waves have a higher frequency than those from the transmitter. The increase in frequency sensed by the receiver is doubled because the reflected waves are also compressed into a shorter distance, thus decreasing their wavelength and increasing apparent frequency further. For clarity the incident and reflected waves are shown as parallel beams though in reality they are superimposed. T = transmitter, R = receiver.

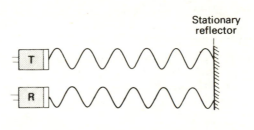

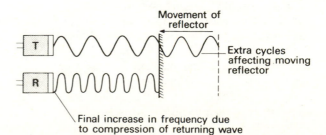

Since the signal is within the audible range the output can be made to drive a loud-speaker or earphones. The resulting sound often proves vividly descriptive. For example pulsatile flow in a blood vessel sounds like a high-pitched murmur whilst movements of the fetal heart sound very like fetal heart sounds.

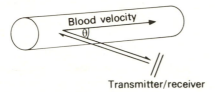

Blood velocity

θ

Transmitter/receiver

Fig. 9.11. Use of Doppler principle to measure flow in a blood vessel.

The application of the Doppler principle is not restricted to the detection of movements in the direction of the beam. When the ultrasound beam is at an angle θ to the direction of movement (Fig. 9.11) the resulting frequency shift is given by

$$f_r - f_o = \frac{2f_o v \cos \theta}{c}$$

When making comparisons between blood flow in different vessels it is therefore necessary to ensure that due account is taken of the angle between the beam and the direction of blood flow. Note that when the beam is at right angles to the motion of the reflecting surface $\cos \theta = \cos 0° = 1$. Furthermore, small departures from a right angle (e.g. $\cos 10° = 0.98$) cause relatively small errors in $f_r - f_o$.

CLINICAL APPLICATIONS

In most simple Doppler-shift instruments, separate transmitting and receiving crystals are mounted side by side in a hand-held probe. Although the receiver senses echoes from both static and moving objects the output is related to frequency shift so that static reflections are not detected. Although the direction of movement can be derived from the direction of the frequency shift

this requires somewhat complicated signal processing. In most inexpensive instruments the output is therefore restricted to an indication of the velocity of movement, but there is no indication of its direction.

One application of this type of instrument is the detection of fetal heart movements. These are almost always present by 12 weeks. Doppler monitoring of fetal heart rate during labour is now widely practised, since it is greatly superior to the simple stethoscope.

Another application is the sensing of flow in blood vessels, for example in determining the patency of a peripheral vessel after suspected thromboembolism (Yao 1972), or in sensing the onset of systolic flow in indirect blood pressure measurement. In the latter application the small transducer head is placed over a peripheral artery with the ultrasound beam aligned at an angle of about 45° with the long axis of the artery. As the cuff is deflated the systolic point is marked by an audible signal related to the intermittent flow through the vessel.

The Doppler technique can also be used to sense the movement of the arterial wall under a sphygmomanometer cuff so that systolic and diastolic points can be established (p. 175). The output signal from most Doppler units is complex because there are usually many components of flow moving at different speeds and directions within the ultrasonic beam. In simple instruments, for example those designed to detect the presence of air emboli in the bloodstream or the presence of flow in an artery, the output is conveniently presented by loudspeaker or earphone, for pulsatile flow produces a sound which aptly mimics the pulsatile flow of blood through an orifice. However, for more complex applications it is necessary to analyse the Doppler signal into its frequency components and also to indicate the direction of flow. An instrument utilizing these techniques is currently being evaluated for measuring aortic flow, the beam being directed backwards and downwards from the suprasternal notch so that it views the flow profile in the transverse part of the aorta. It is hoped that measurements of early systolic acceleration and peak flow velocity will provide a continuous noninvasive indication of myocardial performance. However, it should be noted that quantification of flow in terms of litres per minute can only be achieved if the cross-sectional area of the aorta is known from accurate radiographic or other ultrasound measurements (Gross & Light 1974; Hanson & Bilton 1978).

Recently, pulsed-Doppler techniques have been introduced into blood-flow measurements. These have the advantage that the depth and cross-sectional area of the vessel can be identified as well.

OTHER USES OF THE DOPPLER TECHNIQUE

The capacity to record movements of the heart muscle and valves, together with quantitative measurements of flow in major blood vessels introduces an extra dimension into the assessment of cardiovascular performance. Doppler techniques have been extended to include the measurement of gas volumes (p. 200) and the detection of air emboli during surgery (Maroon, Edmonds-Seal & Campbell 1969).

References

GROSS G. & LIGHT L.M. (1974) Non-invasive intra-thoracic blood velocity measurement in the assessment of cardiovascular function. *Biomedical Engineering*, **9**, 464.

HANSON G.C. & BILTON A.H. (1978) Clinical experience with transcutaneous aortovelography: preliminary communication. *Journal of the Royal Society of Medicine*, **71**, 501.

MAROON J.C., EDMONDS-SEAL J. & CAMPBELL R.L. (1969) An ultrasonic method for detecting air bubbles. *Journal of Neurosurgery*, **31**, 196.

TRAILL T.A. & GIBSON D.G. (1977) Echocardiography for measuring ventricular performance. *British Journal of Clinical Equipment*, **2**, 125.

YAO S.T. (1972) Ultrasound in the transcutaneous assessment of blood flow. *British Journal of Hospital Medicine*, **8**, 521.

Further reading

MCDICKEN W.N. (1976) *Diagnostic ultrasonics, principles and use of instruments*. London: Crossly, Lockwood, Staples.

WELLS P.N.Y. (1977) *Ultrasonics in clinical diagnosis 2nd Edition*. Edinburgh: Churchill Livingstone.

WELLS P.N.I. (1977) *Biomedical ultrasonics, principles and use of instruments*. London: Academic Press.

Chapter 10
Measurements Using
Radioactive Substances

Patients are commonly encountered in whom the diagnosis has been established or confirmed by the use of radioactive isotopes. Furthermore a number of radioactive techniques have now been automated to a degree which permits the doctor to use them in clinical measurement with no more difficulty than performing a haemoglobin estimation or a simple urine analysis. Some understanding of the basic principles underlying these measurements and their possible applications is therefore desirable.

Basic concepts

ATOMIC STRUCTURE

All atoms consist of a *nucleus* surrounded by an *outer system* of orbiting electrons. The nucleus of all the elements except hydrogen consists of two types of particles of virtually identical mass: protons and neutrons. Each orbiting electron has a mass which is about one two-thousandth that of a proton. Each proton possesses a single positive charge and each electron a single negative charge, whilst neutrons possess no charge. When the atom is in its normal state the number of protons in the nucleus balances the number of electrons in the outer system so that the atom is electrically neutral.

ATOMIC STRUCTURE AND CHEMICAL PROPERTIES

Elements are characterized by the number of protons in the nucleus, the number being specific for each element. Thus hydrogen has one proton, helium two, lithium three and so on (Fig. 10.1). The number of protons is indicated by the *atomic number* (Z). However the chemical properties of an element are determined by the number of electrons in the outer structure. It is convenient to consider the electrons as orbiting within a series of well-defined concentric orbits or 'shells'. Each shell is designated by a number, the principal quantum number, which determines the most stable configuration of the atom. The greatest stability occurs when each shell contains $2n^2$ electrons. In the inner or K-shell this condition is achieved when there are two electrons present, in the L-shell the number is 8, the M-shell 18, the N-shell 32 and so on. For example, helium has two electrons in the K-shell whilst neon has 2 in the K-shell and 8 in the L-shell. Both of these

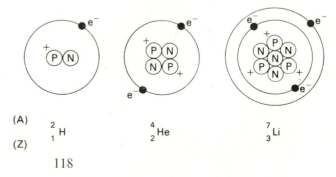

Fig. 10.1. Structure of hydrogen, helium and lithium atoms. A = Mass number (sum of weights of protons plus neutrons) Z = atomic number (number of protons in nucleus).

(A)

$^2_1$H $^4_2$He $^7_3$Li

(Z)

elements have their full complement of electrons and are chemically inert. Elements with an incomplete shell are chemically reactive. Thus lithium, sodium and potassium all have one electron in their outer shell and readily surrender this to become positively-charged ions Li^+, Na^+, and K^+. Elements with a deficiency of one electron in the outer shell, such as chlorine, bromine and fluorine readily accept an electron and become stable, negatively-charged ions (Cl^-, Br^-, F^-). The configuration of the electrons in the outer shell thus determines the chemical relationships displayed in the periodic table of the elements.

Electrons may be shared as well as transferred. Thus hydrogen has one electron in the K-shell and shares this with another hydrogen atom so that hydrogen normally exists as the molecule H_2. Similarly two oxygen atoms will pool 4 of their outer shell electrons to create an L-shell of 8 electrons, whilst two nitrogen atoms will share a total of 6 electrons.

Within each shell there may be one or more energy levels which electrons can take up. If an electron moves from a higher to a lower energy level, either within the shell or by transferring to another shell, then energy is emitted. This is manifested as an *emission spectrum*. An *absorption spectrum* is the reverse process.

ISOTOPES

The simplest atom, that of hydrogen, is made up of one proton and one electron and contains no neutrons. All the other atoms contain a variable number of neutrons which alter the mass of the atom but do not affect its chemical properties. Atoms of an element which contain the same number of protons and electrons but a different number of neutrons are called isotopes of that element (Fig. 10.2). Because they contain the same number of protons and electrons they are chemically indistinguishable from each other.

Table 10.1. Percentage of stable isotopes of hydrogen, carbon, nitrogen and oxygen found in nature.

Isotope	Number of protons	Number of neutrons	Mass number	%
^1H	1	0	1	99.99
^2H	1	1	2	0.01
^{12}C	6	6	12	98.9
^{13}C	6	7	13	1.1
^{14}N	7	7	14	99.63
^{15}N	7	8	15	0.37
^{16}O	8	8	16	99.76
^{17}O	8	9	17	0.04
^{18}O	8	10	18	0.20

Most naturally-occurring elements exist as mixtures of isotopes (Table 10.1). These are known as *stable isotopes* because the configuration of the nucleus does not cause it to break down. However, the number of stable configurations of protons and neutrons is limited, and there are many configurations which are unstable and in which the nuclei tend to disintegrate in various ways. These are known as *unstable isotopes* or *radionuclides*; since their disintegration is associated with the release of radiation energy or charged particles they are said to be *radioactive*. Although some

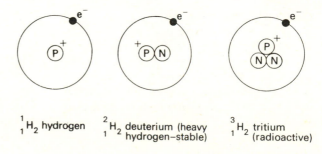

Fig. 10.2. Isotopes of hydrogen. $^1_1H_2$ hydrogen $^2_1H_2$ deuterium (heavy hydrogen–stable) $^3_1H_2$ tritium (radioactive)

radioactive isotopes with long half-lives, such as ^{226}Ra or ^{40}K, occur naturally, the majority of radioisotopes are manufactured by nuclear reactors or by particle accelerators such as the cyclotron. Conventionally, isotopes are identified by placing a superscript *mass number* (A), which designates the total number of protons and neutrons in the nucleus, before the chemical symbol. For example both ^{127}I and ^{131}I have 53 protons but ^{127}I has 74 neutrons whilst ^{131}I has 78 neutrons in the nucleus. In some texts both the mass number and the *atomic number* (the number of protons in the nucleus) are given, but the latter is placed as a subscript before the chemical symbol (Fig. 10.2).

Types of radiation

The disintegration of the nucleus may be accompanied by the emission of particles, or energy, or both.

Alpha-radiation

This consists of heavy, positively-charged particles equivalent to two protons in charge, associated with two further units of mass, making four units of mass in all. They are thus identical with helium nuclei. Emission of an alpha-particle results in the formation of an element with an atomic number two less and an atomic weight of four less, than the original element. For example, the initial breakdown of radium leads to the formation of radon:

$$^{226}_{88}\text{Ra} \rightarrow {}^{222}_{86}\text{Rn} + \alpha\text{-particle } ({}^{4}_{2}\text{He}).$$

Because of their considerable mass, alpha-particles do not have a high velocity. They are easily absorbed by passage through a fraction of a millimetre of Perspex or body tissue, or a few centimetres of air. However, they are extremely harmful to biological tissues so that radioisotopes emitting alpha-particles are not employed in the clinical situation.

Beta and positron radiation

The majority of isotopes decay by the emission of particles which have a mass equal to that of the electron. These particles carry a single unit of charge which is usually negative (beta particles) but may be positive (positrons).

Radioisotopes with an excess of neutrons usually decay by the emission of a negatively-charged beta particle which is identical with the electron. By the loss of a unit of negative charge the nucleus effectively replaces a neutron by a proton; the resulting nucleus is that of an isotope of the element with the next *higher* atomic number in the periodic system. For example the decay of the phosphorous isotope ^{32}P forms stable sulphur:

$$^{32}_{15}\text{P} \rightarrow {}^{32}_{16}\text{S} + ({}^{\ 0}_{-1}\beta)$$

In a similar manner many neutron-deficient radioisotopes decay by the emission of a positively-charged particle or positron, thereby reducing the atomic number of their atoms by 1 unit. For example ^{18}F decays to form an isotope of oxygen:

$$^{18}_{9}\text{F} \rightarrow {}^{18}_{8}\text{O} + ({}^{\ 0}_{+1}\beta).$$

Whilst beta-particles are less easily absorbed than alpha-particles their range is still less than a few millimetres in body tissues or Perspex. The marked absorption of beta-radiation by the body renders external detection of its presence in body tissues difficult so that radioisotopes which emit only beta-radiation are most commonly used for tracer studies in which the radioactivity is measured in samples removed from the body.

Gamma radiation

Usually, the emission of the beta-particle is not able to dissipate all the energy that is released during the nuclear rearrangement, and the excess is radiated as gamma-radiation. Gamma-radiation is electromagnetic radiation of very short wavelength and is identical with X-rays, though the method of production differs. In a nuclear disintegration there is always a specific amount of energy released, depending on the original and final configurations, so that the energy levels of gamma-radiation released by a given radionuclide are characteristic of that substance. More than one kind of rearrangement may occur, in which case more than one level of energy may be emitted. Gamma-radiation with a high energy penetrates many centimetres of tissue and is often called 'hard' radiation; conversely 'soft' radiation has a low energy and poor penetrating power.

Neutrons

These are produced in a cyclotron and are now being used in both therapy and measurement. Their biological effect depends on their velocity. When a fast moving neutron collides with the nucleus of another atom, it disrupts it, producing secondary particles which are radioactive. Large radiation doses can therefore be given to tissue in tumour therapy, whilst measurement of the quantity of various constituents of the body can be undertaken by the technique of neutron activation (see below).

UNITS OF MEASUREMENT

The *amount* of radioactivity in a substance is defined in terms of the rate at which that substance is disintegrating. A substance undergoing 3.7×10^{10} disintegrations per second contains 1 *curie* (Ci) of radioactivity. This unit has been in use for many years but has now been replaced by the SI unit, the *Becquerel* (Bq). Since the Becquerel is equal to 1 disintegration per second, $1\,\text{Ci} = 3.7 \times 10^{10}\,\text{Bq}$. A measure of X-ray or gamma-ray emissions is given by the quantity known as *exposure*. This defines the intensity of X-rays or gamma-rays in terms of the amount of ionisation they produce in air. The unit is the *roentgen*: this is the exposure of X- or gamma-radiation which produces 2.58×10^{-4}

coulombs per kilogram of air (1.61×10^{15} ion pairs per kilogram of air). This unit is used for the calibration of instruments which determine X-ray or gamma-ray intensity by measuring the amount of ionisation produced in air.

Of great clinical importance is the unit of *absorbed dose*. This is a measure of the energy transferred to a substance by beta and other radiation, as well as by X-ray or gamma-ray radiation. The old unit of absorbed dose is the *rad*: this is equal to 100 ergs per gram of material. The SI unit of absorbed dose is the *Gray* (gy) which is equal to 1 Joule per kilogram ($= 10^7$ ergs per kilogram $= 100$ rad). Note that the absorbed dose due to an exposure of 1 roentgen depends on the energy of X-ray or gamma-ray radiation and on the type of material being irradiated. In body tissue one roentgen produces about 0.85–0.95 rad.

The biological effects produced by different types of ionising radiation such as X-rays, neutrons or alpha particles differ from one another quantitatively rather than qualitatively. For example a given amount of chromosome damage may result from an absorbed dose of one rad given by neutrons or, say, 10 rads given by X-rays. When persons are liable to be exposed to a mixture of different radiations it is convenient to use units which will sum up the overall effect of the radiation exposure on the organism. Such equivalent doses are expressed in *rems* (roentgen *equivalent for man*). This method of expressing radiation dosage is less rigorous than the other units already referred to for it depends on a somewhat arbitrary choice of quality factors for different types of radiation. However, it is a convenient method of expressing radiation dosage when dealing with problems of radiation protection.

Another aspect of radiation dosage which must be considered is the distribution of radioactivity within the body. Some isotopes are distributed throughout the body (for example in the bloodstream) so that the distribution of radiation mirrors the distribution of blood flow. Other isotopes may be localized in a particular organ such as kidney or thyroid. This is then called the *critical organ* for that isotope. Beta-particles are almost completely absorbed by body tissues so that a critical organ receives a high dose of radiation. Gamma rays, however, transfer less of their energy to the tissues and so are relatively less damaging than beta-radiation.

The energy of any radiation is defined in terms of the electron volt (eV): this is equal to the energy of an electron accelerated through 1 volt ($= 1.6 \times 10^{-19}$ joules). Most radiations used in medical work have energies between a few keV (thousand electron volts) and 1 MeV (million electron volts).

These quantities are related in a complex manner to the number of 'counts' which may be recorded from instruments which detect radiation. A radioactive source emits in all directions, and the proportion of its emissions which reaches a detecting device depends on the geometric relationship between the two. If the detector is visualized as occupying a finite area on the surface of an imaginary sphere with the source at its centre, the radioactive flux which will impinge on the detector will depend not only on the area of the detector but will also vary inversely as the square of the radius of that sphere, which is, of course, the distance between the source and the detector. The amount of absorption of radiation which takes place between the source and the detector also modifies the amount of the radiation detected, and this depends on its energy and on the medium through which it is passing. In some cases even a thin Perspex window may effectively absorb the radiation. For this reason detectors of quite different designs are needed to match different applications.

HALF-LIFE

At any moment the rate of disintegration is dependent on the total number of atoms which have a potential for disintegration. Radioactive decay is therefore exponential,

and analogous to such processes as the passive emptying of the lungs and the metabolism or excretion of many drugs. The rate at which an exponential process is taking place is usually described by the time constant (Chapter 2). However in the case of radioactive decay the rate is customarily defined by the half-life. This is the time it takes for the radioactivity to fall to one half of its initial value.* A knowledge of the half-life enables one to calculate the activity at any future time once the activity at any stated time has been determined, for it takes just as long for the remaining half of the activity to fall by half (to one quarter of the initial value) and as long again to fall to an eighth of the initial value.

Radioisotopes disintegrate at very different rates. Half-lives vary from thousands of years, in the case of some naturally-occurring radioisotopes, down to a few seconds for some artificially-produced radioisotopes. The rate of decay is quite characteristic of the isotope and cannot be altered by any physical or chemical process. However it is important to distinguish this *physical* half-life of the radioisotope from the *biological half-life*.

The latter term is used to describe the disappearance of a substance from a particular organ or tissue, in which case it will depend on metabolism and blood flow; alternatively it may refer to the rate of disappearance from the whole body, in which case it will depend on excretion. The combination of physical and biological half-lives is known as the *effective half-life*. If the physical, biological and effective half-lives are given by T_p, T_b and T_e then

$$\frac{1}{T_e} = \frac{1}{T_p} + \frac{1}{T_b}.$$

Detection of radiation

Radiation may be detected by chemical change, by ionization or by conversion to

---

* It must be emphasized that the half-life is *not* half the time taken for all the activity to disappear for, with an exponential change, the process is only complete in infinite time.

another form of energy such as light or sound.

PHOTOGRAPHIC FILM

Radiation has an action on photographic film which is similar to that of light, the degree of darkening depending on the intensity (or quantity) of the radiation and its energy (or quality). Photographic detection is, of course, the basis of radiodiagnosis, but it is also used for monitoring the dose of radiation received by radiation workers. For this purpose a strip of photographic film is incorporated in a specially-designed badge. Such badges should be worn by all personnel exposed to radiation hazards and the films should be assessed and replaced at regular intervals. A third use of photographic detection is in autoradiography, a technique in which the distribution of injected radioactivity is recorded by placing a slice of tissue in contact with a photographic film until the film has received adequate radiation exposure. When the film is developed it contains an image which is related to the distribution of radioactivity in the tissue slice. The technique has been used to show the time course of the distribution of muscle relaxants and other drugs in whole body slices of small experimental animals such as rats.

IONIZATION CHAMBER

When radiation passes through a gas, some of the electrons of the gaseous atoms are dislodged so that positively-charged ions and free electrons are formed. These can be collected on negatively- and positively-charged plates (cathode and anode) and so used to generate an electrical current, the magnitude of which depends on the intensity and energy of the radiation. In this type of instrument the voltage difference between the plates is comparatively low so that no secondary ionizations are induced (see below). Such an instrument is known as an ionization chamber. It is chiefly used for assaying diagnostic and therapeutic quanti-

ties of radioisotopes prior to administration to patients, and also for measuring the radiation produced by X-ray machines.

GEIGER (GEIGER-MÜLLER) COUNTER

By raising the voltage across the plates it is possible to accelerate the free electrons produced by the radiation to such speeds that they themselves produce further ionization by collision with other atoms. This process repeats itself many times so that a given quantity of radiation produces a very large electrical signal which can be measured easily, but whose size is no longer related to the energy of the radiation which produced it. This is the basis of the Geiger counter.

The counter consists of a tube filled with a gas such as argon or helium. The positively-charged anode is a thin wire situated in the centre of the tube and the negatively charged cathode is often a metal screen adjacent to it. An organic vapour or halogen gas (quenching gas) is added to the argon to prevent the production of spurious pulses. For a short time after a discharge is initiated the tube fails to react to further radiation so that there is always a short period during which further ionizing radiation will not be detected. For this reason a 'dead time' correction factor must be applied when counting rates are high. Geiger counters are very sensitive to beta-radiation (free electrons and positrons) but are relatively insensitive to gamma-radiation.

SCINTILLATION DETECTORS

This form of detector utilizes the emission of light induced by radiation in luminescent materials. The detector consists of a crystal of a substance such as sodium iodide activated with a very small amount of thallium iodide (Fig. 10.3). The crystal is contained in a light-proof case and produces a brief flash of light (half-life about $2\,\mu s$) whenever it receives energy from a disintegration. The intensity of the light

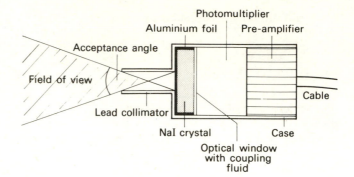

Fig. 10.3. Essential features of a scintillation detector.

emitted by the crystal (i.e. the number of photons produced) is proportional to the energy of the absorbed radiation. The outside of the crystal is usually faced with a thin layer of aluminium foil which tends to prevent the entry of low energy beta-rays; it also reflects the light flashes from the crystal towards a photomultiplier tube which is optically coupled to the opposite side of the crystal. The photomultiplier contains a photocathode. This consists of a thin layer of semi-conductor material such as antimony–caesium, which produces an electron whenever a certain number of photons impinges on it. The number of electrons produced by the photocathode is thus proportional to the energy of the absorbed radiation. The electrons from the photocathode pass to a series of dynodes which produce an increasing cascade of electrons, thus multiplying the original signal many times. The final pulse of electrons is collected on an anode and passed to a pre-amplifier situated within the detector unit. This provides a much stronger voltage pulse which is not degraded by electrical interference during its passage to the processing unit. Since the magnitude of this pulse is proportional to the energy of the radiation absorbed in the crystal, it is possible to select pulses originating from radiation of a given energy and so to count only the radiation emitted by a particular radioisotope. Since many radioisotope techniques utilise a mixture of isotopes, this facility greatly increases the versatility of the detector.

Scintillation detectors are most common-ly used for detecting gamma radiation from various parts of the body. In order to limit the field of view a lead collimator is added to the front of the crystal. Heavy shielding is also provided round the side of the crystal to ensure that it only receives radiation from the area for which the collimator is designed (Fig. 10.3). However, care must be taken to ensure that stray radiation does not reach the photomultiplier end of the crystal for this is often inadequately shielded.

Well-counters

In certain circumstances it is necessary to measure gamma activity in small samples removed from the body. This is usually accomplished by using a specially adapted scintillation detector known as a well-counter. This consists of a sodium iodide crystal with a well at its centre. The sample is placed in a small tube within the well so that counts are received from both the bottom and sides of the sample. This greatly increases counting efficiency. Because of the small amounts of radioactivity in the sample, well-counters must be completely shielded from external radiation and are correspondingly heavy. Although some high energy beta-radiation from the sample may penetrate to the crystal most beta-particles are absorbed by the sample tube.

Liquid scintillation counting

The principle of scintillation detection is also used in the measurement of beta-radiation from tissues and blood samples removed from the body, the most common pure beta-emitting radionuclides being ^{14}C and ^{3}H. In this case a liquid scintillator which is compatible with the sample to be examined is mixed with it so that the light flashes occur within the tube containing the sample and scintillator. These are then detected by a pair of photomultipliers which are situated on either side of the sample tube.

PROCESSING THE SIGNAL

The electrical output from a Geiger–Muller detector usually passes to a *discriminator* which rejects the electronic noise (i.e. pulses below a certain height) before the signals are processed further. Signals from a scintillation detector are sometimes processed similarly but more commonly are subjected to pulse-height analysis. A pulse-height *analyser* rejects all signals above and below pre-set limits (*the gate-width*) and so enables pulses originating from selected energies of radiation to be passed to a *scaler* which counts the pulses accumulated over a period of time. The pulse-height analyser or discriminator may also be connected directly to a *ratemeter* which continuously registers the number of impulses received per unit time. The output from the ratemeter may be recorded as an analogue signal on a chart recorder, or a digital output of the number of counts recorded in pre-set periods of time can be recorded on paper or magnetic tape using a *multiscaler*.

Since radioactive decay is a random process it is subject to statistical inference. This topic is dealt with in the later chapters on statistics and in the Appendix to this Chapter.

METHODS OF LOCALIZING RADIOACTIVITY

There are basically two methods of localizing radioactivity within the body—those in which the detector moves and those in which the detector is stationary.

Moving detector systems

The simplest localization technique is profile scanning in which a single, shielded and collimated detector is moved linearly over the region of interest. Usually the movement of the detector is controlled mechanically, the transit of the detector being recorded on one axis of a chart recorder whilst the count rate is displayed on the other axis. This type of scan has been used for the localization of thyroid metastases and in the measurement of the vertical gradient of ventilation and perfusion in the lung. In an extension of this method the scanner is caused to move to and fro across the area of interest but is moved laterally by a fixed amount at each traverse so that a rectangular area is eventually covered by the scan (Fig. 10.4).

This technique has been widely used for lung, brain and liver scanning. The method tends to be slow because the scanning speed

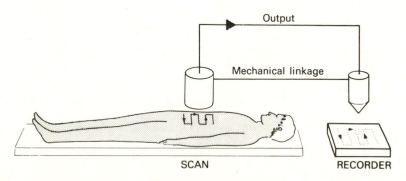

Fig. 10.4. Principle of operation of a rectilinear scanner.

is limited by the necessity to accumulate sufficient counts at each point on the scan but, by using a carefully focussed collimator, good resolution of detail can be obtained. The display of such scans may be accomplished by printing the count-rate distribution as a series of monochrome dots on paper. A grey-scale image is thus built up along the parallel scan lines, the final image appearing rather like a coarse television screen picture. A similar image may be produced by photographic recording. An alternative mode of display relates the count rate to the colours of the visible spectrum. Thus areas with high count rates may be displayed by red dots whilst areas with lower count rates are displayed in 'cooler' colours such as green or blue.

Fixed detector systems

A number of detectors may be formed into a regular array and so collimated that each detector covers a segment of the area of interest. This method has been used for regional lung function measurements, for measuring cerebral blood flow washout curves, and for measuring whole body radioactivity. It has the advantage that the counters record continuously from the same area so that high numbers of counts can be obtained rapidly. This permits the method to be adapted to measure variations in regional count rates with time, for example during respiratory manoeuvres.

However, spatial resolution is limited by the number of counters which can be mounted within a given area.

The gamma camera represents a modification of this system. In the original camera, developed by Anger & colleagues in 1958, a conical collimator was designed with a single small hole so that the radiation from different areas of the subject impinged on different parts of a large flat disc of sodium iodide, the principle being similar to that employed in the pin-hole camera. The spatial resolution of the image was then recorded by integrating the output from a number of photomultipliers which viewed the opposite side of the crystal. In modern versions of this instrument the single hole in the lead block is replaced by about 1000 or more narrow parallel holes in a lead plate which is some 5 cm thick and may be up to 40 cm in diameter (Fig. 10.5). The sodium iodide crystal is situated immediately behind the collimator. Each area of the crystal is affected only by radioactivity emanating from a source lying along the axis of one of the holes in the lead plate so that the image is built up by the flashes of light occurring in the relevant areas of crystal. Behind the crystal there is an array of photomultiplier tubes. Although there may be as many as 64 of these in some cameras, the number can be considerably less than the number of holes in the collimator. Spatial resolution of each flash is then obtained by coordinating the informa-

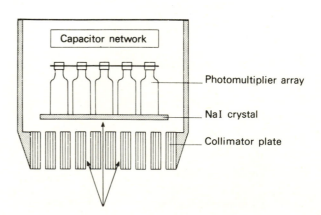

Fig. 10.5. Structure of a gamma camera.

tion received from several photomultipliers by a condenser network, the position of a light flash being identified by the relative amounts of light arriving at the different photomultipliers.

The image may be formed on an oscilloscope screen where it may be photographed whilst the camera is operating. The signals received from the camera may require considerable processing before they are finally displayed, so that the camera is operated in conjunction with a computer and the information is stored on disc or magnetic tape. Images may then either be printed out by the computer using different symbols for different count rates, so that a grey-scale image is produced, or may be displayed on a TV screen in either grey-scale or colour. Further computer manipulation permits designated areas of the image to be selected for further analysis (Fig. 10.6). The gamma camera has the advantage that it provides good images of reasonably large areas of

the body and that scanning times are short enough to permit very fast variations in count rate (e.g. respiratory manoeuvres) to be recorded. The machine performs best with relatively low energy gamma rays, since high energy rays penetrate the lead between the holes in the collimator and so impair resolution.

Another development of the gamma camera is the positron camera used with positron-emitting isotopes. When a positron comes to rest in an absorbing medium it combines with an electron and the two particles are annihilated to produce two gamma-ray quanta each of 0.51 MeV energy which are emitted from the point of interaction in exactly opposite directions. Coincidences between pairs of annihilation gamma rays can be detected by two scintillation detectors placed on opposite sides of the subject. With this instrument it is possible to localize the point of interaction very precisely: it is also possible to obtain

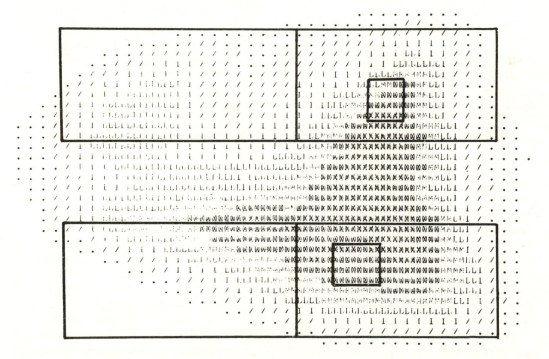

Fig. 10.6. Computer print out from gamma camera showing activity in right lateral view of thorax of supine dog. The head is to the left. Areas such as those demarcated by the rectangles can be subjected to further analysis e.g. to determine regional ventilation washout curves.

images of radioactivity distributions in planes at different depths within the subject (Fig. 10.7).

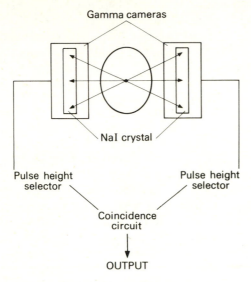

Fig. 10.7. Principle of a positron camera.

PROTECTION AGAINST RADIATION HAZARDS

When using radioactive substances, hazards arise in two ways. There may be exposure to radiation during use, or there may be inhalation or ingestion of material which is retained in the body, giving rise to prolonged exposure of some tissues to radiation.

The magnitude of the external hazards depends on the nature of the radiation, the source strength and the duration of exposure. Radionuclides emitting only soft beta-radiation constitute less of an external hazard than gamma-emitters. The dose can be controlled by shielding and distance, the dose diminishing inversely as the square of the distance. Ingestion hazards depend on the half-life of the radionuclide, on the types and energies of its emissions, on the degree of retention in the body (biological half-life), and whether or not the radionuclide is concentrated in specific tissues.

These factors have been taken into account in a classification of the toxicity of isotopes which is published in the 'Codes of Practice'. Two of the codes are of relevance to medical workers: 'Code of practice for the protection of persons against ionising radiations arising from Medical and Dental Use' (HMSO 1972) and 'Code of practice for the protection of persons against Ionising Radiations in Research and Teaching' (HMSO 1972). The safety aspects of all projects must be approved by an 'Appointed Safety Officer'. The administration of radioactive material to patients is controlled, and in the United Kingdom, must be approved by the Department of Health.

In the control of hazards from external radiation, it is of prime importance not to handle isotopes directly. A suitable container or screen should be interposed between the source and any personnel. It is, however, permissible to maintain a sense of proportion. The chief hazard from tracer doses of a few microcuries may be the risk of dropping the lead screening bricks on your foot! When even microcurie amounts of unsealed isotopes are handled, surgical rubber gloves should be worn and washed before being removed. Smoking, eating and drinking, licking labels, etc. should also be avoided.

Applications of radioisotope techniques in clinical measurement

Radioisotopes may be used in patients for therapy or for measurement purposes. In the therapeutic field the isotope may be used as an external source of radiation (e.g. radium or the cobalt teletherapy unit), or it may be used as an internal agent. Examples of the latter use are the instillation of radioactive gold into the peritoneum to treat secondary carcinomatosis, or the administration of radioactive iodine which is concentrated in the thyroid gland. In the measurement field there are four main types of application: the measurement of body composition; metabolism, turnover and function studies; localization studies; and measurements of circulation and blood flow.

In most of the measurement applications the radioisotope is used as a tracer substance, the behaviour of which is believed to be similar to the normal constituent in the system under study. The tracer must therefore satisfy certain criteria. First, it should not affect the behaviour of the system being studied. Second, it should be identical with the substance it represents in terms of its physical, chemical and biological properties so that its behaviour accurately reflects that of the subject of interest. Third, if the isotope is being used to label a compound, the label should remain attached to the parent compound, or to the part of it being studied, throughout the period of study. Fourth, the isotope should be easily detectable, should produce minimal radiation hazard to both target organs and the whole body, and its half-life should be appropriate to the planned investigation.

The characteristics of some commonly-used isotopes are given in Table 10.2.

BODY COMPOSITION

A known quantity of the isotope is injected into the space and allowed to mix throughout that space. When mixing is complete the volume of the space can be calculated by dividing the amount injected by the concentration of the diluted sample. Thus for a volume of indicator V_1 of initial concentration C_1 diluted in a volume V_2 to a concentration C_2:

$$C_1 \times V_1 = C_2 \times (V_1 + V_2)$$

V_1 is usually small and can be neglected when considering the final volume so that

$$V_2 = V_1 \times \frac{C_1}{C_2}.$$

If the concentration of the natural substance in V_2 is determined by chemical analysis the total quantity of the substance in the compartment may be calculated.

This technique is used in measuring blood volume and the various fluid and electrolyte spaces within the body. These spaces or compartments may not correspond with obvious anatomical spaces and are therefore more correctly referred to as 'dilution volumes'. Although they are not clearly defined, studies of these spaces have contributed greatly to our understanding of a number of pathological conditions. However, dilution analysis is subject to many errors which limit the interpretation of the results. For example, mixing may be delayed by a sluggish circulation: alternatively the volume of distribution of the tracer may be reduced by a severe decrease in regional blood flow or by a physical barrier to diffusion. Another problem is that the tracer may leak out of the compartment during the equilibration period. For example, radioactive serum albumin may be lost from the circulation due to increased permeability of the capillaries during shock, whilst continuing haemorrhage may also cause loss of tracer attached to albumin or to red cells.

Blood volume

This may be measured by labelling red cells with ^{51}Cr or by labelling albumin with ^{125}I or ^{131}I. All these isotopes are gamma-emitters but the energy emitted by ^{125}I is less than that emitted by ^{131}I so that less shielding is required in the counting ap-

Table 10.2. Characteristics of some commonly used radionuclides.

Non-diffusible indicators	Half-life	Energy of principal gamma emission
^{51}Cr	28 days	320 keV
^{131}I	8.1 days	364 keV
^{125}I	60 days	27 keV
^{133}In^{m}	100 min	393 keV
^{99}Tc^{m}	6 hours	140 keV
Diffusible indicators		
^{133}Xe	5.3 days	81 keV
^{85}Kr	10 years	514 keV
^{81}Kr^{m}	13 s	190 keV
^{24}Na	15 hours	1.4 & 2.8 MeV
^{42}K	12.5 h	1.5 MeV

paratus: this reduces the cost of commercial equipment.

When using ^{51}Cr the red cells are withdrawn from the patient and labelled by incubation with the isotope. The background activity is measured in a sample of the patient's blood and the activity of the labelled red cells determined before injection. The cells are then injected intravenously. After allowing 10 minutes for mixing within the circulation a blood sample is withdrawn from the other arm and the activity measured. A similar technique is used with labelled albumin but since there are no incompatibility problems commercially available radioactive iodinated human serum albumin may be used (Lewis & Szur 1967). Several semi-automatic blood volume measuring systems are available commercially. However it should not be forgotten that although these machines are called blood volume computers, they actually measure a dilution volume, usually an iodine-dilution volume. These are not necessarily comparable, since the sample of blood drawn from a peripheral vessel has a different haematocrit from the haematocrit of the whole body, and therefore does not contain a truly representative quantity of isotope. If the haematocrit of the sample is measured and a normal value of the whole-body/venous haematocrit ratio is assumed, the true blood volume can be calculated from the formula:

$$\text{blood volume} = \frac{\text{plasma volume}}{(1 - \text{haematocrit}) \times (0.91)}.$$

Failure to make this correction is only one of many errors in methodology that render the measurement of blood volume potentially very inaccurate (Heath & Vickers 1968).

Interpretation may be further complicated by sequestration of part of the circulating blood volume in states of shock or as a result of cardiopulmonary bypass. Nevertheless, the measurement of blood volume may prove useful when assessing a patient for surgery since blood volume is often reduced in cachectic conditions, after pro-longed diuretic therapy and in patients with a phaeochromocytoma.

Other body spaces

An example of this type of measurement is the exchangeable sodium space. In this case radioactive sodium (e.g. in the form of ^{24}NaCl) is injected, and the radioactivity in plasma determined to give the dilution volume. Since the exchange of sodium throughout the pool is slow, it is usual to delay sampling until 18–24 hours after injection by which time it is assumed that mixing will be complete. Corrections must be made for physical decay, since the half-life of ^{24}Na is only 15 hours, and also for the excretion of sodium in the urine.

Other spaces commonly measured are total body water using tritiated water (^{3}H), and extracellular fluid volume using the isotopes ^{35}S-labelled sulphate or ^{85}Br (in NaBr) (Pain 1977).

The size of body compartments can also be determined by the whole body counting of naturally occurring isotopes (e.g. ^{40}K) or by the use of in vivo neutron activation analysis. In the latter technique the whole body is bombarded with neutrons which generate radioisotopes of a number of substances present in the body. These isotopes may be detected by whole body counting. The technique is very complex and the analysis subject to many possible errors. Nevertheless, the technique is useful for certain specific measurements, e.g. changes in total body calcium or sodium (Lambie 1980).

TURNOVER, ORGAN FUNCTION AND METABOLIC STUDIES

Radioisotopes can be used to label substances such as iron or vitamin B_{12} so that their absorption and excretion can be measured. Gastric emptying time can be measured by ingesting a standard meal labelled with a suitable tracer, whilst clearance of secretions from the lung can be followed by sequential imaging of the lung after inhalation of a radioactive aerosol.

Other substances tend to localize in certain organs of the body. For example, the thyroid takes up the thyroid hormone, T_3, labelled with radioactive iodine, whilst the progressive accumulation of labelled red cells in the spleen indicates active cell destruction in that organ.

LOCALIZATION: IMAGING TECHNIQUES

The greatest advance in the application of radioisotopes to medical practice over the past decade has been the development of imaging techniques using the rectilinear scanner or the gamma camera. Although the images so obtained often have inferior definition when compared with those obtained by standard radiographic techniques, there is usually less radiation hazard. Furthermore, the scans not only reveal the size, location, configuration and gross internal architecture of the feature of interest but can often provide information about cellular function as well. Most imaging techniques do not yield quantitative information and are described very briefly. However some techniques provide a quantitative measurement of regional blood flow and are therefore described in more detail either here or in Chapter 16.

Brain

Although computer-assisted tomography (the CAT scanner) has revolutionised the diagnosis of space occupying lesions in the brain, there are a number of lesions which are not visible on the CAT scan but which can be visualised by nuclear imaging techniques. The most commonly-used radionuclide is Technetium 99^m pertechnetate*.

* The superscript ^{m} indicates that the isotope is in a metastable state. This is a comparatively stable excited state which decays into a more stable lower energy state with the emission of gamma rays. Thus $^{99}Tc^m$ decays to ^{99}Tc, the half-life being 6 hours.

Provided uptake by the choroid plexus has been blocked by prior administration of potassium perchlorate this substance only accumulates in those parts of the brain where there has been a breakdown of the blood–brain barrier. It thus produces an increase in radioactivity in tumours, abscesses and many other intracerebral lesions, although in some instances (e.g. subdural haematomata) it may be several days before the abnormality of the blood–brain barrier becomes sufficiently marked to produce an abnormal scan.

Radioisotopes can also be used to obtain cerebral angiograms. A bolus of radioactivity is injected into a peripheral vein and the resulting image recorded using a gamma camera. Although, the detail is inferior to that obtained by conventional cerebral angiography the technique is relatively non-invasive and may yield useful information concerning flow in major vessels.

Liver and spleen

Radionuclides which localize in the reticulo-endothelial cells are now generally used, $^{99}Tc^m$-labelled sulphur colloid being the most popular isotope. This has a particle size of approximately 0.01 μm and so is taken up by the reticuloendothelial system in the liver, spleen and bone marrow. Space occupying lesions completely replace the reticuloendothelial cells so that the lesions appear as 'cold spots' on the scan. Other agents such as 1^{131} Rose bengal can be used to define the gall-bladder, whilst the use of $^{99}Tc^m$ labelled denatured red cells, which are sequestered in the spleen, permits this organ to be differentiated from liver.

Kidney

Radionuclides can be used to measure total renal function or the function of each kidney separately.

Traditionally renal function has been considered to consist of two entities, glomerular filtration and tubular secretion, which were measured by the clearance of inulin (for glomerular filtration rate) and para-amino hippuric acid (for the effective renal plasma flow). Examples of the radioisotopes used for measuring glomerular filtration rate are ^{51}Cr-EDTA and ^{99}Tc^m-DTPA, whilst ^{131}I-hippuran is used for effective renal plasma flow. These isotopes are injected intravenously and their activity in blood samples is then estimated for a period of several hours after the injection.

The function of each kidney can be measured by following the activity-time curve over each kidney after the injection of ^{131}I-hippuran. This can be done by placing separate scintillation detectors over each kidney or by recording the radioactivity on a gamma camera. The resultant curve is termed a renogram and is discussed further on p. 216. Static and dynamic imaging of the kidneys is also used to localize lesions, detect obstruction to urine outflow and to assess changes in renal perfusion.

Other compounds such as ^{197}Hg chlormerodrin are primarily concentrated by tubular cells, have long residence times in the kidney, and are therefore suitable for static imaging.

Heart

There are three main uses of radioisotopes in the evaluation of cardiac pathology. These are angiocardiography, the determination of regional ventricular function, and the distribution of myocardial blood flow.

Radioisotope angiocardiography is performed by injecting a bolus of radioactive isotope into a peripheral vein and recording its passage through the central circulation with a gamma camera over the ensuing 30 seconds or so. This is termed 'first pass' radioisotope angiography to distinguish it from the imaging of the cardiac blood pool after the isotope has been completely mixed within the circulation. The radioisotope most commonly used is ^{99}Tc^m either as pertechnetate, or attached as a label to human serum albumin or to autologous red cells. The technique is used to detect intra-cardiac shunts or other congenital defects and is particularly valuable as a preliminary diagnostic tool in infants in whom cardiac catheterization is technically difficult.

Some quantitative information can be derived from the angiogram by picking out areas of interest with a computer light-marker and then replotting the localized curves of activity against time. For example, it is possible to estimate left ventricular ejection fraction by measuring the variation in radioactivity over the left ventricle between systole and diastole.

Some of the limitations of the first pass technique have been overcome by imaging the precordium after the tracer has equilibrated throughout the blood pool, the images being collected at specific points in the cardiac cycle by triggering the gamma-camera from the ECG signal. This is known as gated cardiac blood pool data acquisition since the 'gate' is only opened to permit the camera to record data at fixed points in the cardiac cycle. Initially, the gates were of 50- to 70-m sec duration and were linked to the R-wave and the downslope of the T-wave to signal ventricular end-diastole and end-systole respectively. Providing the cardiac rhythm was stable images of these two points in the cycle could be accumulated over a period of several hundred heart beats. The technique has now been extended to produce multiple gated images which can then be viewed in the form of a continuous loop movie, similar to the conventional cine-angiogram. However the gamma camera images show both ventricles, atria and great vessels simultaneously. The technique permits very small abnormalities in wall movement to be detected and, since the radioactivity persists in the blood pool for several hours, it is possible to make repeated studies of the effects of drugs or exercise on myocardial dynamics. The images can also be subjected to quantitative analysis to measure regional differences in wall movement or to determine ventricular ejection fraction.

The third application, the measurement of

regional blood flow, has expanded enormously in recent years as a result of developments in the surgical treatment of myocardial ischaemia. The techniques can be divided into those in which the isotope is injected via a catheter into the root of the aorta or directly into the coronary arteries, and those in which it is injected intravenously.

The two techniques utilizing catheter injection are based on the use of either labelled microspheres or inert gases. The microspheres consist of small aggregates of human serum albumin labelled with a radioisotope such as $^{99}Tc^m$, $^{133}In^m$ or ^{131}I. These are injected as a bolus and distribute throughout the myocardium in proportion to the regional blood flow. Since the particles are small they impact in the arterioles where they remain until absorbed by the normal phagocytic processes over the ensuing 6–24 hours. The proportion of arterioles obstructed by the microspheres is small so that the haemodynamic effects of the injection are minimal.

The two inert gases used are ^{133}Xe and $^{81}Kr^m$. Both are dissolved in saline, the xenon being delivered as a bolus and the krypton as a continuous infusion. The xenon is imaged during its first pass through the circulation and is then excreted by the lungs. The $^{81}Kr^m$, however, has a half-life of only 13 seconds and can therefore be delivered as a constant infusion.

The techniques based on intravenous injections of the radioisotope may again be subdivided into two: those in which the isotope is concentrated in normal myocardium and those in which it is concentrated in necrotic areas. The former technique (negative imaging) shows the ischaemic zone as an area with diminished radioactivity (cold spot) whilst the latter shows it as a positive image (hot spot).

The radioisotopes most commonly used for negative imaging are ^{43}K, ^{81}Rb and ^{201}Th. These are taken up into normal muscle by the usual metabolic processes and give a measure of the relationship between regional myocardial metabolism and blood flow. Thus their uptake can be blocked by a reduction in blood flow or by disordered cellular metabolism. Although negative imaging yields results during the first few hours after an infarction it cannot differentiate between old and new myocardial damage, cannot be used for serial imaging, is relatively expensive and has inappropriate energy levels for optimal gamma camera imaging. Many centres therefore utilize positive imaging for the diagnosis of myocardial infarction. The most commonly-used isotope has been $^{99}Tc^m$ labelled pyrophosphate. However, although these techniques improve the accuracy of diagnosis they not infrequently yield false-positive or false-negative results (Serafini, Gilson & Smoak 1977; Editorial, *British Medical Journal* 1978).

Pulmonary ventilation and pulmonary blood flow

The radioactive methods may be divided into those employing 'very soluble' or 'poorly soluble' gases, the 'solubility' in this context referring to the ease with which these gases are absorbed into the pulmonary capillary blood (West 1977). The soluble gases are oxygen and carbon dioxide. The most suitable isotopes of these gases have very short half-lives and so have to be piped directly from the cyclotron to the laboratory. To measure the distribution of pulmonary blood flow the patient is seated between a number of detectors covering different regions of the chest. A breath of radioactive gas is then inhaled and the counting rates are observed whilst the breath if held. The rate of fall of activity during the breath-holding period is proportional to the blood flow in the area of lung being scanned by the counters.

The relatively insoluble isotopes are ^{133}Xe and $^{13}N_2$. Although $^{13}N_2$ is less soluble than ^{133}Xe, and therefore contributes less to tissue radioactivity, it has a short half-life and has to be prepared in a cyclotron. Its use has therefore been restricted to special centres. ^{133}Xe has a half-life of 5.3 days and can be used as a gas or as a solution in saline. There are a number of different techniques which utilize this isotope. In one, the dissolved xenon is injected as a bolus through a catheter in the superior vena cava. When the gas reaches the pulmonary capillaries, it is evolved into the alveoli because of its low solubility. If the subject holds his breath during this period, the rate of rise of radio-activity counted over the chest provides a measure of pulmonary blood flow. In practice, the lung is scanned either with multiple stationary counters or with moving counters during the breath-hold. The result-ing graph of count rate against position is related both to the regional blood flow and to the regional lung volume. To eliminate the geometrical factors, a second scan is made after the subject has rebreathed the xenon in and out of a bag. This ensures that all the alveolar gas is uniformly labelled and the resulting scan shows the record which would have been obtained if all the alveoli had been evenly perfused. The difference between the first and second scans therefore represents regional differ-ences in blood flow. Usually, however, the ordinates of the first scan are divided by the second, so that an arbitrary scale of blood flow per unit alveolar volume is obtained.

If it is only necessary to measure the distribution of ventilation the lung can be scanned after a single breath of xenon. Again regional lung volume can be obtained by scanning the lung after rebreathing the xenon, so that ventilation per unit volume can be obtained.

Another imaging technique is based on the inhalation of $^{81}Kr^{m}$ gas (Fazio & Jones 1975). This isotope has a half-life of about 13 seconds and is continuously evolved from a column containing the parent radioisotope rubidium-81, the generator itself having a half-life of about $4\frac{1}{2}$ hours. The advantage of using this radioisotope is that no special breathing manoeuvres are required. The patient simply inhales the radioisotope from an oxygen mask and the image is recorded when equilibrium has been achieved (usually after 1–2 minutes). The amount of activity entering a lung region depends on the radioactivity of the gas mixture and on the regional ventilation. The quantity leav-ing the region is governed by the regional washout rate (ventilation per unit lung volume) and the natural decay of the iso-tope. Since the half-life is very short, regional count rates depend mainly on regional ventilation. The technique therefore pro-vides a simple and rapid way of detecting areas of regional underventilation. The technique is often combined with the injection of albumin microspheres to provide an image of regional blood flow, thus enabling abnormalities of both ventila-tion and perfusion to be detected with minimal disturbance to the patient. The combination is particularly useful for the detection of abnormalities such as pulmon-ary emboli.

For surveys of other imaging techniques readers are referred to Matin 1977; Ell, Williams & Todd-Pokropek 1978; Critch-ley 1978; Britton 1978; Wainwright & Maisey 1978a, b.

CIRCULATION AND BLOOD FLOW STUDIES

Methods are available for determining cardiac output, and the perfusion of organs and other tissues, There are three main principles (see Chapter 16).

Constant injection indicator dilution

This can be applied to organs with single inflow and outflow channels from which samples can be obtained. The indicator is injected continuously at a known rate (F_1) and known concentration (C_1), care being taken to ensure that the indicator is thoroughly mixed with the flowing blood. A sample is then withdrawn at a constant rate from a site downstream and its concen-tration (C_2) is measured. If the rate of flow past the injection point is F_2, F_1 is small compared with F_2, and no indicator is lost between the points of injection and sampling, then at equilibrium:

$$F_1 \times C_1 = F_2 \times C_2$$

or
$$F_2 = \frac{F_1 \times C_1}{C_2}$$

Bolus indicator dilution

A bolus of radioactivity is injected into the blood flowing into an organ. The bolus must be thoroughly mixed with the blood by passing it through a mixing chamber, such as the right heart. A 'dilution curve' of the outflow activity is then obtained by withdrawing a blood sample at a constant rate and passing it through a coil within a scintillation detector. The flow can be calculated from the curve and the radioactivity of a single blood sample (p. 211).

Clearance methods

An isotope is injected into the tissue and its rate of clearance by the tissue blood flow is monitored. The clearance may be a simple monoexponential expression. This can only occur where there is effectively no bar to diffusion between the tissue and the blood and therefore no delay in the transfer of the isotope. Frequently, the situation is more complex: more sophisticated methods of analysis are then required. However a simple measure such as the 'half-time of clearance' (the time taken for the radioactivity to fall to half its initial value) allows useful statements to be made for, as a first approximation, the blood flow is equal to 0.693 divided by the half-time of clearance. Methods using inert gas clearance have proved valuable in measuring the blood flow to organs such as muscle, brain and lung. These are described in detail on pages 215 and 216.

References

BRITTON K. (1978) Radionuclides in renal imaging. *British Journal of Hospital Medicine*, **20**, 140.

CRITCHLEY M. (1978) Radioisotope imaging of the liver and pancreas. *British Journal of Hospital Medicine*, **20**, 129.

Editorial (1979). Myocardial imaging. *British Medical Journal*, **1**, 717.

ELL P.J., WILLIAMS E.S. & TODD-POKROPEK A.E. (1978) The clinical use of diagnostic imaging. *British Journal of Hospital Medicine*, **20**, 119.

FAZIO F. & JONES T. (1975) Assessment of regional ventilation by continuous inhalation of radioactive krypton-81m. *British Medical Journal*, **3**, 673.

HEATH M.L. & VICKERS M.D. (1968) An examination of single tracer, semi-automated blood volume methodology. *Anaesthesia*, **23**, 659.

LAMBIE A.T. (1980) Measurement of sodium and potassium in body fluids. *British Journal of Clinical Equipment*, **5**, 70.

LEWIS S.M. & SZUR L. (1967). Diagnostic uses of radioisotopes. 4: Haematology. *Hospital Medicine*, **2**, 1150.

MATIN P. (1977) *Handbook of clinical nuclear medicine*. London: Henry Kimpton.

PAIN R.W. (1977) Body fluid compartments. *Anaesthesia and Intensive Care*, **5**, 284.

SERAFINI A.N., GILSON A.J. & SMOAK W.M. (1977) *Nuclear cardiology. Principles and methods*. New York: Plenum Publishing Co.

WAINWRIGHT R.J. & MAISEY M.N. (1978a) Nuclear medicine: 4. Cardiac imaging. Part 1 Radionuclide angiocardiography. *Hospital Update*, **4**, 623.

WAINWRIGHT R.J. & MAISEY M.N. (1978b) Nuclear medicine: 4. Cardiac imaging. Part 2. Radionuclide angiocardiography. *Hospital Update*, **4**, 673.

WEST J.B. (1977) *Regional differences in the lung*. London: Academic Press.

Appendix

STATISTICS OF COUNTING*

The moment at which any atom of a radioactive source will decay cannot be predicted. It is a random process, and the behaviour of one atom has no influence on the others. There cannot, therefore, be a 'true' counting rate, but only a mean counting rate. If one were to make many measurements of a radioactive sample and plot the number of times each count was obtained, providing that several hundred counts were recorded on each occasion, the graph would

*The reading of this section may be delayed until the chapters on statistics have been read.

resemble the 'normal' curve, with the peak at the mean counting rate. As such, it is susceptible to statistical inference, as described in Chapters 20 and 21. It will be shown that the spread of a normal distribution curve as measured by the standard deviation, is a representation of the variability of the individual results. When variables can take any value (a continuous distribution), the standard deviation is not related to the mean. However, when the measurements are counts of events, such as radioactive disintegrations, the two parameters are interrelated. It can be seen intuitively that the more counts are recorded on each occasion, the nearer the result is likely to approach the mean count, and the smaller will be the scatter of results and the smaller the standard deviation. In fact, the variance is equal to the mean count, and the standard deviation is therefore equal to the square root of the mean count. This means that as the mean count increases the standard deviation becomes proportionally smaller. For example, a mean count of 100 has a standard deviation of $\sqrt{100}$ or 10, i.e. $\pm 10\%$. A mean count of 10 000

has a standard deviation of 100, or $\pm 1\%$ of the mean. In real life one counts a sample once or twice only, and therefore the mean count is not known, and so the 'true' standard deviation cannot be calculated. However, if the count is sufficiently large, little error is introduced by using the observed count in place of the mean count. For example, a mean count of 10 000 has a standard deviation of $\sqrt{10\,000}$ or 100. We would expect, knowing the properties of the normal curve, that there is a 95% chance that our count is within two standard deviations of the mean count. If our actual count is at the limit, i.e. 10 200 then the standard deviation derived by using this figure would be $\sqrt{10\,200}$ or 101 instead of 100. In this number of counts this is a negligible error.

From a knowledge of the normal distribution one can determine the limits within which the 'true' mean count lies at any desired level of probability. A useful approximation is that there is a 95% probability that the answer lies between the limits: counts recorded $\pm 2 \times \sqrt{\text{counts recorded}}$. This is acceptable when the total number of counts exceeds a few hundred.

Chapter 11
Patient Safety

It should never be forgotten that most monitoring instruments are powered by mains electricity which is extremely dangerous unless properly handled. Electrical power is supplied in the UK at an alternating voltage of 240V r.m.s. with a frequency of 50 Hz and it is important to know what are the effects of passing currents of this frequency through the body.

EFFECTS OF MAINS CURRENT

If a gradually increasing 50 Hz current is passed between left and right finger tips, a slight tingling sensation will be felt at the points of contact when it reaches approximately 1 mA (Table 11.1). The exact threshold depends upon the area of contact; the threshold rising with the area. When the current reaches 10–15 mA, the sensation becomes very painful, and the muscles of the hands and forearms contract tetanically. Since the flexor muscles are stronger, the hands will close, so that if any object were held, rather than touched, it would be gripped tightly. As the current is increased further, the tetanic spasm spreads to the

Table 11.1. The effects of hand-to-hand 50 Hz alternating current.

50 Hz current (mA)	Effect
1	Tingling sensation
5	Pain
15	Severe pain, with local muscle spasm
50	Respiratory muscle spasm
80–100	Dysrhythmias with pump failure, leading to ventricular fibrillation.

thorax, so that the respiratory muscles are affected: currents of this magnitude (around 50 mA) cannot be survived for very long. As the current reaches 90–100 mA, the electrical activity of the heart is disturbed, so that major dysrhythmias with reduction in cardiac output are rapidly followed by ventricular fibrillation.

The effects of a 50 Hz alternating current upon a particular tissue depend upon the current density ($A \cdot m^{-2}$). Thus the threshold of sensation at the fingertips depends on the current passing through each bit of skin rather than the total current. If the contact area is halved whilst the current is unchanged, the current density will be doubled, with a corresponding increase in the intensity of the sensation.

This principle applies to the heart also. Much less current is needed to fibrillate the heart when one of the points of contact is within or on the ventricle itself than when the current is diffused across the whole thorax. Two other factors determine the potential lethality of alternating currents. One is the time for which they are applied, the threshold decreasing as the time increases. The other is frequency. 50 Hz is particularly dangerous: higher frequencies are progressively less so, so that at radio frequencies (> 100 kHz) as used for surgical diathermy, alternating currents have no fibrillating potential.

MAINS SUPPLY

Electrical power usually arrives on the hospital site as a three-phase, 11 000V supply. This means that there are 3 wires, so phased that each sinusoidal voltage is 120° out of phase with the other two. This

137

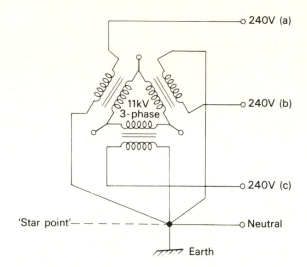

Fig. 11.1. The 3-phase, 11 kV supply is reduced to three 240V supplies by the local substation transformer. The neutral carries current returning from all three 240V supplies.

supply is transformed down to three 240V supplies by a local transformer (Fig. 11.1).

Each 240V supply is of course 120° out of phase with the other two, so that odd things would happen if interconnected electrical devices were powered from different phases. Accordingly, the regulations governing the wiring of operating theatres or intensive care units specify that all the outlets must be connected to the same phase supply. All three secondary windings are connected together (the 'star point') and bonded to earth, to form the neutral connection. The current used by a machine or instrument passes between a live 240V connection and the neutral. The earth bond is an essential safety factor, as it limits the voltages which could develop in the secondary circuit if,

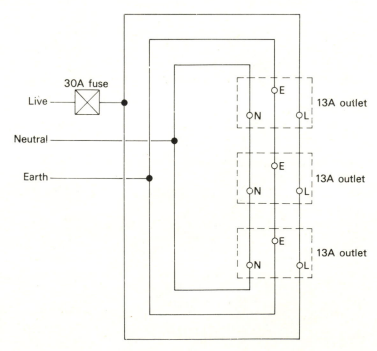

Fig. 11.2. One 30 Ampère ring circuit supplying three 13 Ampère outlets.

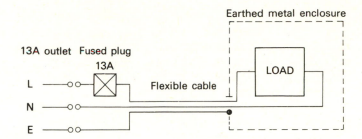

Fig. 11.3. A 'user device' connected to the mains supply.

for instance, the insulation between it and the 11 000V supply were to fail or the transformer were to be struck by lightning.

The 240V power to each theatre is distributed by one or more 'ring main' circuits which are simply loops of wire to which a number of outlets are connected, the live input containing a fuse to protect against overload (Fig. 11.2). Since each outlet terminal connects with the live supply by two routes, the current in the circuit will automatically distribute itself according to the relative loads on the outlets in the ring. The number of outlets in each ring is determined by an assessment of the number of outlets which are likely to be in simultaneous use, together with the likely loads presented by the devices to be used. The neutral connection goes back to the earthed transformer star point and the earth connection goes to a local earth point. It is important to remember that the current returns to the transformer along the neutral wire, not the earth, which is for protective purposes only.

USER DEVICES

Any machine or instrument connected to one of the power outlets contains a 'load'

which is of course electrically live (Fig. 11.3). The load is insulated from the conductive metal enclosure, to which the earth connection is made. This earth connection is the key to the safety of the device. If the insulation deteriorates or is compromised by a short-circuit so that a connection is made between load and enclosure, current will return to the star point via both neutral and earth wires. The current thus produced is called the *leakage current*, and its magnitude depends upon the resistance of the load-to-enclosure connection, and the source potential. If the leakage current is large the line current will exceed the rating of the fuse, causing it to blow and so breaking the circuit. The fuse therefore protects the system from the effects of significant short circuits between the mains and the enclosure. Smaller leakage currents will allow the device to continue to operate but because the earth connection keeps the casing potential down to zero volts it remains safe.

FAULTY EARTHING OF USER DEVICES

If, however, the earth connection is faulty (Fig. 11.4) a very different situation exists.

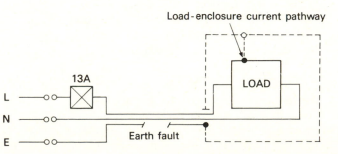

Fig. 11.4. With a load-enclosure current pathway and an earth fault, the device is now highly dangerous.

Since there is no pathway to the star-point via the earth connection, current does not flow, the protective fuse does not blow, and the enclosure remains at the same potential as the leakage source, which may be any potential between ground and 240V. If a person now touches the enclosure, he provides a pathway for the leakage current, which will flow through him to ground and thence back to the star point. The magnitude of the current that flows will depend upon his resistance. If he is standing on an antistatic floor, but touching nothing else, his resistance to ground should be in excess of $20 \text{k}\Omega$, so that, by Ohm's Law, the maximum current which can flow is $240/20 = 12 \text{mA}$. He would receive a painful shock, but would survive. If, on the other hand, he touches the enclosure with one wet hand, and an earthed conductor (such as a cold water tap) with the other, his resistance to earth may now be only $2 \text{k}\Omega$, and he will sustain a lethal electrocuting current of 120mA. Furthermore, since this current is small, the fuse will remain intact, so that the enclosure remains a hazard until the mains supply is switched off.

Gross electrocution can, of course occur without earth faults. If a person simultaneously touches the load and the enclosure, a lethal accident is to be expected. For this reason, it is extremely dangerous to remove any of the protective shielding from any instrument without disconnecting it from the mains supply.

PREVENTIVE MAINTENANCE

Electrical accidents can be minimized by careful maintenance, since the 3-wire mains system is fundamentally safe unless leakage and earth faults occur. To avoid them, both current leakage and earth continuity need to be checked.

Earth leakage

All mains powered devices in patient-care areas should be checked regularly for earth leakage currents. To do this, the engineer removes the earth connection and connects an a.c. ammeter between the enclosure and a good earth. The leakage current which then flows must never exceed 0.5mA. He then reverses the live and neutral connections, and repeats the test. Any device with excessive leakage should not be used until corrected, except in dire emergency. This test should never be carried out by anybody but a qualified electrical engineer, who then accepts responsibility for the safety of the device.

It is possible to detect the presence of leakage currents by a device which detects the difference *between* the currents flowing in the live and neutral wires. This difference current is, by definition, leakage. The detected current can be made to operate a relay, which switches off the supply to the socket. Set at a threshold of, say, 30mA, such a contact breaker will operate very quickly, and may prevent electrocution in a hazardous situation. It is not however very useful to have a theatre socket which refuses to deliver power to a device with high leakage, since a patient's life may depend upon it. For this reason, contact breakers are not used in operating theatres.

Earth continuity

The engineer tests the earth continuity of the device itself by measuring the resistance between the earth pin on the mains plug and the main earth terminal on the instrument. This is usually externally accessible to facilitate testing. The measured resistance should never exceed 0.1 ohm. It is of course possible for the flexible cable to be badly frayed, with one single strand of wire maintaining the earth continuity, so that the resistance test will not detect any abnormality. To guard against this eventuality, the engineer employs the surge test. A current of 25A is passed through the earth pathway for at least 5 seconds. If any part of the pathway is limited to one or two strands, they will rapidly overheat and 'blow' like a fuse, and the current will stop. The combination of surge and resistance tests guards against all likely earth faults, but is only of value if carried out at frequent intervals.

The earth pathway does not, of course stop at the mains plug, but continues to the local building earth point. The continuity of this earth must also be checked periodically. This can be done, after switching the power off, by measuring the resistance between earth and neutral connections on the mains socket (earth-neutral-loop test) and as before, passing a surge current to detect badly frayed or corroded connections.

USER CODE

Although most hazards can be prevented by regular testing and maintenance, the user can create hazards by sheer carelessness. Only when all the staff in patient-care areas are aware of electrical hazards can they be prevented.

They should be aware of the following simple rules:
1   If anyone reports a shock or even a 'tingle' from a device, do *not* touch it to see if they are right: switch off at the wall and call for an engineer.
2   If mains cables are seen to be knotted or frayed, insist on their replacement.
3   Do not allow electrical equipment into a patient-care area which does not satisfy the requirements of Hospital Technical Memorandum (HTM) 8.
4   Keep mains cables as short as practicable, to discourage long lengths of cable coiled on the floor.
5   Never push wheels or castors over mains cables.
6   Do not handle electrical equipment with wet hands.
7   Do not use portable distribution boxes unless you are certain that they are included in the engineers' earth continuity checks.
8   Ensure that preventive electrical maintenance is carried out regularly.

EARTH-FREE MAINS SUPPLY

The conventional live-neutral-earth system, as used in the UK, is relatively inexpensive and if properly maintained is associated with few fatal accidents. In some countries however, the mains supply specified for use in operating theatres and intensive care areas is 'earth free'. With this system the safety margin for all mains-powered devices can be considerably enhanced. An isolating transformer, with a ratio of 1:1 is added to the normal system so that no voltage change occurs. The primary winding of this transformer is connected to the live and neutral wires of the supply and the secondary winding is connected to the supply socket. The secondary circuit is not connected to ground, and is therefore 'earth-free'. (The outlet socket does, of course, have an earth terminal in exactly the same way as a normal live-neutral system.) The advantage of this system lies in the fact that leakage currents do not seek earth since they no longer return to the star point, but to the isolating transformer secondary, which cannot be reached via an earth pathway. Someone touching a 'live' casing of an instrument does not provide a pathway for the leakage current unless, simultaneously, another fault has earthed the secondary circuit. The safety margin is thus very large. It is however necessary to provide a monitoring circuit, called the line isolation monitor, which warns when earthing occurs.

MICROSHOCK

In experiments in both dogs and man, it has been shown that ventricular fibrillation can be induced by very small alternating currents when applied to a small area of the right ventricular endocardium. The actual site of contact is important, since it has been shown that currents in the $100\,\mu A$ range will only induce fibrillation if applied to the ventricle. Atrial contacts require substantially larger currents. The threshold is proportional to the surface area and also related to the time for which the current is passed. As the duration increases, the threshold decreases. The threshold is also dependent on frequency and it is unfortunate that 50 Hz is almost the most lethal frequency. Fibrillation by very small currents has come to be known as 'microshock', as distinct from 'gross electrocution' by externally applied current.

Because of the need to have the necessary current density at a particular site, the microshock hazard only applies to a very few specialized situations. It is necessary to have an electrical contact of low surface area in or on the surface of the heart such as could be achieved by a transvenous pacemaker wire, a cardiac catheter with a terminal electrode, a catheter filled with conductive material such as radio-opaque dye, an implanted but exteriorised pacemaker wire, or a saline-filled central venous catheter. The smallest a.c. current which can produce ventricular fibrillation when applied to a small area of the right ventricular endocardium is probably about 50 μA (Watson, Wright & Loughman 1973). Devices which are to be connected directly to the patient's heart are covered by a leakage standard of 100 μA (DHSS 1969) which is likely to be revised to 50 μA (Hull 1978). Leakage currents may also arise from faults in other equipment and reach the endocardium via a cardiac catheter. For example, in one reported accident, a patient undergoing cine-angiography developed ventricular fibrillation when the motorized syringe pump connected to the cardiac catheter was switched on (Bousvaros, Conway & Hopps 1962). From the published account it is evident that the motor of the syringe was poorly insulated, and the injector not earthed (Fig. 11.5). The patient, on the other hand, *was* earthed by a 'right leg' electrode to the grounded chassis of an obsolete, non-isolated electrocardiograph. The leakage current therefore flowed along the cardiac catheter, through the patient's heart and right leg electrode, to ground. Of course, a leakage current can flow out of the endocardial lead, rather

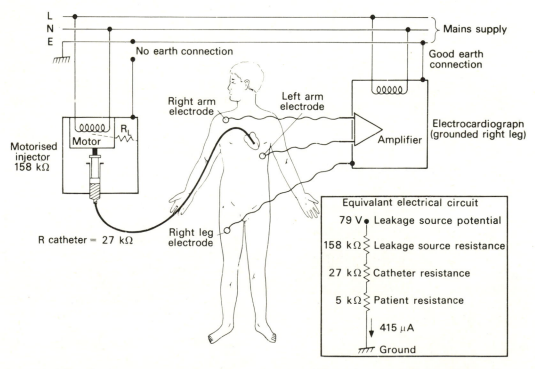

Fig. 11.5. Microshock. (Based on data from Bousvaros *et al.* 1962.) The equivalent electrical circuit is shown on the right.

than into it. Thus if the electrocardiograph had a faulty earth and an excessive leakage current, but the syringe pump a perfect earth, the outcome would have been exactly the same as soon as the syringe pump was connected to the catheter. It is quite likely that the motorized injector would have passed a leakage test for equipment of its type (0.5 mA) although it would have failed the earth test.

It therefore follows that the stringent leakage limits must be applied to all equipment making contact with the patient when an endocardial lead is present. It should in fact be applied to all equipment in the immediate vicinity of all patients who are especially electrically susceptible by virtue of intrathoracic conductors, since lethal leakage currents in the microampère range can be carried by skin contact with staff members. They need only to have one hand on a leakage source and the other holding a pacemaker wire to carry such a current without even being aware of having done so, since the current is below the threshold of sensation. For the special case of the electrically-susceptible patient a stringent code must be observed:

1 All electrical equipment in the vicinity of the patient must conform to a leakage specification of $< 100 \, \mu A$, and if possible $< 50 \, \mu A$. For some years the European Electrotechnical Commission (I.E.C. Committee 62A) has considered the problem of leakage current limits. Their conclusion (incorporated into the new British Standard 5724 on electromedical safety), is that all equipment in the immediate vicinity of the electrically susceptible patient should have a normal leakage current of $< 10 \, \mu A$, rising to no more than 50 μA under fault conditions.

2 Wherever possible, such equipment should be battery operated, thus avoiding 50 Hz leakage currents altogether.

3 All electrical circuits making contact with the patient must be electrically isolated from earth.

4 All electrical equipment in the susceptible zone should, wherever possible, be coated with resistive material, so as to limit earth pathways produced by hand to hand contacts.

5 Pacemaker leads or catheters must only be handled with gloved hands. Never hold the lead in one hand, and touch an oscilloscope or any other mains powered equipment with the other.

6 Earth-free mains supplies will not in themselves provide sufficient protection against microshock, but will greatly reduce the magnitude of any leakage current, and therefore increase the safety margin.

EXPLOSION HAZARDS

Electrical sparks are a major potential source of ignition for explosive anaesthetic mixtures. They may be due to the discharge of static electrical charges or to the make or break of electrical circuits which are carrying voltages well below those of the mains. The energy of the spark which will cause ignition depends on the particular mixture. A spark with an energy of 1 μJ is the safe upper limit (Macintosh, Mushin & Epstein 1963).

Other possible instrumental sources of hazard include the heated stylus of certain kinds of recorders and, of course, sparking in the mains switches themselves.

The principal safety factor is distance. The components of anaesthetic mixtures rapidly become diluted by diffusion so that at a distance of 10 cm from the expiratory valve or other major leak from a breathing circuit, mixtures are not ignitable. A distance of 25 cm is therefore recommended as a safe distance for siting equipment which is not gas proof. Vapours which are much heavier than air may pool on horizontal surfaces in special circumstances, for example, when the liquid anaesthetic is spilled directly. Again, however, at a distance of more than 10 cm above the surface, the mixture of vapour in air is not ignitable.

Where high concentrations of oxygen are being employed, not only are flammable anaesthetic mixtures much more dangerous, but other materials will ignite and burn furiously. Fires have been attributed to the plastic components in ultrasonic nebulizers, to plastic masks and tubing, and to drape materials. The same hazard arises in connection with hyperbaric oxygen.

Where electrical current components are in, or within 5 cm of a gas path which contains an anaesthetic or oxygen-enriched mixture, IEC 62A recommends construction to a stringent standard which ensures that sparks with an energy greater than $1 \mu J$ cannot occur. Such equipment is to be marked APG (Anaesthetic Proof G). A less-stringent standard (AP) can be adopted for equipment which can be operated between 5 and 25 cm of anaesthetic circuits (BS 5724).

References and further reading

BOUSVAROS G.A., CONWAY D. & HOPPS J.A. (1962) An electrical hazard of selective angio-cardiography. *Canadian Medical Association Journal*, **87**, 286.

DOBBIE A.K. (1972) Electricity in hospitals. *Biomedical Engineering*, **7**, 12.

Department of Health and Social Security (1969) *Hospital Technical Memorandum No. 8*, London, HMSO.

HAHN C.E.W. (1980) Electrical hazards and safety in cardiovascular measurements. p. 605 in *The circulation in anaesthesia*. Ed. C. Prys-Roberts. Oxford: Blackwell Scientific Publications.

HULL C.J. (1978) Electrocution hazards in the operating theatre. *British Journal of Anaesthesia*, **50**, 647.

BS5724. *Safety of Medical Electrical Equipment.* Part I General Requirements (1979).

LEEMING M.N. (1973) Protection of the electrically susceptible patient. *Anesthesiology*, **38**, 370.

MACINTOSH R., MUSHIN W.W. & EPSTEIN H.G. (1963). *Physics for the Anaesthetist*, 3rd edn., p. 374. Oxford: Blackwell Scientific Publications.

WATSON A.B., WRIGHT J.S. & LOUGHMAN J. (1973). Electrical thresholds for ventricular fibrillation in man. *Medical Journal of Australia*, **1**, 1179.

Part 2
Specific Measurements

Chapter 12
The Measurement of Pressure

This chapter deals with the general principles of devices used to measure pressure, the specific applications being dealt with in subsequent chapters.

UNITS USED IN PRESSURE MEASUREMENT

Pressure is defined as force per unit area. The SI unit of pressure is the newton per square metre ($N \cdot m^{-2}$) or pascal (Pa). However, this unit is too small for most physiological applications. The kilopascal (kPa) which is 1000 times larger has therefore been adopted for most physiological measurements. In meteorology and many commercial applications it has been agreed that a still larger unit, the bar, should be used. The bar is a derivative of the c.g.s. system in which the unit of pressure was dynes per square centimetre ($dyne \cdot cm^{-2}$). A bar was 10^6 $dyne \cdot cm^{-2}$. The newton ($kg \cdot m \cdot s^{-2}$) is 100 000 times larger than a dyne ($g \cdot cm \cdot s^{-2}$), but the square metre is 10 000 times larger than a square centimetre. Thus, the pascal (newton per square metre) is 10 times as big as the dyne per square centimetre. 10^5 Pa is therefore equal to 10^6 $dyne \cdot cm^{-2}$, or 1 bar. 10^5 Pa is 100 kPa and since a standard atmosphere is 101.325 kPa this is equivalent to 1.013 bar or 1013 mbar. The bar is obviously more convenient for the measurement of pressures in compressed gas cylinders.

These units have now officially replaced the older units of pressure which related the measurement to the pressure exerted by the atmosphere or to the height of a column of fluid which the pressure would support. The pressure exerted by the atmosphere will support a column of mercury 76 cm

(approximately 30 inches) high. Since the density of mercury is 13.6 times the density of water, this is equivalent to a column of water $76 \times 13.6 = 1033$ cm (34 feet) high. If the cross-sectional area of the water column is one square centimetre, the pressure is $1033 g \cdot cm^{-2}$ or $1033 kg \cdot m^{-2}$. This is equivalent to 14.7 pounds per square inch ($lb \cdot in^{-2}$ or psi). Since weight is the product of mass times the acceleration due to gravity ($981 cm \cdot sec^{-2}$ or $32 ft \cdot sec^{-2}$) and since the latter varies slightly in different parts of the world, the height of the liquid column supported by one standard physical atmosphere will also vary with the site of measurement. Furthermore, the density of the liquid will vary with temperature, so that the height of a fluid column supported by a given pressure will be temperature-dependent as well. It is for these reasons that an attempt is being made to replace the older units with SI units which are not affected by such factors. Conversion factors between old and new units are shown in Table 12.1.

When measuring large pressures it is customary to refer them to atmospheric pressure. Such measurements are usually termed *gauge* pressures for the reading on the gauge will be zero when the measured pressure is atmospheric and the reading on the gauge at other pressures will define how much the pressure is above or below atmospheric. In certain applications it is desirable to measure the pressure with respect to a true zero pressure (i.e. a vacuum). Such measurements are termed *absolute* pressures. Thus atmospheric pressure is zero gauge pressure or 1 atmosphere absolute (1 ATA) whilst a gauge pressure of 1 atmosphere (101.325 kPa or 760 mmHg) is 2 atmospheres (202.65 kPa or

Table 12.1. Conversion factors relating the most commonly used units of pressure

	dynes·cm⁻²	kPa	g·cm⁻²	kg·m⁻²	lb·in⁻²	mmHg 0°C (torr)	in. Hg 0°C	cm H₂O 20°C	in. H₂O 20°C	mbar
1 atmosphere (physical)	1 013 250	101.325	1033.227	10 332.27	14.696	760	29.921	1035.08	407.513	1013.250
1 bar	1 000 000	100	1019.716	10 197.16	14.504	750.062	29.530	1021.545	402.18	1000
1 kPa	10 000	1	10.197	101.972	0.145	7.501	0.295	10.215	4.022	10
1 mmHg 0°C (torr)	1333.224	0.133	1.359	13.595	0.019	1	0.039	1.362	0.536	1.333
1 cm H₂O 20°C	980.638	0.091	0.998	9.98	0.014	0.734	0.029	1	0.394	0.979
1 lb·in⁻²	68 947.58	6.895	70.307	703.07	1	51.715	2.036	70.433	27.73	68.948

−101·3	0	101·3	202·6	kPa	
−1	0	1	2	atmospheres	GAUGE
−760	0	760	1520	mmHg	

0	101·3	202·6	303·9	kPa	
0	1	2	3	atmospheres	ABSOLUTE
0	760	1520	2280	mmHg	

| 101·3 | 0 | | kPa | |
| 760 | 0 | | mmHg | VACUUM |

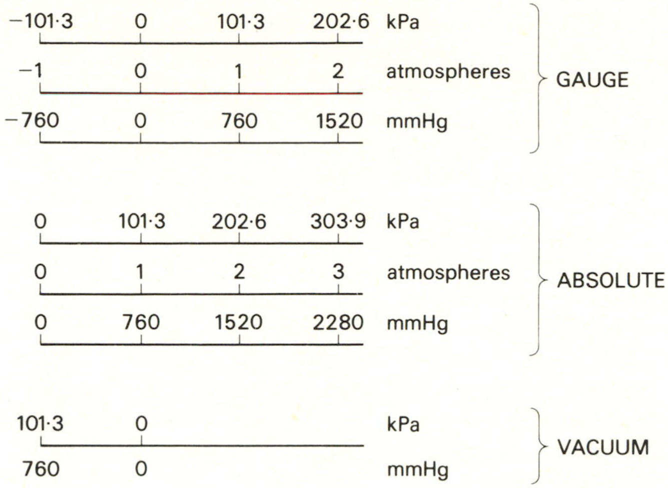

Fig. 12.1. Comparison of scales for measuring pressure.

1520 mmHg) absolute (2 ATA). Absolute pressures are most commonly used in hyperbaric medicine and in vacuum technology. However, in the latter application a *vacuum* pressure is often quoted (Fig. 12.1).

Instruments used for measuring pressure

The principle of the liquid manometer is best illustrated by considering the simple physics involved. The force exerted by a column of fluid is the product of mass times the acceleration due to gravity (g). However, the mass of the liquid column is the product of the volume of the fluid times its density. Therefore the force produced by a column of fluid

= volume × density × g

= height × cross-sectional area of liquid
   × density × g.

Since pressure = force per unit area, the pressure exerted by a column of fluid

$$= \frac{\text{height} \times \text{cross-sectional area} \times \text{density} \times g}{\text{cross-sectional area}}$$

= height × density × g.

The pressure is thus independent of the *width* of the fluid column. It is equally true, therefore, that pressure is independent of the *shape* of the fluid column.

There are two main types of liquid manometer. An example of the first type is the mercury barometer (Fig. 12.2). In this device there is a virtual vacuum above the mercury so that the height of the mercury column indicates *absolute* pressure. In the second type the tube is open at both ends (Fig. 12.3). Since the top is open to atmosphere the height of the fluid column indicates the amount by which the pressure exceeds atmospheric, i.e. *gauge* pressure.

When using U-tube manometers it is important to remember that the pressure is given by the difference in height between the two menisci, and not the distance between each meniscus and the zero point.

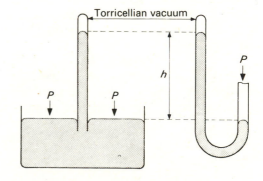

Fig. 12.2. Mercury manometer yielding measurements of absolute pressure (e.g. barometer). P = applied pressure; h = pressure measured.

In single tube manometers the height of the column is measured from the meniscus in the reservoir. This falls as the fluid is forced up the tube so that a fixed scale graduated in millimetres will not accurately reflect the true difference between the two menisci. The error can be minimized by making the cross-sectional area of the reservoir large in relation to the cross-sectional area of the tube. Alternatively the scale length can be shortened to allow for the fall in reservoir level. Both methods of correction are commonly employed in mercury sphygmomanometers.

An error in the measurement of pressure by liquid manometers may arise from the surface tension of the liquid. With most liquids, the curvature of the meniscus is concave upwards. The surface tension thus causes the position of the meniscus to be higher than it should be. If the two limbs of a liquid manometer are of equal diameter, surface tension forces are the same in each limb and so cancel each other. However if the diameters differ an error may be introduced because surface forces exert a greater effect in a narrow tube than in a wide one*. Surface forces become important if the tube is less than about 1 cm in diameter. With most liquids, surface forces cause the meniscus to be higher than it should be. However, the meniscus of mercury is concave downwards and this causes a negative error in the reading in narrow tubes. In a tube 6 mm in diameter surface forces cause a water meniscus to be 4.5 mm too high whilst a mercury meniscus would be 1.5 mm too low.

The sensitivity of liquid manometers can be increased in a number of ways. The most obvious method is to use a liquid of low density, such as alcohol or liquid paraffin.

---

* The height (h) to which a liquid of surface tension σ and specific weight w is raised in a tube of diameter d is

$$h = \frac{4\sigma \cos \theta}{wd}$$

where θ is the angle of contact between liquid and solid.

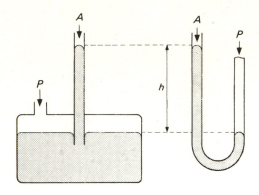

Fig. 12.3. Mercury manometer yielding measurements of gauge pressure (e.g. sphygmomanometer). P = applied pressure; A = atmospheric pressure; h = measured pressure.

Another method is to incline the tube so that the vertical movement of the meniscus is amplified (Fig. 12.4). In such an *inclined plane* manometer great care must be taken to level the baseplate accurately before taking a reading. Yet another way of increasing sensitivity is to use a *differential liquid manometer* (Fig. 12.5). Two nonmiscible liquids of slightly different density are placed in opposing limbs of a U-tube, the quantities of each liquid being adjusted so that a meniscus is formed close to the top of one limb of the U. If the pressure to be measured is now applied to this limb the meniscus will be displaced downwards.

If the two reservoirs at the top have a large diameter compared with the diameter of the connecting tube a large movement

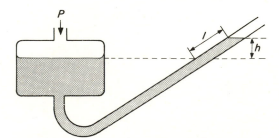

Fig. 12.4. Inclined plane manometer. The small pressure P produces a small difference in height between the two menisci (h) but this is amplified on the scale (l).

of the boundary meniscus between the two liquids can occur without there being much difference in height between the fluid levels in the two reservoirs. If this slight difference

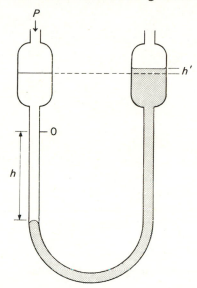

Fig. 12.5. Differential liquid manometer. $P =$ applied pressure; $h =$ measured pressure. h' is small in relation to h because of the difference in diameter between the manometer tube and reservoirs.

in height is ignored it can be seen that the movement of the boundary meniscus will be inversely related to the difference in density between the two liquids.

$$\Delta P = h(d_1 - d_2)g$$

where $\Delta P =$ the pressure difference to be measured,

$\quad h =$ the movement of the meniscus,

$\quad d_1$ and d_2 are the densities of the two liquids

Therefore:

$$h = \frac{\Delta P}{(d_1 - d_2)g}.$$

Hence, sensitivity can be increased by using two liquids of very similar density. By an extension of this analysis, which takes into account the difference in height between the liquid in the reservoirs, it is possible to show that sensitivity is also increased by

making the reservoir large in relation to the diameter of the connecting tube.*

The sensitivity of a manometer can be decreased by filling the closed end of the U-tube with a gas (Fig. 12.6). The movement of the meniscus is then governed by the height and density of the liquid column and the balancing pressure exerted by the compressed gas. The latter can be calculated by the application of Boyle's Law. This type of manometer is used for measuring such high pressures that the length of the mercury column would become unmanageable.

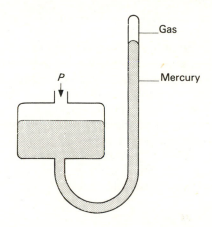

Fig. 12.6. Liquid manometer containing gas for measurement of high pressures.

MECHANICAL PRESSURE GAUGES

Bourdon gauge

This type of manometer is usually used for measuring high pressures. However it can also be adapted for the measurement of temperature (p. 265) and flow (p. 194).

The gauge consists of a coiled tube which is flattened in cross-section (Fig. 12.7).

* The full equation is

$$\Delta P = wh\left(d_1\left(1 + \frac{a}{A}\right) - d_2\left(1 - \frac{a}{A}\right)\right)$$

where $w = 9.81 \times 10^3$ N·m^{-3}, whilst a and A are the cross-sectional areas of the narrow and wide sections of tube (Douglas 1975).

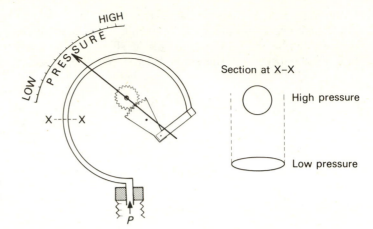

Fig. 12.7. Bourdon gauge. The increase in pressure causes the tube to become more circular in cross-section. This tends to straighten the coiled tube and so moves the needle across the dial.

One end of the coil is anchored to the case and connected to the source of pressure, whilst the other end is closed and attached to a mechanism which drives the pointer across the dial. The application of pressure to the inside of the tube causes the cross-section to become more circular. This causes the coiled tube to straighten. Since one end is fixed, the other unwinds, and so moves the pointer across the dial.

Aneroid gauge

A metal bellows is often used to sense lower pressures. Expansion of this bellows is detected by a lever mechanism which amplifies the movement and drives the pointer across the scale (Fig. 12.8). Aneroid

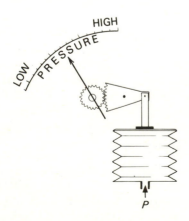

Fig. 12.8. Aneroid gauge.

gauges are commonly used for measurement of blood pressure or for monitoring the pressures developed by mechanical ventilators.

Diaphragm gauge

Most physiological pressure measurements are now made by sensing the movement of a flexible diaphragm. This movement can be sensed directly or converted into electrical energy for subsequent processing and display.

METHODS OF SENSING DIAPHRAGM MOVEMENT

Direct

The movement can be detected by attaching a thread or lever to the centre of the diaphragm, the other end being connected to a pointer or writing arm. This arrangement is not very sensitive and possesses marked inertia.

Optical

An improved method of sensing the movement of the diaphragm (used by many of the early physiological workers) is shown in Fig. 12.9. A small mirror is attached to one side of the diaphragm. When the diaphragm is stretched by the application of pressure it becomes curved and the mirror is rotated.

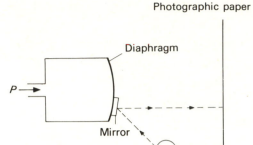

Photographic paper

Diaphragm

$P \rightarrow$

Mirror

Light

Fig. 12.9. Use of a mirror to sense the movement of a transducer diaphragm.

The displacement of the mirror is recorded by causing it to reflect a beam of light onto moving photographic paper. Great sensitivity is possible since the light path can be lengthened by reflecting it back and forth between fixed mirrors. However the relationship between the applied pressure and the movement of the diaphragm is only linear over a narrow range so that the diaphragm must be sufficiently stiff to limit the degree of curvature produced by the applied pressure.

Electromechanical

In most diaphragm gauges used for sensing dynamic pressures the movement of the diaphragm is sensed by a device which converts the mechanical energy imparted to the diaphragm into electrical energy. The resulting electrical output has the enormous advantage that it may be processed in many different ways to yield signals which are suitable for recording or display. Thus, it may be amplified to increase the sensitivity of the instrument; it may be differentiated to give the rate of change of pressure; or it may be digitized to facilitate subsequent processing by a digital computer. Any device which converts energy from one form to another is known as a *transducer*; since a pressure transducer converts pressure energy into electrical energy it is often called an *electromanometer*.

Physical principles of electromechanical transducers

Some electromechanical transducers are designed to convert electrical energy into mechanical energy. Examples are the electric motor, the loudspeaker or the piezoelectric crystal used in the generation of ultrasound. However in the present application we are concerned with transducers which convert mechanical energy into electrical energy. The mechanical energy may cause movement which may then be sensed by a *displacement* transducer. If the tendency to movement is opposed by the transducer, a force is generated so that the instrument becomes a *force* transducer. In the case of a *pressure* transducer it is the force per unit area which is sensed by the movement of the diaphragm. The relationship between the applied pressure and movement of the diaphragm is governed by the stiffness of the diaphragm. A relatively stiff diaphragm is necessary because undue distortion of the diaphragm causes the response to become nonlinear and because the frequency response of the transducer is intimately related to the stiffness of the diaphragm. Although many methods have been developed for sensing diaphragm movement the following are those most commonly employed in commercially available pressure transducers.

OPTICAL

The movement of the diaphragm is sensed by reflecting a beam of light off the silvered back of the diaphragm onto a photoelectric cell. As the diaphragm is pressurized the silvered surface becomes convex. This causes the reflected light beam to diverge so that the intensity of light sensed by the photoelectric cell decreases and its electrical output falls. If both sides of the diaphragm are silvered and two light beams are reflected on to opposing photoelectric cells, the sensitivity can be greatly increased.

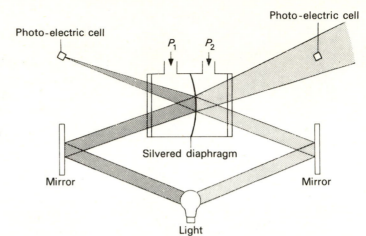

Fig. 12.10. Optical defocussing manometer. The curvature of the diaphragm produced by the difference between pressures P_1 and P_2 causes one beam of reflected light to converge and the other to diverge, thus altering the relative intensities of the light beams sensed by the two photoelectric cells.

This forms the basis of the optical defocusing manometer (Fig. 12.10).

The reflection technique has been exploited successfully for intravascular pressure measurement. The diaphragm is situated at the end of a fibre-optic bundle contained within a cardiac catheter. Light is transmitted down one section of the fibre-optic light path and transmitted back via another, the intensity of the reflected beam being sensed by a photoelectric cell placed at the external end of the fibre-optic bundle. Such a transducer has a high frequency response and completely eliminates the risk of microshock for there are no electrical components within the catheter (Lekholm & Lindström 1969).

WIRE STRAIN GAUGE

When a wire is stretched or compressed it undergoes a change of electrical resistance, the change in resistance being produced by changes in the length and diameter of the wire and by changes in the atomic structure of the metal (Baldwin 1979). In the *unbonded* wire strain gauge (now almost uniquely represented by the Statham range of strain gauges) the resistance wire is stretched between a fixed point and a movable block attached to the diaphragm. The resistance wires are arranged in two sets so that the application of pressure stretches one set and compresses the other (Fig. 12.11). The

difference in resistance between the two sets is measured by a Wheatstone bridge system, so that the output voltage is proportional to the displacement of the diaphragm (Chapter 3). The actual output voltage depends on the voltage used to energise the bridge but a typical output voltage would be $150\,\mu V \cdot kPa^{-1}$ $(20\,\mu V/mmHg)$ at 10 volts excitation. In some strain gauges the resistance wires are formed into a zig-zag pattern and cemented to the back of the diaphragm to form a *bonded* strain gauge (Fig. 12.12). The resistance elements in this type of gauge may also be etched out of a sheet of foil and bonded to the diaphragm by cement. Bonded gauges are considerably more robust but are subject to hysteresis and often have an inferior frequency response.

Since the resistance of the strain gauge element is affected by temperature it is important to choose a metal which possesses

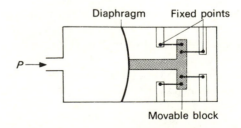

Fig. 12.11. A strain gauge using wire resistance elements.

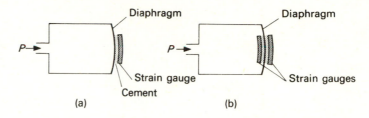

Fig. 12.12. Bonded strain gauges. a. Single. b. Double. Increasing the curvature of the diaphragm stretches one gauge and compresses the other.

a low temperature coefficient of resistance. The effects of temperature can also be cancelled by using two gauges of equal dimensions in the opposite arms of the Wheatstone bridge. For example, if two gauges are bonded onto opposite sides of the diaphragm both will be equally affected by changes in temperature but one will be stretched and the other compressed, thus providing a difference in resistance which is proportional to the deflection of the diaphragm. By putting two gauges on each side and incorporating them in a 'full bridge' arrangement sensitivity can be doubled (Fig. 12.13).

SILICON STRAIN GAUGE

In recent years other types of strain gauge have been developed. In one of these, the silicon bonded strain gauge, an extremely thin slice of a silicon crystal is bonded onto the back of the diaphragm. The silicon crystal changes resistance as it is compressed or expanded when the diaphragm changes shape. By suitably 'doping' the silicon crystal with elements such as phosphorus or boron it is possible to produce gauges with either positive or negative change in resistance characteristics. If these are mounted in parallel and incorporated in all

four arms of a Wheatstone bridge great sensitivity can be achieved. Although such gauges may be fifty times more sensitive than comparable wire strain gauge elements they are very temperature-sensitive and also tend to suffer from nonlinearity. However, improvements in technology have now reduced these disadvantages.

Another type of silicon strain gauge utilizes a silicon diaphragm with a number of silicon gauges etched into the back of the diaphragm. Although the gauge elements are temperature sensitive they are mounted beside temperature-sensitive elements of opposing coefficient so that the thermal effects are fully compensated. Such gauges have a high sensitivity and can produce an output of $2\,\text{mV} \cdot \text{kPa}^{-1}$ (or $25\,\text{mV}/100\,\text{mmHg}$). The diaphragm is very stiff so that the gauge has a high natural frequency and is very resistant to the application of excess pressure. These transducers can be made very small and have been incorporated in the tip of a cardiac catheter.

CAPACITANCE

The diaphragm of the pressure transducer is used as one plate of a capacitor, the second plate being fixed. Movement of the

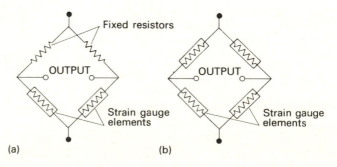

Fig. 12.13. a. Strain gauge half-bridge circuit. b. Full bridge circuit.

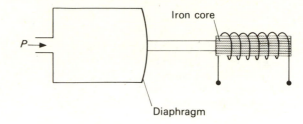

Fig. 12.14. Variable inductance transducer.

diaphragm varies the distance between the plates, and this varies the charge which can be carried by the capacitor. This is sensed by a Wheatstone bridge circuit energized by an alternating current. This type of transducer can be made very sensitive with a high frequency response but it is also much affected by ambient temperature variation. This renders it relatively unstable.

INDUCTANCE

The inductance of a coil can be varied by changing the position of a core of magnetic material lying within the magnetic field of the coil (Fig. 12.14). The magnetic core is attached to the diaphragm and the inductance of the coil is measured by making it part of a Wheatstone bridge circuit which is energized by an alternating current.

A more common form of inductance transducer is that employing a differential transformer (Fig. 12.15). The core is placed between the two secondary windings of a transformer. These are wound in opposite directions so that when the core is situated symmetrically between them the a.c. voltage induced in the secondary coils is equal in magnitude but opposite in phase. There is therefore zero output. If the core is now

displaced by movement of the diaphragm the voltage in one coil will exceed that in the other and an output voltage will appear at the terminals. If the core is moved in the opposite direction the output will be equal in voltage but opposite in phase. By using a phase-sensitive rectifier (which changes the a.c. signals to d.c.) an appropriate d.c. voltage will be produced.

SINGLE-ENDED AND DIFFERENTIAL PRESSURE TRANSDUCERS

Most pressure transducers are designed to measure a pressure applied to one side of a diaphragm, the other side of the diaphragm being at atmospheric pressure. These are termed *single-ended* transducers. However there are a number of occasions on which it is necessary to measure the difference between two pressures. This is most conveniently done by applying the two pressures to the opposite sides of the diaphragm. A transducer which is designed for this mode of operation is known as a *differential* transducer. Most differential pressure transducers are designed to measure the difference in pressure between two gases (for example the difference between airway and oesophageal pressure or the difference in

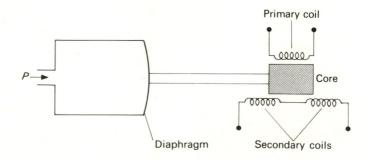

Fig. 12.15. Differential transformer transducer. The output signal appears across the secondary coils.

pressure between the two sides of a pneumo-tachograph screen (p. 196). Some transducers are designed to accept liquid on one side but can only tolerate gas on the opposite side because liquid would damage the sensing mechanism. Such transducers may be used for measurements of transmural pressure differences within the thorax (i.e. the difference between intravascular and oesophageal pressure). In some circumstances (e.g. the differential pressure method of measuring cardiac output, p. 204) it is necessary to compare two liquid pressures. This can usually only be achieved by using two carefully-matched single-ended liquid pressure transducers.

SOME CLINICAL APPLICATIONS OF PRESSURE MEASUREMENT

In the respiratory system pressure measurement is used in the measurement of respiratory mechanics or as a monitor during mechanical ventilation. A measurement of intrathoracic pressure is required for determining lung compliance. In experimental situations this may be obtained by measuring the pressure inside a partially-inflated balloon inserted into the pleural space. However in clinical work it is usually determined by passing a 10-cm long 1-cm diameter, balloon into the lower third of the oesophagus. The balloon is made of rubber and is attached to a 1-mm internal diameter rigid catheter which has several lateral holes at the tip. The balloon is inflated with a small quantity of air so that the membrane is lifted away from the holes in the catheter, but is nevertheless able to respond to changes in the negative pleural pressure without stretching the membrane. The pressure is then recorded with a sensitive pressure transducer (Gibson & Pride 1976).

Pressure measurements in the gastro-intestinal tract can be obtained by the use of an air-filled balloon or by a water-filled catheter. Similar techniques can be used to measure intra-uterine pressure. However care is necessary to ensure that the catheter is flushed at regular intervals and that it does not perforate the uterine wall (Steer 1977). Catheter-tip transducers have also been used but are expensive. Intracranial pressure measurements have proved valuable in monitoring patients with brain damage. Three techniques are used. The most popular method is direct measurement of intraventricular pressure using a fine catheter inserted into a lateral ventricle. However it is sometimes difficult to locate the ventricle and recourse must then be had to supratentorial subarachnoid pressure monitoring. In this technique the pressure is measured through a saline-filled metal screw which is mounted in a drill hole in the skull. The third approach is to measure the pressure from the epidural space either by inserting a tambour or fluid-filled adaptor into the space or by placing the transducer diaphragm against the dura. Unfortunately it takes some time for the recorded pressure to equal C.S.F. pressure and if an implanted transducer is used, it is difficult to recalibrate it (McDowall 1976; Miller 1978).

Pressure measurements in the cardiovascular system are dealt with in the next two chapters. However, pressure transducers may also be used to detect the pulsations of the apex beat or carotid artery in several noninvasive techniques for estimating myocardial function (Reitan 1978). Furthermore the microphones used in phonocardiography are acting as pressure detectors to sense pressure variations due to sound waves.

References

BALDWIN A. (1979) Transducers. *British Journal of Clinical Equipment*, **4**, 32.

DOUGLAS J.F. (1975) *Solution of problems in fluid mechanics*. Part 1, p. 14. London: Pitman Publishing.

GIBSON G.J. & PRIDE N.B. (1976) Lung distensibility. The static pressure volume curve of the lungs and its use in clinical assessment. *British Journal of Diseases of the Chest*, **70**, 143.

LEKHOLM A. & LINDSTRÖM L. (1969) Opto-
electric transducer for intravascular measurements of pressure variations. *Medical and Biological Engineering*, **7**, 333.

McDOWALL D.G. (1976) Monitoring the brain.
Anesthesiology, **45**, 117.

MILLER J.D. (1978) Intracranial pressure monitoring. *British Journal of Hospital Medicine*, **19**,
497.

REITAN J.A. (1978) Noninvasive monitoring. Page
85 in *Monitoring in Anesthesia*. Eds L.J.
Saidman & N.T. Smith. New York: John
Wiley & Sons.

STEER P.J. (1977) Monitoring in labour. *British
Journal of Hospital Medicine*, **17**, 219.

Chapter 13
Direct Measurement of Intravascular Pressure

Although noninvasive methods of measuring arterial and venous pressure may be satisfactory in routine clinical practice they often prove inadequate in the acute situation. Direct measurements of arterial pressure are usually indicated when sudden, large changes of blood volume are anticipated (aortic graft or other major surgery); when rapid and extreme changes of pressure are likely (operation for phaeochromocytoma or controlled hypotension during surgery); when the shape of the arterial wave form can provide useful information (assessment of cardiac contractility or aortic valve disease); and when myocardial function is disturbed by dysrythmias, myocardial infarction or open-heart surgery.

Direct measurements of central venous or pulmonary artery wedge pressures are of use during transfusion in patients with severe anaemia, haemorrhage, or other forms of shock; in patients with acute heart failure and in those undergoing cardiac surgery; and when deciding whether the sudden onset of hypotension is caused by a decreased venous return or cardiac failure.

Although liquid manometers have been used for measuring mean arterial pressure they·are now only employed in central venous pressure measurement. However, even in this application there is a tendency to replace them by electromanometers, for the display of the venous waves and respiratory fluctuations provides a continuous confirmation of the patency of the catheter and may also provide diagnostic information (e.g. tricuspid incompetence).

Liquid and aneroid manometers

Central venous pressure

Catheters may be inserted into central veins through the median cubital, axillary, subclavian, internal or external jugular or femoral routes, and are then connected to the sensing system with a bridge of saline. The simplest sensing system is a saline manometer. This is connected to an intravenous infusion set by a three-way tap so that the patient can be connected directly to the manometer, to a flushing solution, or to both. It is an advantage to add 1000 i.u. (10 mg) of heparin to each litre of flushing solution to minimize clotting in the catheter. There should always be a dependent loop of tubing between the manometer and the patient to minimize the risk of air embolus.

The zero on the manometer scale should first be adjusted to lie on the same horizontal plane as the patient's right atrium. The surface marking for the right atrium (Fig. 13.1) is the junction of a line running

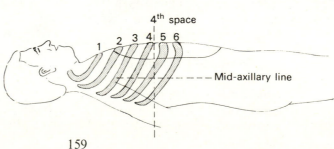

Fig. 13.1. Zero reference point for central venous pressure measurement.

159

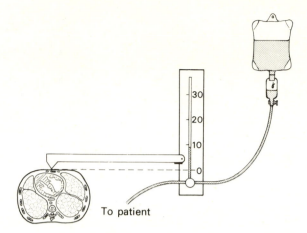

Fig. 13.2. Use of a hinged arm to set the manometer zero. The arm folds back into the stand when not in use. The manubriosternal junction is being used as a reference point.

To patient

in the coronal plane half-way between the xiphoid and the dorsum of the body, and a line drawn at right angles to the fourth interspace where it meets the sternum (Winsor & Burch 1945). In some circumstances it is simpler to use an alternative fixed point such as the manubriosternal junction (angle of Louis) but in these circumstances due allowance must be made for the difference in level. When the manubriosternal junction is used the measured pressure will be 0.5–1.0 kPa (5–10 cmH$_2$O) lower than that recorded using the true reference point at atrial level (Debrunner & Bühler 1969). Since the normal venous pressure is 0–0.6 kPa (0–6 cmH$_2$O) when referred to the atrium, negative values will often be obtained when the manubriosternal junction is used as the reference point.

There are several methods of aligning the zero on the scale with the right atrium. The simplest is to use a hinged arm which is permanently fixed to the manometer stand (Fig. 13.2). When this arm is lowered it impinges on a stop which maintains it at right angles to the stand and which thus ensures that the tip of the arm is aligned with the manometer zero. The stand is then raised or lowered until the tip of the arm is opposite the reference point and clamped in position on the drip pole. To avoid errors the manometer stand must be kept vertical. An alternative method is to align the two zero points by means of a spirit

level. Optical sights on the manometer stand have also been used but again these must be kept horizontal by means of a spirit level. For greatest accuracy a hydrostatic method should be used. One method utilizes a closed loop of intravenous drip tubing which is half filled with liquid containing a small quantity of dye. One side of the loop is fixed to the manometer stand parallel to the lower part of the manometer tube whilst the other side of the loop is held opposite the zero point on the patient. The menisci within the loop remain at the same horizontal level and thus provide a clear and accurate indication of the true zero level (Fig. 13.3). An alternative method is to utilize the saline bridge itself as a hydrostatic zero. This is illustrated in Fig. 13.4.

When a zero position has been set and the central venous line has been flushed through, the manometer is filled from the reservoir. The three-way tap is then turned to connect the manometer to the vein. The saline meniscus should fall fairly rapidly and should stabilize at the venous pressure. It is normally possible to see a small respiratory fluctuation (up to several cmH$_2$O with a deep breath) and, under some circumstances, venous pulsations in time with the heart beat are also visible. The absence of a respiratory swing indicates that the catheter is situated peripherally or is blocked, and that the measurement is not acceptable. Occasionally the recorded

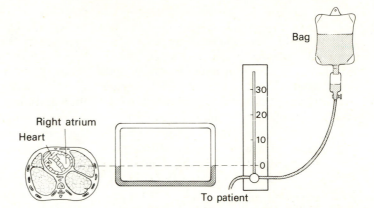

Fig. 13.3. Use of a closed loop of coloured liquid to set manometer zero. The two menisci remain at the same horizontal level.

pressure is found to be higher than expected or marked cardiac pulsations are observed. This may be due to passage of the catheter into the right ventricle or pulmonary artery and may be corrected by withdrawing the catheter. Another little-recognized but major error occurs if the cottonwool filter at the top of the manometer becomes wet and obstructs the free flow of air in and out of the tube.

In order to check the patency of the catheter it is advisable to fill the manometer tube before each reading and then to observe the fall of the saline when the flushing line is excluded from the circuit. An alternative method is to set the three-way tap so that the flushing line, manometer and venous catheter are all interconnected. A slow drip of flushing solution is then maintained throughout the period of measurement. This does not affect the manometer reading if the flushing rate is in the region of 10 drops per minute and the resistance of the catheter is in the normal range.

Fig. 13.4. Hydrostatic method of adjusting manometer zero. The three limbs of the manometer system are filled with saline and lowered below the patient whilst the end of the patient limb is held opposite the zero reference point. The three-way tap is then turned to connect the manometer and patient tube and the manometer tube raised slowly whilst saline is allowed to drip out of the patient tube. The level of saline in the manometer limb remains at the level of the outlet from the patient limb; the manometer tube is raised until the saline meniscus is opposite the zero on the scale and the saline ceases to flow out of the patient limb. The manometer tube is then clamped to the stand.

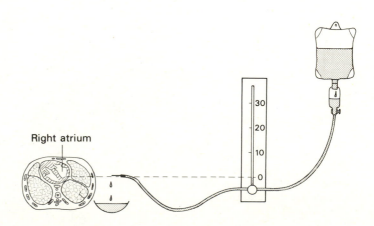

ARTERIAL PRESSURE

Although saline manometers have been used to monitor arterial pressure in some units, they have not been widely used because the manometer tubing is inconveniently long. Furthermore the arterial pulsations are damped by the large volume displacement and inertia of the saline column, so that only mean pressures can be displayed. Mercury manometers have been used to reduce the height of the manometer column but these also have a high inertia. In addition it is difficult to sterilise the mercury and there is always a risk of mercury emboli.

An aneroid blood-pressure manometer gauge may also be used for monitoring mean arterial pressure, providing the bellows is sterilized and no liquid is allowed to enter the gauge (Fig. 13.5) (Zorab 1969). This is a useful technique, particularly in an emergency, and for monitoring during transfer of a patient from one electronic recording system to another.

Electromanometers

Although catheter-tip pressure transducers are now available they are expensive and their use is generally restricted to situations in which a high frequency response is essential. For routine measurements the lumen of the vessel is connected to the pressure transducer by a fluid-filled catheter. The fluid and the diaphragm of the transducer then constitutes a system which will oscillate in simple harmonic motion. The fluid and the mass of the diaphragm represent the oscillating mass, while the compliance of the diaphragm, the tubing and any air bubbles in the system represent the spring. Such a system can only record the pressure and waveform accurately if certain physical conditions are satisfied. To understand the underlying principles it is first necessary to discuss the fundamental characteristics of any waveform.

FOURIER ANALYSIS OF COMPLEX WAVEFORMS

No matter how complicated the waveform, it can always be analysed mathematically as being the sum of a series of much simpler waveforms. The simple waveforms are called sinusoids or sine waves and are generated by any body oscillating in simple harmonic motion. Sine waves are found in many naturally occurring radiations (e.g. electromagnetic radiations such as light or sound) and may be produced artificially (e.g. alternating current). When analysing a complex waveform it is found that it con-

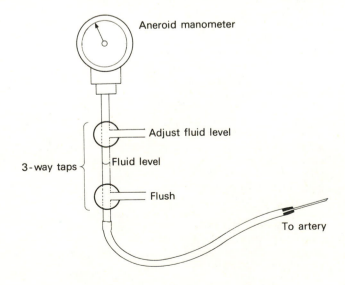

Fig. 13.5. Aneroid gauge used for recording mean arterial pressure. The fluid level should be aligned with the zero reference point.

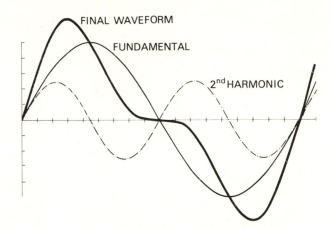

Fig. 13.6. Fourier analysis of a simple waveform; resolution into fundamental (first harmonic) and second harmonic.

tains a *fundamental* frequency and a series of *harmonics*. The fundamental frequency is the lowest frequency sine wave present in the waveform and, in the case of the arterial pulse, would be equal to the pulse rate. This is often called the first harmonic. The second harmonic is a sinusoidal waveform with a frequency twice that of the fundamental or first harmonic, whilst the third harmonic has a frequency three times that of the fundamental and so on. Figure 13.6 shows the effect of combining the first harmonic (the fundamental) and the second harmonic which, in this instance, is roughly half the amplitude of the first. The two waves are *in phase*; that is to say they are moving in the same direction and pass through zero amplitude together. As already pointed out on page 9 quite a different final waveform would result if the harmonics had the same amplitude but were out of phase. In a complex waveform there may be significant contributions from up to 30 harmonics. Since the lower harmonics tend to have the greatest amplitude, a rough approximation to the arterial pressure waveform can often be obtained by reproducing the fundamental and the first eight to ten harmonics. In the case of the arterial waveform at 70 beats per minute this would require a frequency response which is undistorted up to $(70 \times 10)/60 = 11.7\,Hz$. In order to reproduce pulse rates up to 140 beats per minute a flat frequency response up to $20\,Hz$ is required. However, for extremely accurate recording of complex waveforms it is necessary to be able to record a greater range of harmonics. Thus, to record the maximum rate of rise of left ventricular pressure (dP/dt max) it may be necessary for the transducer system to respond accurately up to $30\,Hz$ or even higher. In general the sharper the waveform (i.e. the more rapid the rate of change in pressure) the greater the number of harmonics and the higher must be the frequency response. A square wave has, in theory an infinite number of harmonics and is therefore the most difficult waveform to record accurately (McDonald 1974).

FREQUENCY RESPONSE

A recording system must accurately reproduce both the *amplitude* and *phase difference* of each harmonic present in the waveform. To achieve this it is necessary to design a system with a high *undamped natural frequency* (resonant frequency) and then to apply the correct amount of *damping*.

Undamped natural frequency

A simplified recording system together with its mechanical analogue is shown in Fig. 13.7. Pressure is applied to a column of fluid connecting the blood to the elastic transducer diaphragm. In the mechanical analogue the force is applied to a mass which simulates the inertia of the fluid in

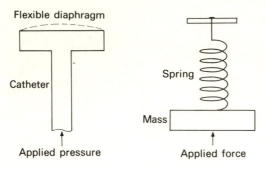

Fig. 13.7. Principle of electromanometer recording system with its mechanical analogue.

the catheter whilst the diaphragm is simulated by a spring. If the mass is set in motion by suddenly applying a force to its under surface it will oscillate up and down in simple harmonic motion, the frequency of oscillation being governed by the mass and the stiffness of the spring. The un-damped natural frequency of this oscillation (f_0) is given by the general formula:

$$f_0 = \frac{1}{2\pi}\sqrt{\frac{S}{M}}$$

where S is the stiffness of the spring (applied force/displacement) and M is the mass of the oscillating body. From this formula it can be seen that the natural frequency of oscillation will be highest when the spring is stiff and the mass is small.

This formula can also be applied to a catheter-transducer system, S referring to the stiffness of the diaphragm and M the mass of fluid in the catheter and transducer. It would then appear that the natural frequency would be highest when the diaphragm was as stiff as possible, and the volume of the oscillating fluid was as small as possible. Furthermore since the mass term is contributed by the fluid in both the catheter and the transducer it would seem that a small volume should be contained in both.

However, these assumptions are not true, for they do not take into account the velocity of fluid movement along the catheter. This not only affects the amount of kinetic energy which has to be imparted

to the fluid column but also alters the viscous resistance to fluid flow.

The essence of any oscillating system is the continual interchange between energy in two forms; in this case it is between the kinetic energy of the mass in motion, and the potential energy of the deformed spring. Now the kinetic energy of the mass in motion is $\frac{1}{2}mv^2$ where m is the mass and v is the velocity. It thus takes more energy to make any given mass of fluid oscillate in a narrow tube than in a wider tube, because it has to reach a higher velocity in the narrow tube. (This ignores the effect of friction, which will be discussed later.) Since the velocity is inversely proportional to the cross-sectional area of the tube, the mass term in the equation must be adjusted by dividing the mass of each part of the system by the square of the cross-sectional area of that part. The cross-sectional area of the transducer diaphragm and dome is much greater than that of the catheter so that the velocity of fluid movement within it is much less than the velocity of fluid movement within the catheter. Indeed, for all practical purposes the mass of fluid in the transducer may be ignored.

The true mass of fluid in the catheter is $\pi r^2 \times l \times \rho$ where r is the radius of the catheter, l is the length and ρ (pronounced 'roe') is the density of the liquid. Since this is usually saline, which has a density close to 1, it may be ignored. Thus the 'equivalent mass' of the saline in the catheter (i.e. the quantity of fluid which is affected by the square of the velocity) is given by the equation:

equivalent mass

$$= \frac{\text{true mass}}{(\text{cross-sectional area})^2}$$

$$= \frac{l \times \pi r^2}{\pi r^2 \times \pi r^2} = \frac{l}{\pi r^2}.$$

If this mass is substituted for M in equation (1) we get:

$$f_0 = \frac{1}{2\pi}\sqrt{\frac{\pi r^2 S}{l}}.$$

Thus the undamped resonant frequency of a catheter-transducer recording system is highest when the diaphragm is stiff and when the catheter is short and wide. Note that the stiffness of the diaphragm in this formula is defined by the elastic modulus stress/strain, i.e. applied force/displacement. In the manufacturer's literature the stiffness of the diaphragm is usually given in terms of the volume displacement in mm^3/kPa or $mm^3/100\,mmHg$. This is the reciprocal of the elastic modulus. Therefore, if the volume displacement or compliance of the system is C then

$$f_0 = \frac{1}{2\pi}\sqrt{\frac{\pi r^2}{l \times C}}.$$

An additional factor which must be considered is the frictional resistance to fluid flow through the catheter. This is the principle factor producing damping. If laminar flow is assumed, Poiseuille's equation* indicates that the resistance to flow is directly proportional to the length of the tube and to the viscosity of the fluid, and inversely proportional to the fourth power of the radius. Once again it is apparent that the minimal hindrance to the flow of fluid in the catheter will occur when the catheter is short and wide and when the viscosity is low. It is therefore apparent that the least amount of damping will be obtained when the velocity of fluid movement is reduced by a low volume displacement transducer and a wide catheter. However, it is important that the catheter has rigid walls for any elasticity in the catheter will increase the compliance of the whole system and so decrease f_0.

* For a Newtonian fluid under conditions of laminar flow the equation is

$$\dot{Q} = \pi \frac{(P_1 - P_2)r^4}{8\eta l}$$

where $\dot{Q}$ = flow, $(P_1 - P_2)$ = difference in pressure, r = the radius of the tube, l = the length of the tube and η = the coefficient of viscosity.

Determination of resonant frequency and damping

If an undamped catheter-transducer system is artificially oscillated by applying a sinusoidal pressure of constant amplitude but gradually increasing frequency (e.g. with a sinusoidal pump) it yields an electrical signal similar to that shown in Fig. 13.8. At low frequencies the amplitude of the output signal remains constant indicating that the system accurately follows the input pressure waveform. However, as frequency is increased further the output signal increases in amplitude, the peak of the response occurring at the resonant frequency of the catheter-transducer system. At still higher frequencies the amplitude of the response declines towards zero due to the increasing magnitude of the viscous and inertial forces already described. It is apparent that errors in the amplitude of the recorded waveform will be minimal if the resonant frequency of the system is well above the significant harmonics in the input waveform, but that the amplitude of a waveform will be exaggerated when any of its contained frequencies are close to the resonant frequency of the system. When the resonant frequency is less than any of the important harmonics there will be attenuation of the waveform due to damping.

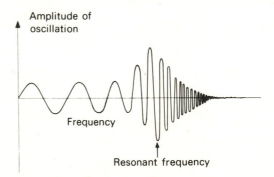

Fig. 13.8. Amplitude of oscillation of a diaphragm in a catheter-transducer system as the applied frequency is increased. The amplitude is maximal at the resonant frequency of the system but at higher frequencies the diaphragm fails to follow the applied pressure.

The effects of damping are best illustrated by applying a single step change in pressure to the catheter-transducer system and recording the response. This is conveniently done by pressurizing a thin rubber balloon to about 6 or 7 kPa (50 mmHg) and then bursting it with a red-hot wire (Fig. 13.9). The response is shown in Fig. 13.10. In a system with no damping the system would oscillate at the undamped natural frequency and there would be no decrease in the recorded oscillations with time ($D = 0$). In a system with minimal damping ($D = 0.2$) the recorded signal falls rapidly, overshoots the base line and is then followed by a series of oscillations of decreasing amplitude. The frequency of oscillation is close to the undamped natural frequency of the system and the rate at which the amplitude decreases gives a measure of the amount of damping (Gabe 1972). If damping is excessive the recorded signal falls slowly and takes some time to reach the baseline. However, there is no overshoot. With care it is possible to adjust the damping so that the output signal falls more rapidly but overshoot is just avoided. In this state the system is said to be *critically damped*

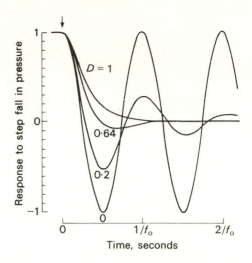

Fig. 13.10. The response of a catheter-transducer system to a step fall in pressure generated by the apparatus shown in Fig. 13.9. Results are shown for four values of the damping factor (D): Undamped ($D = 0$); Slightly damped ($D = 0.2$); Critically damped ($D = 1$); damping 64% of critical ($D = 0.64$). The time scale is in terms of the reciprocal of the undamped natural frequency (after Gabe 1972).

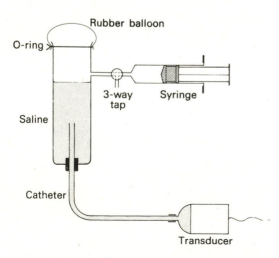

Fig. 13.9. Generation of a square wave fall in pressure for testing catheter-transducer system ('pop test'). The pressurized balloon is burst with a red-hot needle or lighted match.

($D = 1$). All of these situations are obviously undesirable, for on the one hand the system responds rapidly but overshoots, and on the other hand the amplitude of response is correct but the speed of response is too slow.

In the underdamped state pressures with a frequency close to the resonant frequency will be exaggerated whilst in the overdamped state high frequency oscillations will be damped out so that the true pressure change will be underestimated (Fig. 13.11). However, it is found that if the damping of the system is carefully adjusted a recording can be achieved in which overshoot is minimal and yet the speed of response is only slightly reduced. This point is reached when the overshoot is 7% of the original deflection. The damping is then 64% of critical ($D = 0.64$) (Fig. 13.10). This represents the best compromise that can be obtained between speed of response and accuracy of registration of the amplitude of the pressure trace. When the damping is

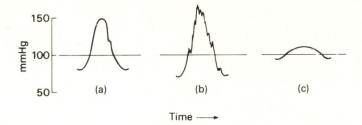

Time ⟶

Fig. 13.11. Errors in arterial pressure waveform caused by inadequate frequency response of catheter-transducer system. a. Correct waveform: optimally-damped system with adequate frequency response. b. Underdamped system with low resonant frequency resulting in exaggeration of high frequency transients. Systolic pressure overestimated and diastolic pressure underestimated. c. Overdamped system due to presence of air bubble or partial blockage of catheter. This results in underestimation of systolic pressure and overestimation of diastolic pressure. Note that the mean pressure is the same in all recordings (13.3 kPa or 100 mmHg).

adjusted in this manner and the response to a sinusoidal pressure signal of increasing frequency is measured, it is found that the amplitude of the recorded oscillation remains within 2% of the input signal up to a frequency which is about two-thirds that

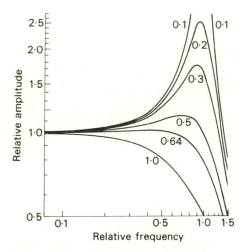

Fig. 13.12. Effect of damping on the amplitude of the recorded signal. The horizontal axis indicates the signal frequency expressed as a fraction of the natural resonant frequency of the system. The figures by each curve indicate the damping factor (D). $D = 0.1$ indicates gross underdamping whilst $D = 1$ indicates critical damping. When the damping factor is 0.64 there is less than 2% distortion in the recorded amplitude of the signal up to about two thirds of the resonant frequency (after Gabe 1972).

of the undamped resonant frequency of the system. At higher frequencies the amplitude of response gradually decreases, there being no resonant zone. With underdamped or overdamped systems amplitude distortion occurs at much smaller fractions of the natural resonant frequency (Fig. 13.12). Optimal damping thus ensures that maximal use is made of the natural resonant frequency of the system.

Phase shift

The accurate registration of a pressure wave depends not only on the correct reproduction of the amplitude of the harmonics but also on the reproduction of the correct *phase difference* between them.

Since all recording systems possess inertia they impose a time delay on the recorded signal. This delay is usually not important as long as it is applied equally to all the components of the wave so that the original phase relationships between the harmonics are maintained. Since the length of a wave is inversely related to its frequency it is only possible to achieve an equal time delay for each harmonic if the phase lag is directly proportional to the frequency of the wave (Fig. 13.13). However, in recording systems the phase lag is a function not only of frequency of the wave but also of the amount of damping present in the system

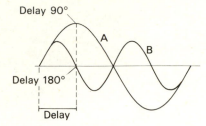

Fig. 13.13. Waveform B has twice the frequency of waveform A. To ensure that an equal time delay is applied to both waveforms the phase lag must be 90° with waveform A and 180° with waveform B, i.e. phase lag must be proportional to the frequency of the harmonics.

(Fig. 13.14). All waves having a frequency equal to the undamped natural frequency of the system are delayed by 90° whatever the degree of damping, but at other frequencies the phase lag is only linearly related to the frequency when damping is about 64% of critical. It is thus apparent that both amplitude and phase distortion are minimal when damping is adjusted to this figure. However, it must be remembered that although the shape of the waveform is accurately reproduced when damping is

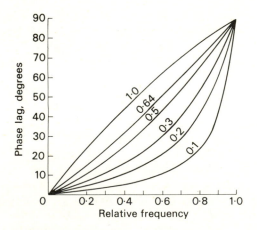

Fig. 13.14. Relation of phase shift to damping. Phase shift is directly related to frequency when damping is about 64% of critical ($D = 0.64$). Relative frequency is the ratio of the applied frequency to the undamped natural frequency of the system (after Gabe 1972).

64% of critical, the whole waveform is slightly delayed. This delay is only of importance in certain specialized measurements, for example, when the pressure measurement is being related to an electrophysiological event in the cardiac cycle.

PRACTICAL CONSIDERATIONS

It will be apparent that one way of overcoming the problems inherent in arterial pressure measurement is to choose a pressure recording system with an extremely high undamped natural frequency. The only transducer with these characteristics is the catheter-tip transducer which may have an undamped natural frequency of 25–40 kHz. Since this is many times greater than the frequency of the tenth harmonic of an arterial pressure waveform, amplitude and phase distortion will be minimal. However, such transducers are still somewhat delicate and expensive so that for most applications it is necessary to use a standard catheter-transducer system.

Although a standard pressure transducer may itself have an undamped natural frequency of 100 Hz or more the addition of the catheter, tap and arterial cannula may reduce the resonant frequency very considerably. Moreover the frequency response which may be achieved in a laboratory is not often reproduced under clinical conditions. The most frequent source of error is the presence of air bubbles. As the pressure changes from systolic to diastolic the bubbles change in volume, and with even quite a small bubble the volume of saline that flows in and out of the catheter in response to this volume change may be greater than the volume change due to the displacement of the transducer diaphragm. Since this extra flow has to take place during the same period, the velocity of the flow is increased, thus increasing the effective mass of the system. This has two effects. It lowers the resonant frequency of the system, and may bring it below the frequencies which are being measured, and it increases the damping. These effects do not depend on the bubble being in the catheter, and are just the same if it is in the transducer. It is of the greatest practical importance, therefore, to avoid bubbles anywhere in the system. In the most stringent applications the catheter-transducer system is flushed with boiled saline for several hours before use to promote absorption of the bubbles.

A second cause of damping is the elasticity of the walls of the catheter. Soft catheters distend in response to the pulse wave and so have the same effect as an air bubble. Attaching the transducer directly to the arterial cannula greatly improves the reproduction of the waveform.

A further cause of damping is clotting in the arterial cannula. This is minimised by maintaining a slow flow (4 ml/hr) of flush solution through the catheter using a pressurized reservoir and fine capillary* or by flushing with 0.5 ml aliquots of solution at hourly intervals. It must also be remembered that the narrowest parts of the catheter-transducer system are usually the arterial cannula and the orifices inside taps and that the use of a relatively wide bore cannula (minimum size 20 S.W.G. in adults) and wide bore taps greatly improves the frequency response of the system (Shapiro & Krovetz 1970).

It is important to use the correct technique of arterial cannulation. It has been shown that thrombotic complications in the artery are greatly reduced by using a parallel-sided, 'Teflon' cannula of small size (Bedford 1977; Davis and Stewart 1980). The shape and size of the cannula permit some blood to flow past the cannula and the material appears to be the most inert currently available. A 20 S.W.G. catheter is small enough to minimize arterial and ischaemic damage and yet large enough to permit accurate registration of pressures.

Finally, it must be remembered that the display or recording system must have a

*A suitable device is the 'Intraflo', Sørenson Research Company 2505 South West Temple, Salt Lake City UTAH 84115.

frequency response which exceeds that of the catheter-transducer system. A good heated-stylus recorder is usually adequate for the routine monitoring of arterial and venous pressure. However, for adequate registration of left ventricular end-diastolic pressure or left ventricular $dP/dt\ max$ it is necessary to employ a photographic, ultraviolet or ink-jet recorder.

Adjustment of damping

Damping of the system can be increased both hydrostatically and electrically. It can be increased hydrostatically by inserting an additional constriction in the line (Gabe 1972) or by allowing the velocity of flow in the catheter to rise by inserting a compliant tube into the system (Latimer & Latimer 1974). Electrical damping is used more commonly and is achieved by passing the electrical signal arising from the moving diaphragm through frequency-selective circuits. It must be emphasized however, that manipulation of electronic controls cannot put back frequencies that were lost on their way to the transducer. Regular flushing to prevent clotting and to remove air bubbles is essential.

Correctly damping is less important when the natural frequency of the transducer is high in relation to the frequencies being recorded. With a number of modern transducers which have a very small compliance and with the catheter-tip transducer, correct damping is of relatively little importance since the undamped natural frequency is very much higher than the frequencies of interest. However, when the natural frequency is closer to the applied frequencies, only a critically-damped system will be accurate. When the natural frequency is so low that important harmonics of the pressure wave correspond with it, over-damped systems produce a smaller error than underdamped ones. Since it is difficult to measure, still less control, the damping, it is common practice to increase the damping if the record looks 'spiky', the assumption being that this is due to the higher

frequency harmonics being near the resonant frequency.

This approach, while pragmatic, is making the best of what may be a very bad job.
If accuracy is important one must make
some evaluation of the frequency response
in the prevailing conditions. This can be
done by observing the response to a sudden
stepwise change (Gabe 1972) or to an increasing frequency sine-wave generator as
already described (McCutcheon, Evans &
Stanifer 1972; Asmussen, Lindström &
Ulmsten 1975). Providing the undamped
response is adequate further damping can
then be added electronically.

CHOICE OF APPARATUS FOR
INTRAVASCULAR PRESSURE
MEASUREMENT

In order to obtain a high natural frequency,
designers of transducers for arterial pressure
recording have been developing stiffer and
stiffer diaphragms with smaller volume displacements.

Most of the standard strain gauge transducers have a volume displacement of
$1-5 \times 10^{-5}$ mm$^3 \cdot$ kPa^{-1} (0.01–0.04 mm^3/
100 mmHg) whilst the internal volume of the
transducer dome is about 1 ml. When a
pressure of 13.3 kPa (100 mmHg) is applied
to this volume of saline it reduces its volume
by about 0.006 mm^3. Since this represents
about half the volume displacement of the
transducer it is apparent that the only way
to secure a further reduction in volume
displacement is to decrease the volume of
fluid in the dome. Volumes as low as 0.2 ml
have now been achieved in some silicon
strain gauge transducers. Since these devices
give a high electrical output for a given
deflection it has been possible to reduce
the volume displacement to 1.3×10^{-7}
mm$^3 \cdot$ kPa^{-1} (0.0001 mm^3/100 mmHg). This
results in an undamped natural resonant
frequency of 5 kHz. A still higher undamped
natural frequency (25–40 kHz) is obtained
with the catheter-tip transducers where the
diaphragm is very small and is in direct
contact with the blood.

In general, a stiffer diaphragm has to be
paid for by a reduced sensitivity of the
system. A stiff diaphragm must result in a
smaller movement for a given pressure
change, and no matter what method is used
to sense the movement, a smaller change of
that quantity will result. A high frequency
response, and a sensitive system, are therefore mutually incompatible characteristics.

Venous pressure measurements require
high sensitivity, but very little high-
frequency capability, and transducers with a
higher volume displacement may be used.
When the shape of the waveform is of
importance, as in arterial tracings, one needs
a high frequency response, and for this a
low volume displacement is essential. If the
shape of the waveform is not of crucial
importance, and it is only desired to record
the systolic and diastolic pressures, a flat
response up to 10 Hz will give figures within
5% of the correct figure, despite amplitude
and phase distortion.

FLOW-GUIDED PULMONARY ARTERY
CATHETERIZATION

Flexible catheters may be passed from the
venous system into the pulmonary circulation under fluoroscopic control as in the
standard procedure of cardiac catheterization. However in many clinical situations it
is more convenient to use flow-guided
catheters which float into the pulmonary
artery under the influence of the blood flow
returning to the lungs. A number of different
catheters have been designed for this
application (Fife & Lee 1965; Bradley 1964)
but the one most commonly employed is the
Swan-Ganz (Swan et al. 1970). This catheter
has a small balloon at its tip. It is passed into
the superior vena cava via an antecubital or
internal jugular vein (Civetta & Gabel 1972)
and the balloon then partially inflated with
0.5 ml of air. The main channel of the
catheter is connected to a pressure transducer and the tip of the catheter is allowed
to float into the right atrium. Another
0.5 ml of air is added to inflate the balloon

fully and the catheter then allowed to float into the pulmonary artery, its progress being monitored by the pressure waveforms detected by the transducer. When the catheter is wedged it is fixed firmly to the skin and its position checked by deflating the balloon. This should yield a recording of pulmonary artery pressure. It is important to ensure that the tip lies in a large pulmonary artery (wedge pressure should only be obtained when the balloon has been fully inflated) and it is advisable to check that the catheter is not partially coiled up in the ventricle by taking a chest X-ray. The balloon should only be inflated whilst wedge pressure is being recorded to minimize the danger of pulmonary infarction.

The catheter can be used to obtain wedge and pulmonary artery pressures. Whilst frequency response is not important when measuring mean wedge pressures, satisfactory pulmonary artery pressures can only be recorded with a low volume displacement transducer. However, artefacts caused by oscillations of the tip of the catheter in the pulmonary artery are not infrequent. Mean pulmonary artery wedge pressure correlates well with mean left atrial pressure when there is no pulmonary vascular disease (Lappas et al. 1973). However pulmonary wedge may be up to 15 mmHg higher than left atrial when the tip of the catheter is situated in the nondependent part of the lung and a positive end-expiratory pressure of more than $5 \, cmH_2O$ is applied (Roy et al. 1977). It is believed that this error is due to closure of alveolar vessels in the upper zones of the lung at high transpulmonary pressures. Pulmonary artery diastolic pressure also correlates well with mean left atrial pressure when pulmonary vascular resistance is normal. However, the estimate becomes inaccurate when there is pulmonary vascular disease (e.g. due to pulmonary thromboembolism, chronic bronchitis, severe mitral valve disease or fibrotic infiltration of the lung) or when the heart rate exceeds 115/min (Forsberg 1971). Of course, it must also be remembered that left atrial pressure does not necessarily reflect the filling pressure of the left ventricle when mitral valve disease is present (Jenkins, Bradley & Branthwaite 1970).

The Swan–Ganz catheter may also be used to sample mixed venous blood. This provides a most useful guide to the adequacy of tissue oxygenation (Tenney 1974). However, care must be taken to ensure that contamination of the sample with left atrial blood is avoided by partial withdrawal of the catheter and by the use of a low sampling flowrate (Shapiro et al. 1974). A modified version of the catheter is available with thermistor probes for thermodilution cardiac output measurement (see Chapter 16).

References

ASMUSSEN M., LINDSTRÖM K. & ULMSTEN U. (1975) A catheter manometer calibrator—a new clinical instrument. *Biomedical Engineering*, **10**, 175.

BEDFORD R.F. (1977) Radial artery function following percutaneous cannulation with 18 and 20 guage catheters. *Anesthesiology*, **47**, 37.

BRADLEY R.D. (1964) Diagnostic right-heart catheterisation with miniature catheters in severely ill patients. *Lancet*, **ii**, 941.

CIVETTA J.M. & GABEL J.C. (1972) Flow directed-pulmonary artery catheterization in surgical patients: indications and modifications of technic. *Annals. of Surgery*, **176**, 753.

DAVIS F.M. & STEWART J.M. (1980) Radial artery cannulation. A prospective study in patients undergoing cardiothoracic surgery. *British Journal of Anaesthesia*, **52**, 41.

DEBRUNNER F. & BÜHLER F. (1969) 'Normal central venous pressure', significance of reference point and normal range. *British Medical Journal*, **3**, 148.

FIFE W.P. & LEE B.S. (1965) Construction and use of self-guiding right heart and pulmonary artery catheter. *Journal of Applied Physiology*, **20**, 148.

FORSBERG S.Å. (1971) Relations between pressure in pulmonary artery, left atrium, and left ventricle with special reference to events at end diastole. *British Heart Journal*, **33**, 494.

GABE I.T. (1972) Pressure measurement in experimental physiology. *Cardiovascular fluid dynamics*. Chapter 2, Editor D.A. Bergel. London: Academic Press.

JENKINS B.S., BRADLEY R.D. & BRANTHWAITE M.A. (1970) Evaluation of pulmonary arterial end-diastolic pressure as an indirect estimate of left atrial mean pressure. *Circulation*, **42,** 75.

LAPPAS D., LELL W.A., GABEL J.C., CIVETTA J.M. & LOWENSTEIN E. (1973) Indirect measurement of left-atrial pressure in surgical patients—pulmonary-capillary wedge and pulmonary-artery diastolic pressures compared with left-atrial pressure. *Anesthesiology*, **3,** 394.

LATIMER R.D. & LATIMER K.E. (1974) Continuous flushing systems. A critical review. *Anaesthesia*, **29,** 307.

MCCUTCHEON E.P., EVANS J.M. & STANIFER R. (1973) *Evaluation of miniature pressure transducers in chronically implanted cardiovascular instrumentation,* editor E.P. McCutcheon. New York: Academic Press.

MCDONALD D.A. (1974) *Blood flow in arteries.* *2nd Edn.* London: Arnold.

ROY R., POWERS S.R., FEUSTEL P.J. & DUTTON R.E. (1977) Pulmonary wedge catheterization during positive end-expiratory pressure ventilation in the dog. *Anesthesiology*, **46,** 385.

SHAPIRO G.G. & KROVETZ L.J. (1970) Damped and undamped frequency responses of underdamped catheter manometer systems. *American Heart Journal*, **80,** 226.

SHAPIRO H., SMITH G., PRIBBLE A.H., MURRAY J.A. & CHENEY F.W. (1974) Errors in sampling pulmonary artery blood with a Swan–Ganz catheter. *Anesthesiology*, **40,** 291.

SWAN H.J.C., GANZ W., FORRESTER J., MARCUS H., DIAMOND G. & CHONETTE D. (1970) Catheterization of the heart in man with use of a flow-directed balloon-tipped catheter. *New England Journal of Medicine*, **283,** 447.

TENNEY S.M. (1974) A theoretical analysis of the relationship between blood and mean tissue oxygen pressures. *Respiration Physiology*, **20,** 283.

WINSOR T. & BURCH G.E. (1945) The phlebostatic axis and phlebostatic level, reference levels for venous pressure measurements in man. *Proceedings of the Society for Experimental Biology and Medicine*, **58,** 165.

ZORAB J.S.M. (1969) Continuous display of the arterial pressure. A simple manometric technique. *Anaesthesia*, **24,** 431.

Further reading

GERSH B.J. (1980) Measurement of intravascular pressures. p. 511 in *The Circulation in Anaesthesia*, ed. C. Prys-Roberts. Oxford

Chapter 14
Indirect Methods for Measuring Arterial Pressure

Although tonometric devices have been developed to measure arterial pressure by recording the deformation of the skin surface over a small superficial artery in response to applied pressure, the majority of indirect methods are still based on the occlusion of a major artery by the Riva–Rocci type of cuff (Riva–Rocci 1896). In the standard technique the systolic and diastolic points are detected by auscultation of the Korotkoff sounds (Korotkoff 1905). Although there are many alternative techniques for recognizing the systolic point the only other methods which provide a reliable indication of diastolic pressure are those which detect sound energy at lower than audible frequencies, or which detect the movement of the arterial wall by the use of a second cuff or ultrasound.

RIVA-ROCCI CUFF AND AUSCULTATION OF KOROTKOFF SOUNDS

Although this technique is generally believed to correlate reasonably well with direct measurements in the majority of patients, there are a number of occasions on which there are gross discrepancies between the two methods, particularly in the determination of the diastolic point (Berliner *et al.* 1960).

Procedure

The cuff is wound closely round the upper arm (which should be at heart level) and the site of the brachial artery is identified by palpation. The cuff is then inflated to 33–40 kPa (250–300 mmHg) and deflated at a rate of about 1 kPa (10 mmHg) per

second so that a rough estimate of the systolic point is obtained by palpation. (This precaution is necessary because in some hypertensive patients there is a 'silent zone' between systolic and diastolic points and inadequate cuff inflation might cause the observer to mistake the return of the sounds for the systolic point.) The cuff is then inflated to about 4 kPa (30 mmHg) above the estimated systolic point and deflated at a rate of about 0.3 kPa (2 mmHg) per second whilst the observer listens over the brachial artery. The systolic point is marked by the sudden appearance of clear, tapping sounds which are synchronous with the heart beat (Phase I, Fig. 14.1). As cuff deflation continues a palpable pulse appears at the wrist (usually about 1 kPa (5–10 mmHg) below the audible systolic point) and the sounds then become somewhat quieter (Phase II). In some patients the sounds disappear completely (the 'auscultatory gap') whilst in other patients there may be little reduction in the intensity of

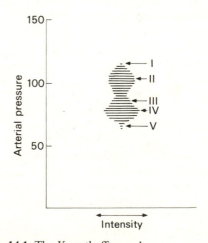

Fig. 14.1. The Korotkoff sounds.

the sound. As the diastolic point is approached the sounds usually become louder and develop a tapping quality (Phase III). They then suddenly become muffled (Phase IV) and usually disappear altogether about 1 kPa (5–10 mmHg) below the point of muffling (Phase V), although in high output states and in exercise, the sounds may not disappear until cuff pressures approach zero.

The physical basis of the method

Riva–Rocci described the idea of using an inflatable cuff to occlude the artery in two papers published in 1896, but he used a cuff which was only 5 cm wide. The pressure in such a narrow cuff was often not transmitted fully to the underlying artery and it was von Recklinghausen who suggested in 1901 that the cuff should be 12 cm wide. However at this time the systolic pressure was determined by palpation of the pulse distal to the cuff and the only method of determining diastolic pressure was to use an aneroid gauge to observe the pulsations transmitted to the cuff between the systolic and diastolic points (Hill & Barnard 1897). It was in December 1905 that N. C. Korotkoff, a Russian surgeon, first reported the auscultatory method of measuring blood pressure indirectly (Booth 1977).

The method of production of the Korotkoff sounds is still not fully agreed but a reasonable conceptual model is that turbulent flow makes the arterial wall vibrate excessively and that this vibration is amplified by resonance of the tissue in the arm. When the cuff pressure lies between systolic and diastolic pressure and the arterial pressure rises during systole, the transmural pressure difference (across the vessel wall) is greatly reduced. Under these conditions turbulent flow can readily induce gross vibrations in the vessel wall. Just below the systolic point the sounds have both low and high frequency components although the former predominate. The high frequency components become particularly marked during phase III and disappear abruptly as Phase IV is reached leaving only the low frequency components.

Accuracy of the method

The sudden appearance of the Korotkoff sounds during cuff deflation corresponds closely with directly-measured systolic pressure though the indirect measurement usually gives values which are slightly lower than direct measurements. Unfortunately the correlation between the two measurements of diastolic pressure is not so good. In the United Kingdom the diastolic pressure is generally assumed to correspond with Phase IV, and a similar recommendation has been made by the Postgraduate Education Committee of the American Heart Association (Kirkendall et al. 1967). However, a number of important epidemiological studies both in the United States and the United Kingdom have since utilized Phase V (Hunyor, Flynn & Cochineas 1978).

In some patients there is little difference between the two phases. In others Phase V may be 1.5 kPa (10 mmHg) or more below Phase IV and sometimes there is no Phase V, the sounds persisting until the cuff pressure is zero. The average difference between Phase IV and Phase V values is about 0.8 kPa (5 mmHg). This is not important for most clinical purposes but is important in epidemiology, for example when studying the need to treat patients with mild hypertension, when such a difference might significantly alter the distribution of patients between groups.

The arguments in favour of using Phase IV are: 1, that the point of muffling should theoretically agree with diastolic pressure; 2, that a gradual disappearance of the sounds at Phase V is much more difficult to identify than a change in their character, since the point of disappearance will depend on the position and efficiency of the stethoscope and on the observer's acuity of hearing; 3, that in high output states and after exercise the fifth phase may not occur until the cuff is completely deflated.

The advocates of Phase V argue: 1, that

Phase V is usually much closer to true diastolic pressure than Phase IV; and 2, that it can be accurately determined in the majority of patients with better agreement between observers. Since Phase IV is on average 1 kPa (8 mmHg) higher than directly-recorded diastolic pressure whilst Phase V is on average only 0.3 kPa (2 mmHg) higher, and since there is better agreement amongst observers, it would seem reasonable to use Phase V as the true diastolic point. However, in situations in which there is a wide discrepancy between the two phases it is probably wise to adopt the World Health Organisation (1962) recommendation to record both phases, e.g. 18.7/10.7/6.7 kPa (140/80/50 mmHg).

Sources of error

Unfortunately most of the sound energy in the Korotkoff sounds occurs at or below the lower end of the audible frequency range (Whitcher 1968) and in hypotension or certain arteriosclerotic conditions the sounds may become difficult to hear (Pederson & Vogt 1973; Taguchi & Suwangool 1974). Apart from the problems inherent in the use of the Korotkoff sounds the most common sources of error are the use of the wrong size of rubber cuff, zero and calibration errors in aneroid manometers and leaks from the pneumatic system which prevent a slow and controlled deflation of the cuff.

It is generally agreed that the rubber cuff need not encircle the arm if it is placed directly over the artery (Burch & Shewey 1973). However, misplacement is difficult to avoid so it is wise to use a cuff which is long enough to encircle the arm completely. Most cuffs in common use measure about 12 × 23 cm. However, Conceiçao, Ward & Kerr (1976) found that over 82% of 500 subjects had an arm circumference exceeding 24 cm and in 8% the circumference exceeded 32 cm. Furthermore, since there was a direct relationship between the required cuff size and body weight, a cuff 36 cm long would have been required to

encircle 99% of arms. A short cuff causes readings to be too high (Simpson et al. 1965) whilst overlapping of a long cuff does not cause error. There thus appears to be a strong case for utilizing a 12 × 35 cm cuff for adults.

The width of the cuff is also important, for too narrow a cuff gives too high a reading, and too wide a cuff may give too low a reading. King (1967) found that when the cuff completely encircled the arm a width above 11 cm was not critical though increasing width could compensate to some extent for a deficiency in length. The World Health Organisation (1962) recommends a cuff 14 cm wide. As a rough guide the cuff should cover approximately two-thirds of the length of the upper arm or its width should be about 20% greater than the diameter of the arm. Recommended cuff widths are therefore: adult arm 12–14 cm; 4–8 years 9 cm; 1–4 years 6 cm; neonate 2–5 cm; adult leg 15–18 cm.

Other methods of detecting Korotkoff sounds

These may be detected by a microphone placed over the artery, and then amplified and transmitted to a loudspeaker. Unfortunately extraneous noise and movement artefacts are difficult to eliminate. A better approach is to sense the high energy in the frequency range just below the audible level and then to convert this into an audible signal. Such an instrument has proved useful when the Korotkoff sounds were difficult to detect (Wallace, Carpenter & Evins 1975). A number of other semi-automated instruments have been manufactured but the agreement with direct measurement of pressure is not impressive (Hunyor et al. 1978).

OTHER METHODS USING THE RIVA-ROCCI CUFF

Doppler technique

The most recent advance in the indirect measurement of blood pressure is based on the application of the Doppler-shift principle using ultrasound (p. 115). In the simplest application a small Doppler probe is placed over an artery which lies distal to an occluding cuff. As flow commences during cuff deflation a difference in frequency develops between the transmitted and reflected ultrasound, the shift being related to the velocity of blood flow towards or from the transducer. The magnitude of the frequency shift is within the audible frequency range and is conveniently presented to the listener by loudspeaker or headphones. The sound resembles a loud, high-pitched, cardiac murmur and changes in character when flow becomes continuous at the diastolic point (Kazamias *et al.* 1971). This technique is particularly useful in neonates and in clinical situations when the Korotkoff sounds are difficult to hear, and although the position of the transducer is quite critical, the detection system is quite cheap.

A more sophisticated technique (Kirby, Kemmerer & Morgan 1969) utilizes the Doppler principle to detect movements of the arterial wall under the cuff. A commercial development of this method (Arteriosonde, Roche) has an array of 3 MHz transducer crystals contained within a flat plastic case which is hinged in the middle. Each section of the case contains both transmitting and receiving crystals and measures about 2 cm × 2 cm × 0.2 cm thick. The case is attached to the inside of an occluding cuff by 'Velcro' tape. The brachial artery is identified by palpation and the transducer carefully positioned to lie over the artery so that when the cuff is wound round the arm the transmitting and receiving surfaces of the two transducers are aligned in a radial direction towards the artery (Fig. 14.2). It is essential that the transducer is 'coupled' to the skin by a layer of silicone gel, which prevents excessive reflections. Both cuff and transducer are connected to the instrument, together with a conventional inflation bulb. When the cuff is inflated, the pressure is indicated by two digital displays. The pressure is lowered by

opening the bleed valve, and the frequency shift signal listened to by loudspeaker or earphones.

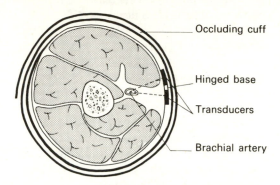

Fig. 14.2. Transverse section of the arm to show the position of the ultrasonic transducers used in the 'Arteriosonde'.

When the cuff pressure falls to systolic pressure, the pulse wave just reaches the distal margin of the cuff, and the arterial lumen snaps open very briefly, vibrating as it does so. This movement produces a Doppler shift in the reflected ultrasound, and therefore a Doppler signal, which is electronically conditioned so as to lie in the audible range. The signal is similar in quality to the first Korotkoff sound, but should not be confused with it, as the sensor is in no way an 'electronic stethoscope'. A softer, lower frequency sound is also heard when the artery closes. As soon as the operator hears the Doppler signal he presses a button on the deflation valve. This locks one of the digital pressure displays which thus records the cuff pressure at the systolic end-point. Deflation is then continued, and the changing quality of the Doppler signal noted. As cuff pressure approaches diastolic, the high frequency opening signal softens, and the closing signal occurs progressively later in the cardiac cycle. At diastole, the opening signal merges with, and becomes indistinguishable from, the closing signal. The button is pressed again, and the cuff pressure is held on the second digital display so that the systolic/diastolic pressures are now displayed together. The bleed valve is fully opened, and the cuff deflated. (The Doppler detector is switched off automatically as the pressure falls to zero, so that switching on/off between readings is unnecessary.) Providing that a cuff of the appropriate size has been correctly positioned and that the arm is at heart level, the 'Arteriosonde' gives readings which are very close to the intra-arterial pressure at the same site.

The Arteriosonde is also available as a fully automatic blood pressure monitor with a recorder output. In this machine the cuff is inflated by a pump at preset intervals and the systolic and diastolic end-points determined by electronically sensing the changing frequency spectrum of the Doppler signal. Complicated artefact rejection systems are incorporated and the machine displays an alarm indication if the signals are affected by excessive noise. Good agreement is obtained with directly measured systolic pressure, but in most clinical situations the automatic Arteriosonde appears to read diastolic pressure about 1 kPa (7.5 mmHg) higher than that revealed by direct recording (Hochberg & Salomon 1971). However in induced hypotension this difference has not been observed (Poppers, Epstein & Donham 1971).

The method has proved satisfactory in children (Zahed et al. 1971), in low output states (Kazamias et al. 1971) and has also been found to be extremely useful in very noisy situations (e.g. helicopter transport) when conventional methods cannot be used (Stegall, Kardon & Kemmerer 1968). It has also proved invaluable in epidemiological studies of blood pressure since it greatly reduces subjective error. However, care is necessary in use. The transducers must be accurately positioned and adequately coated with ultrasonic coupling medium. The cuff must be inflated well above systolic pressure and the bleed rate carefully adjusted. The arm should be kept as still as possible and electrical interference minimized. It is difficult to obtain satisfactory readings in patients with atrial fibrillation or other dysrythmias, and when diathermy

is being used. Most patients also find that the repeated inflation of the cuff seriously disturbs their sleep.

Although there have been suggestions that ultrasound may produce tissue damage the energy output of this machine is less than 50 mW·cm^{-2} at a frequency of 3 MHz. This is well within the levels considered safe for humans.

Other techniques for detecting the onset of systolic flow

One method utilizes a piezo-electric crystal to detect the pulsations over a distal artery. In another method, forearm pulsations are detected by a mercury-in-rubber strain gauge (Greenfield, Whitney & Mowbray 1963). Arterial pulsations may also be sensed by a detector placed over the pulp of the finger. The latter method has the further advantage that the cuff can be placed round the finger instead of the arm, although the cuff and detector should be separated by at least one joint. It is particularly important to consider the position of the cuff in relation to the heart when using finger cuffs, for the hydrostatic pressure between the cuff and the heart contributes to the pressure in the vessels in the finger. Since 10 cm in height is equivalent to a pressure difference of 1 kPa or 7.5 mmHg, the blood pressure in the dependent finger will be 4–6 kPa (30–40 mmHg) higher than that measured with the finger at the level of the heart.

The commonest pulse detector is a photo-electric cell, sensitive to a change in either transmission or reflection of red light. The reflection type can be made very small, attached almost anywhere, and is less prone to interference from incident light. Another common detector system is a partially inflated second cuff; expansion of the part under the second cuff is detected by the movement of air in and out of the cuff which cools a thermistor. Piezo-electric crystals have also been used for detecting finger expansion.

All these techniques, have at one time or another, also been used as the basis of pulse monitors, the pulsations being displayed on a dial or as a flashing light. Unfortunately, most of these methods become inaccurate or cease to function when the blood pressure is low or the periphery is vasoconstricted (Sara & Shanks 1978). Furthermore, under these circumstances the heat produced by light sources is not removed by the bloodstream so that burns may occur.

In neonates the flush method is useful. The arm is raised and milked of blood and the cuff rapidly inflated. The systolic point is then taken to be the pressure at which a skin flush appears. However, this point may often be closer to mean pressure than systolic pressure (Moss *et al.* 1957).

THE OSCILLOTONOMETER

In this method the systolic point is detected by sensing the onset of pulsations distal to the occluding cuff with a second cuff (Von Recklinghausen 1931). Although several makes of oscillotonometer are available, the description will be limited to the Von Recklinghausen 'Scala Alternans Altera' model.

The occluding cuff lies proximal to the sensing cuff and is about 5 cm wide. The sensing cuff is about 10 cm wide and overlaps the outside of the occluding cuff by about 2 cm so that the total width of cuff in contact with the arm is 12–13 cm. Both cuffs and the inflating bulb are connected by separate tubes to a metal block on the side of the instrument. The upper occluding cuff is attached to the part of the block which is uppermost as the oscillotonometer rests horizontally on the table, whilst the *lower* sensing cuff is attached to the nipple on the *lower* part of the block. The inflating bulb with its own discharge valve is attached to the other nipple on the top of the block. There is an adjustable bleed valve on the top of the block and a spring-loaded lever which controls the movement of a rotary control valve within the block (Fig. 14.3). This valve has two positions and determines the interconnections between the cuffs, bleed

valve and the pressure sensing aneroids. The instrument is hermetically sealed and the internal space communicates with the occluding cuff and inflating bulb through the rotary valve. The pressure inside the chamber is sensed by an aneroid (A) which communicates with the atmosphere through a hole in the bottom of the case. A second, more sensitive aneroid (B) is situated slightly above and to one side of (A) and communicates directly with the sensing cuff via a wide-bore channel in the block.

The upper diaphragm of aneroid (B) supports the fulcrum of a lever which is attached at one end to the diaphragm of aneroid (A) and at the other to a mechanism which links it with the pointer indicating the pressure on the dial. The pointer zero can be adjusted by a milled wheel on the side of the case which raises or lowers a baseplate supporting aneroid (B).

To use the instrument the discharge valve on the inflating bulb is closed and the bulb repeatedly compressed in order to inflate the occluding to cuff to a pressure which exceeds the anticipated systolic pressure. Since the control lever is in the 'released' position the air also passes through the wide-bore channels of the control valve to the main chamber and to the tube joining the sensing cuff and aneroid (B). Pressure equilibrium between both cuffs, the main chamber and aneroid B is thus rapidly established. Since the diaphragm of aneroid (B) is in its resting position, the pressure within the cuffs and main chamber is sensed by compression of aneroid (A). This tilts the lever with respect to the fulcrum and so causes the pointer to indicate the chamber pressure on the dial.

To determine the systolic pressure the control lever is pulled towards the operator against the action of the spring. This rotates the control valve so that the bleed valve becomes connected by narrow bore tubes with the occluding cuff and the main chamber and with the wide bore tube connecting the sensing cuff to aneroid (B). The bleed valve is gradually opened until the pointer indicates that the pressure in the

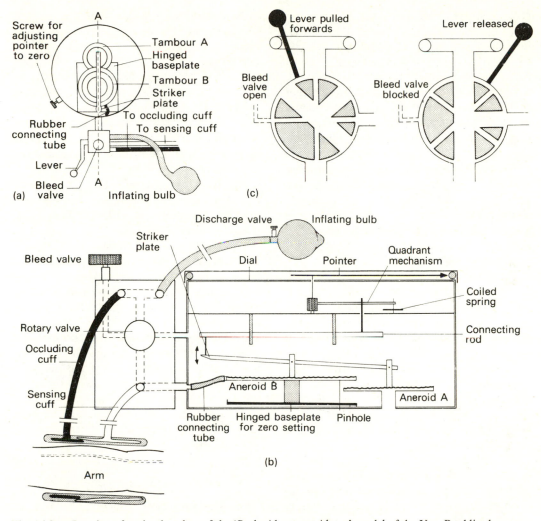

Fig. 14.3. a. Interior of main chamber of the 'Scala Alternans Altera' model of the Von Recklinghausen oscillotonometer. b. Sectional view through A–A. Vertical movement of the striker plate causes the connecting rod to be rotated and this in turn activates the quadrant mechanism which rotates the pointer across the dial. c. The two positions of the rotary valve.

In position 1 (lever released) interconnection is by wide-bore channels so that the pressure indicated on the dial is accurate.

In position 2 (lever forward) interconnection is by fine-bore channels and the bleed valve is connected to all parts of the circuit. The pulse wave is amplified but the absolute pressure indication is inaccurate.

occluding cuff is falling at a rate of about 0.3 kPa (2 mmHg) per second. Small oscillations of the pointer are observed as the pressure falls. These are due to pulse waves striking the upper occluding cuff, producing pressure transients across the diaphragm of aneroid A. Since the occluding cuff does

not allow the pulse wave to reach the lower, sensing cuff, the lever fulcrum on aneroid B remains still, so the observed oscillations are small. When the pressure in the occluding cuff falls to just below systolic pressure, the pulse wave passes the occluding cuff, and strikes the larger sensing cuff. The resulting pressure transient in aneroid (B) raises the fulcrum simultaneously with compression of aneroid A, whilst the fine bore interconnections prevent rapid equalisation of pressure. At this point the pressure swings in aneroid B are larger than those in the main chamber because of the relative disparity between the volumes of the two cuffs and the two chambers, the small occluding cuff discharging through a narrow tube into the large main chamber whilst the larger sensing cuff discharges through a wide tube into the relatively small volume of aneroid (B). Furthermore aneroid (B) has a higher compliance than aneroid (A) thus further amplifying the pressure swings displayed by the pointer.

Partial or complete occlusion of the small holes in the valve by dirt or valve lubricant may cause the pressure in the main chamber or in aneroid (B) to be much higher than it should be. This results in wild swings of the pointer when the lever is released and is a frequent source of error with this instrument. Similar errors may occur if the occluding cuff pressure is reduced too quickly, for this also results in a gross imbalance in pressure between the occluding and sensing systems.

To measure diastolic pressure the lever is once again pulled forward and the deflation of the occluding cuff continued. The oscillations of the pointer usually increase slightly and then suddenly decrease when the diastolic point is reached. This indicates that the artery is remaining open throughout the pulse cycle, so that the impact of the pulse wave is greatly diminished. The lever is released and diastolic pressure read from the scale. Both cuffs are then completely deflated by opening the discharge valve on the inflating bulb.

It has been suggested that the relative position of the cuffs does not matter. This problem was investigated by Corall & Strunin (1975). They found that positioning the sensing cuff proximal to the occluding cuff did not produce an error in the reading if the cuffs were old, but it did produce an error if the cuffs were new. However, most experienced anaesthetists would agree that there are enough sources of error in blood pressure measurement without adding yet one more!

It can be seen that the instrument utilizes the same underlying mechanisms as other indirect methods of blood-pressure measurement. It is therefore prone to the same sources of error. It tends to be least accurate at high pressures, and low pulse pressures. It performs at its best in the presence of moderate hypotension associated with peripheral vasodilation. Fortunately, these are the conditions in which it most often used.

An automated instrument utilizing the oscillometric principle (the Dynamap) has recently been introduced. This utilizes a single cuff of standard dimensions. The cuff is automatically inflated and deflated at pre-set rates and the cuff pressures continually sensed with a pressure transducer. The pressure fluctuations within the cuff are analysed by a microprocessor and the heart rate, systolic, diastolic and mean pressures are displayed digitally. The instrument is easy to use, for there is no separate detector, and it appears to produce accurate results in shock states.

THE TRIPLE CUFF METHOD

This method was originated by de Dobbeleer in 1963 and was based on the observation that the pulse wave travels more slowly through a partially compressed artery. One cuff was used to occlude the artery and two distal cuffs sensed the time lag in transmission of the pulse wave by transmitting puffs of air to a sensitive thermistor. Although the machine was marketed (Godart Haemotonograph) subsequent investigation showed the principle of diastolic detection to be invalid since there was, in fact, no sudden phase shift at the diastolic point.

References

BERLINER K., FUJIY H., HO LEE D., YILDIZ M. & GARNIER B. (1960) The accuracy of blood pressure determinations: a comparison of direct and indirect measurements. *Cardiologica*, **37**, 118.

BOOTH J. (1977) A short history of blood pressure measurement. *Proceedings of the Royal Society of Medicine*, **70**, 793.

BURCH G.E. & SHEWEY L. (1973) Sphygmomanometric cuff size and blood pressure recordings. *Journal of the American Medical Association*, **225**, 1215.

CONCEIÇAO S., WARD M.K. & KERR D.N.S. (1976) Defects in sphygmomanometers: an important source of error in blood pressure recording. *British Medical Journal*, **1**, 886.

CORALL I.M. & STRUNIN L. (1975) Assessment of the Von Recklinghausen oscillotonometer. *Anaesthesia*, **30**, 59.

GREENFIELD A.D.M., WHITNEY R.J. & MOWBRAY J.F. (1963) Methods for the investigation of peripheral blood flow. *British Medical Bulletin*, **19**, 101.

HILL L. & BARNARD H. (1897) A simple and accurate form of sphygmomanometer or arterial pressure gauge contrived for clinical use. *British Medical Journal*, **2**, 904.

HOCHBERG H.M. & SALOMON H. (1971) Accuracy of an automated ultrasound blood pressure monitor. *Current Therapeutic Research*, **13**, 129.

HUNYOR S.N., FLYNN J.M. & COCHINEAS C. (1978). Comparison of performance of various sphygmomanometers with intra-arterial blood pressure readings. *British Medical Journal*, **3**, 159.

KAZAMIAS T.M., GANDER M.P., FRANKLIN D.L. & ROSS J. (1971) Blood pressure measurement with Doppler ultrasonic flowmeter. *Journal of Applied Physiology*, **30**, 585.

KING G.E. (1967) Errors in clinical measurement of blood pressure in obesity. *Clinical Science*, **32**, 223.

KIRBY R.R., KEMMERER W.T. & MORGAN J.L. (1969) Transcutaneous Doppler measurement of blood pressure. *Anesthesiology*, **31**, 86.

KIRKENDALL W.M., BURTON A.C., EPSTEIN F.H. & FREIS E.D. (1967) Recommendations for human blood pressure determination by sphygmomanometers. Report of a subcommittee of the Postgraduate Education Committee, American Heart Association: Recommendations for human blood pressure determinations by sphygmomanometers. *Circulation*, **36**, 980.

KOROTKOFF N.S. (1905) On methods of studying blood pressure. *Izvestiya Imperatorskoĭ Voenno-Meditsinskoi akademii. S. Peterburg*, **II**, 365.

MOSS A.J., LIEBLING W., AUSTIN W.O. & ADAMS F.H. (1957) An evaluation of the flush method for determining blood pressures in infants. *Pediatrics*, **20**, 53.

PEDERSON R.W. & VOGT F.B. (1973) Korotkoff vibrations in hypotension. *Medical Instruments*, **7**, 251.

POPPERS P.J., EPSTEIN R.M. & DONHAM R.T. (1971) Automatic ultrasound monitoring of blood pressure during induced hypotension. *Anesthesiology*, **35**, 431.

RIVA-ROCCI S. (1896) Un sfigmomanometro nuovo. *Gazzetta Medica di Torino*, **47**, 981.

SARA C.A. & SHANKS C.A. (1978) The peripheral pulse monitor—a review of electrical plethysmography. *Anaesthesia and Intensive Care*, **6**, 226.

SIMPSON J.A., JAMIESON G., DICKHAUS D.W. & GROVER R.F. (1965) Effect of size of cuff bladder on accuracy of measurement of indirect blood pressure. *American Heart Journal*, **70**, 208.

STEGALL H.F., KARDON M.B. & KEMMERER W.T. (1968) Direct measurement of arterial blood pressure by Doppler ultrasonic sphygmomanometry. *Journal of Applied Physiology*, **25**, 793.

TAGUCHI J.T. & SUWANGOOL P. (1974) "Pipe-stem" brachial arteries—a cause of pseudo-hypertension. *Journal of the American Medical Association*, **228**, 733.

THICK M.G. & THICK G.C. (1978) Monitoring low blood pressure. A non-invasive technique. *Anaesthesia*, **33**, 726.

VON RECKLINGHAUSEN H. (1901) Über Blutdruckmessung beim Menschen. *Archiv für experimentelle Pathologie und Pharmakologie*, **46**, 78.

VON RECKLINGHAUSEN H. (1931) *Neue Wege zur Blutdruckmessung*. Berlin: Springer Verlag.

WALLACE C.T., CARPENTER F.A. & EVINS S.C. (1975) Acute pseudohypertensive crisis. *Anesthesiology*, **43**, 588.

WHITCHER C.E. (1968) Stethoscope performance in transduction of human Korotkov blood pressure sounds. *Anesthesiology*, **29**, 215.

World Health Organisation (1962) Arterial hypertension and ischaemic heart disease: Preventive Aspects, *Technical Report Series No. 231 : 4*, Geneva, World Health Organisation.

ZAHED B., SADOVE M.S., HATANO S. & WU H.H. (1971) Comparison of automated Doppler ultrasound and Korotkoff measurements of blood pressure of children. *Anesthesia and Analgesia Current Researches*, **50**, 699.

Chapter 15
Measurement of Gas Flow and Volume

The SI unit of volume is the cubic metre (m^3), but it has been agreed that the more convenient unit, the litre ($\simeq 1000 \, cm^3$) may be retained as an alternative. Since flow rate is defined as the volume passing a fixed point in unit time, it is measured in cubic metres (or litres) per second. This concept must be clearly differentiated from the velocity of gas flow. Velocity is the distance moved by a gas molecule in unit time. For a given flow rate, velocity will therefore be higher when the gas is flowing through a narrow tube rather than a wide one. For example, if gas flows at a rate of $1 \, l \cdot s^{-1}$ through a cylindrical tube having a radius of 2 cm and a cross-sectional area (πr^2) of $3.14 \times 2^2 = 12.56 \, cm^2$, then the average velocity of the gas molecules (v) is given by the flow rate divided by the cross-sectional area:

$$v = \frac{1000 \, cm^3 \cdot s^{-1}}{12.56 \, cm^2} = 79.6 \, cm \cdot s^{-1}.$$

If the tube has a radius of 4 cm then:

$$v = \frac{1000 \, cm^3 \cdot s^{-1}}{50.24 \, cm^2} = 19.9 \, cm \cdot s^{-1}.$$

The reverse conversion of velocity to flow rate is accomplished by multiplying the velocity by the cross-sectional area through which the gas passes.

The concept of velocity is important in the context of flow measurement because a number of instruments measure the velocity of flow and not flow rate. If the velocity of all the molecules in the gas or liquid were to be the same there would be no problem in converting the measured velocity to flow rate. Unfortunately this is rarely the case. For example, when flow is laminar, the velocity of particles in the central part of the stream is higher than that of particles situated more peripherally, those next to the wall of the tube being virtually static. This creates a parabolic profile of velocities within the moving gas stream (Fig. 15.1). However, when converting this velocity profile to flow it is not sufficient to average the velocities and then multiply by the cross-sectional area of the tube since the more peripherally-situated layers of gas or fluid have a larger volume than the same thickness of gas or fluid situated more centrally. They therefore contribute proportionately more to the total flow than their velocities would suggest. These complexities impose serious limitations on the use of velocity probes in blood vessels. However, when the velocity profile is essentially flat (as is believed to be the case in the thoracic aorta) the objections are less important.

Flowmeters are standardized by measuring the volume of gas which passes through the meter in unit time, so that methods of measuring gas volumes will be detailed first.

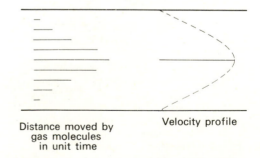

Distance moved by gas molecules in unit time

Velocity profile

Fig. 15.1. Velocity profile during laminar flow in a parallel-sided tube with a constant driving pressure. The axial stream has a higher velocity than the more peripheral streams.

Measurement of volume

Measurements of gas volume are accomplished by collecting the gases in a calibrated spirometer, or by passing the gases through some type of gas meter. Most metering devices are suitable for both continuous or intermittent flows of gas, but if the device is only suitable for use with a continuous flow the gas must first be collected in a Douglas bag and then driven through the device at a steady rate.

SPIROMETERS

Spirometers may be wet or dry. The earliest spirometers were of the wet variety, the appellation referring to the use of a liquid seal between the moving and static parts of the instrument.

The standard *wet spirometers* (e.g. the 300 litre Tissot or the 6 litre Benedict–Roth) consist of a light but rigid cylinder which is suspended inside a larger double-walled container. (Fig. 15.2). The space between the two walls is filled with water to form an air-tight junction. This type of spiro-

meter is suitable for measurements at normal respiratory rates, but at high respiratory rates the inertia of the bell and pulleys and the consequent fluctuations in water-level due to changes in pressure within the bell lead to inaccuracies. For recording at rapid respiratory rates a fast spirometer has been designed. This has a light bell of large diameter, which minimizes the acceleration during rapid breathing, lightweight pulleys and chains, and a large volume of water which minimizes oscillations (Bernstein, D'Silva & Mendel 1952). Dry spirometers are more convenient for clinical work but are more difficult to manufacture. This type of spirometer utilizes a freely moving bellows, which must be carefully folded so that the excursion is linearly related to volume, and which must be accurately counterbalanced by weights or springs so that the internal pressure is always close to atmospheric, whatever the contained volume.

The most popular example of a specialized type of *dry spirometer* is the Vitalograph (Fig. 15.3). This is used for measuring forced vital capacity (FVC), forced expiratory volume in 0.75 or 1 second ($FEV_{0.75}$,

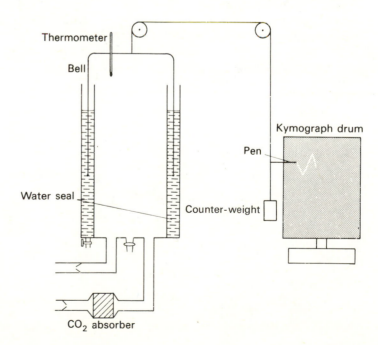

Fig. 15.2. Wet spirometer. The CO_2 absorber is inserted when closed circuit spirometry is used for the measurement of oxygen consumption. The bell is then filled with O_2.

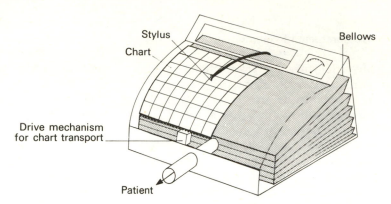

Fig. 15.3. Principle of the
'Vitalograph' spirometer

FEV$_1$) or other indices or airway resistance
such as peak expiratory flow rate (PEFR)
or maximum mid-expiratory flow rate
(MMEF). The patient makes a maximal
forced exhalation into the spirometer
through a wide bore tube, the expansion of
the wedge-shaped bellows being recorded
on a pressure-sensitive chart by a pointed
stylus. To conserve chart space, the movement of the chart along the x (time) axis
only commences when gas begins to flow
into the bellows. The resultant trace represents a volume/time plot of the patient's
expiration. The FVC is the maximal volume
expired. The slope of the line at any point
represents the instantaneous relationship
between volume and time (i.e. flow) and can
be derived by drawing a tangent to the line
at that point (Fig. 15.4). Some of the more
popular measurements used to provide
information about airways resistance are
shown in Fig. 15.5.

There is a small lag between the onset
of expiration and the movement of the stylus

due to preliminary expansion of the bellows.
This is offset by ensuring that the stylus is
aligned with the 'stylus start' position on the
chart before making the measurement. It is
extremely important to ensure that the
patient makes an airtight seal with the
mouthpiece and that the nose is occluded
with a noseclip. The patient must be
actively encouraged to breath out as forcibly
and as rapidly as possible, and the best of
three or four attempts should be recorded.

When bronchospasm is present the
measurement should be repeated after the
administration of a bronchodilator. The
linearity and accuracy of this machine is
remarkably good and its impedance is quite
small (Drew & Hughes 1969). Another type
of dry spirometer for lung function testing
using a square-shaped bellows has been
described by Collins, McDermott &
McDermott (1964).

The construction of dry spirometers
always represents a compromise between
high sensitivity and a low impedance to

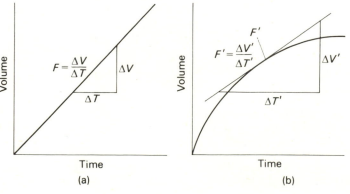

Fig. 15.4. a. Flow (F) is derived
from the volume measured in
unit time. b. Where flow rate
varies rapidly instantaneous
flow at any point (F') is derived
from the tangent of the volume
curve at that point.

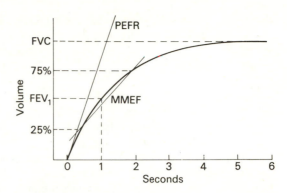

Fig. 15.5. Information which can be derived from record of forced vital capacity. FVC = Forced vital capacity; PEFR = Peak expiratory flow rate at beginning of expiration; FEV_1 = Volume expired in 1 second; MMEF = Average flow rate between 25% and 75% of FVC.

airflow. The greatest sensitivity is achieved when the cross-sectional area of the bellows is reduced, for this produces a bigger movement of the bellows for a given volume change. However, the movement of the bellows is governed by the force applied to the end plate and this, in turn, is a function of the pressure and the area over which it is applied. To cause the end-plate to move in response to a small pressure difference it is therefore necessary to make the end-plate of the bellows large. This, in turn, leads to a loss of sensitivity. In more sophisticated dry spirometers the problems are overcome in two ways. In one type of spirometer (the 'wedge' spirometer) the cross-sectional area of the bellows is made very large (sometimes almost 1-m square) but the relatively small movement of the bellows is sensed electronically (Fig. 15.6a). This not only enables

the amplitude of the recording to be adjusted to suit the chart width, but also permits further electronic processing of the signal to be carried out. For example the volume signal can be differentiated to yield a flow signal, or the volume expired in a given time can be calculated to provide a digital readout of FEV_1 or FEV_1/FVC. In the second type of instrument (Fig. 15.6b) the bellows is replaced by a piston within a cylinder. The cross-sectional area of the piston is of average size, but its movement is assisted by a servo-controlled motor. This motor responds very rapidly to changes in the electrical output of a device which senses small changes in pressure in the chamber, the motor being so adjusted that at all times it tends to move the bellows into a position where the internal pressure is always close to atmospheric. Needless to say

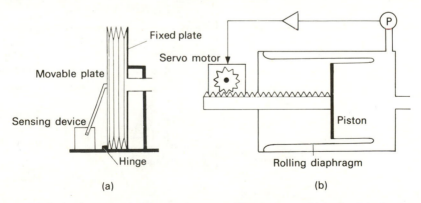

(a)   (b)

Fig. 15.6. a. 'Wedge' spirometer. b. 'Servospirometer. The pressure within the chamber is continuously sensed by the pressure transducer P. When the pressure differs from atmospheric an electrical signal is generated which is amplified and fed to the servomotor. This then moves the piston in such a way that it reduces the pressure towards atmospheric. The seal between the piston and the cylinder is achieved with a sleeve of rubber which creates a 'rolling diaphragm'.

both these types of spirometer are much more expensive than the simpler instruments.

GAS METERS

Gas meters may be wet or dry. *Wet* meters are now rarely used since they need to be kept filled with water and carefully levelled: furthermore, the maximum flow rate which can be tolerated during measurement is limited to about 2.5 litres/min. Such a meter consists essentially of a paddle-wheel, the lower half of which rotates under water. Gas is admitted to the space between two paddle blades and this causes the paddle-wheel to rotate. The gas then passes out through the exit tube. Since the volume of gas isolated in each section of the paddle-wheel is constant, the degree of rotation

of the paddle-wheel is proportional to the volume which has passed. The paddle-wheel is connected to a gear chain which drives a pointer on a dial so that a direct reading is obtained.

Dry gas meters are widely used in the gas industry and have proved useful in medicine since they are portable, accurate and relatively cheap. The meter consists of a box divided into three by two partitions; one partition is horizontal and separates an upper gas inlet and valve compartment from two identical measurement compartments below (see Fig. 15.7). Each of the measurement compartments is further functionally divided by a plastic or leather bellows. Two compound rotary or sliding valves, mounted in the top compartment, direct the gas flow into and out of the four gas chambers thus created. These valves are activated by the

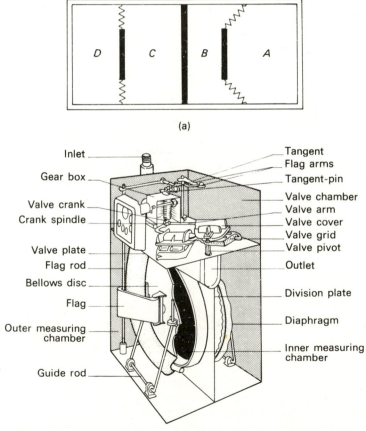

(a)

(b)

Fig. 15.7. a. Coronal section of a dry gas meter. b. Details of mechanism. (From Adams *et al.* 1967; reproduced by kind permission of the Editor of the *British Journal of Anaesthesia*.)

movements of the bellows and are linked together so that the bellows themselves move in fixed relationship to each other. Within each pair of measuring chambers, movement of gas into or out of the inside of the bellows is exactly balanced by an equal volume of gas moving out of or into the chamber surrounding the bellows. Thus, at no time is the gas in the measuring compartments under pressure. The connection between the valves and the bellows ensures that each bellows and its related valves is always 90° out of phase with the other. Thus, apart from the instants when either bellows is at the extreme end of its travel, gas is flowing into or out of all four compartments simultaneously. The movement of the bellows is activated by the pressure of the inlet gas, which need be only two or three centimetres of water (0.2–0.3 kPa): when either of the bellows is at the point of reversal, there is an instant when there is no inlet pressure to that bellows or the surrounding chamber (like top dead centre in the cylinder of an internal combustion engine). A mechanism which relied on a single pair of chambers would be liable to stick at this point: having a second pair, 90° out of phase, mechanically linked to the valve mechanism ensures that when one bellows is reversing at either end of its travel, the other bellows is moving with maximum velocity. This ensures smooth running and reasonably accurate measurements even at low flow rates. In addition to driving the valve mechanism, the movement of the two bellows is linked to a common mechanism which drives a pointer round a scale or provides the motive power for a sequence of clockwork linked dials. The calibration is accurately adjusted to match the excursion of the bellows by altering the length of a tangent arm on the valve mechanism.

The volume which is passed during a complete cycle of a gas meter depends on the size of the meter and this depends on the expected flow which the meter is expected to handle. Two to two and a half litres is a common volume for domestic-sized meters which are suitable for use on mechanical ventilators or in laboratories. This volume, of course, bears no relationship to a complete rotation of the indicator dial. Within the cycle, there may be gross inaccuracies due, for example, to irregular unfolding of a bellows. Once the meter has returned to the same position in the cycle, however, these temporary irregularities have evened out. The greatest accuracy is therefore obtained when the volume to be measured is a multiple of the meter volume. When large volumes are measured, any 'within cycle' inaccuracies are averaged over a large number of cycles. For example, a serious 200 ml irregularity within a cycle would amount to only a 0.44% error in measuring 50 litres, and 0.004% in 500 litres. This increasing accuracy over large volumes has, of course, been the feature which enabled commercial undertakings to sell gas at a profit for over a hundred years. The flow rate also has an influence on accuracy, but even the smallest meters likely to be encountered can be accurate to $\pm 1\%$ over a range of flow rates from 0 to 100 litres min^{-1} if properly adjusted and maintained (Adams *et al.* 1967).

THE DRÄGER VOLUMETER

This instrument is somewhat larger than the Wright respirometer (see below) and responds to airflow in either direction (Fig. 15.8). The registration of volume flow is accomplished by two light, interlocking, dumb-bell-shaped rotors. The meter is more accurate than the Wright respirometer but also more expensive. It is affected by moisture but regains its accuracy when dried out.

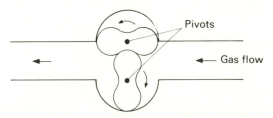

Fig. 15.8. Dräger volumeter.

WRIGHT RESPIROMETER

This device contains a light mica vane which rotates within a small cylinder (Fig. 15.9). The wall of the cylinder is perforated with a number of tangential slits so that the air stream causes the vane to rotate. Flow in the reverse direction impinges on the bottom edge of the vane and so produces no rotational movement. The instrument is therefore unidirectional.

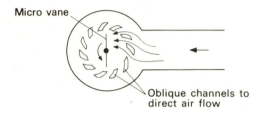

Micro vane

Oblique channels to direct air flow

Fig. 15.9. Wright respirometer. Cross-section (viewed from above).

The rotation of the vane activates a gear chain, which in turn drives the pointer round the dial. By adjusting the relation between the number of rotations of the vane and the volume of gas which has passed through the meter, it has been possible to arrange that the recorded volume approximates closely to the volume of gas which has actually passed through the meter. This calibration is performed with a sinewave pump and is valid for normal tidal volumes and breathing rates, but the meter over-reads at high tidal volumes and under-reads at low tidal volumes due to its inertia. The meter tends to over-read when there is a high peak flow at the beginning of expiration (e.g. during mechanical ventilation) and also overestimates steady flows (Byles 1960; Nunn & Ezi-Ashi 1962).

In a recent version of this instrument the rotation of the vane is detected electronically. The elimination of the gear chain minimizes inaccuracies due to inertia, renders the head less liable to damage from external shocks and reduces inaccuracies due to water condensation (Cox *et al.* 1974). The accuracy of this and two other elec-

tronic respirometers has been evaluated by Conway *et al.* (1974).

Other techniques for measuring gas volumes

INTEGRATION OF THE FLOW SIGNAL

The flow signal from a pneumotachograph (p. 196) or an ultrasonic flowmeter (p. 200) may be electronically integrated with respect to time to yield a volume signal. Although digital methods of integration have greatly increased the accuracy of the procedure there are always problems with baseline drift. This arises from several sources. Firstly, under zero conditions it is difficult to achieve and maintain a zero output from a very sensitive differential pressure transducer because the balance is affected by changes in ambient temperature and by electronic drift. Whilst a small electronic signal resulting from a slight imbalance may not produce any detectable difference in the zero flow baseline, this signal is continually integrated by the integrator and may thus produce significant baseline drift on the volume signal. A second cause of baseline drift in clinical practice is a difference between the inspired and expired volume signals. This arises not only from the actual difference between inspired and expired volumes (due to the unequal volume exchange of oxygen and carbon dioxide and to the uptake or elimination of anaesthetic gases) but also to the difference in composition between inspired and expired gases. These factors cause the inspired and expired signals to differ by about 6%.

These problems, together with changes in resistance of the pneumotachograph head due to the deposition of water vapour or lung secretions, greatly reduce the usefulness of this technique for prolonged monitoring. However, it is possible to overcome these objections by resetting the integrator to zero at the end of each expiration, by heating the head and by applying repeated calibrations.

PLETHYSMOGRAPHY

A plethysmograph is an instrument which is used to measure the change in volume of an organ or limb. The method has been used to record the volume changes of the heart or lungs and also for the measurement of limb blood flow by venous occlusion plethysmography (see p. 203). The traditional method of measuring the change in volume is to seal the organ or limb within a closed container. The container is filled with gas or liquid and the change in volume is then derived from measurements of the volume displaced from the container. In recent years other techniques based on measurements of impedance or capacitance have been introduced. However few approach the accuracy and reliability of the traditional approach.

An important application of plethysmography is in the measurement of changes in lung volume. The standard apparatus for performing this measurement is the *body plethysmograph*. The patient sits in a sealed box and breathes through a tube connected to a pneumotachograph. The change in volume of the lungs can then be measured by one of two different methods. In the *constant pressure* plethysmograph the volume of gas displaced by the breathing movements is measured by a small wedge-shaped spirometer which is connected directly to the interior of the box. In the *constant volume* plethysmograph the change in lung volume creates a change in pressure in the box which is sensed by a sensitive pressure transducer. The relationship between volume and pressure change can then be established by pumping known volumes of air in and out of the box whilst the patient is in the box (Fig. 15.10).

The body plethysmograph can be used for measuring airflow rates and changes in lung volume and can also be used to measure thoracic gas volume. This is a particularly valuable attribute since airway resistance is critically dependent on lung volume and a knowledge of the lung volume at which airway resistance is measured greatly helps the interpretation of the results.

To measure thoracic gas volume (V) the patient makes inspiratory and expiratory efforts against a closed shutter whilst the change in mouth pressure (ΔP) and change in box volume (ΔV) are recorded. During the panting procedure the gas in the lungs is alternately compressed and expanded by the action of the chest muscles. Since there is no flow of gas through the airways, changes in mouth pressure accurately reflect the changes in the pressure of the intrathoracic gas in response to the changes in volume. The change in volume of this gas is measured by the body plethysmograph.

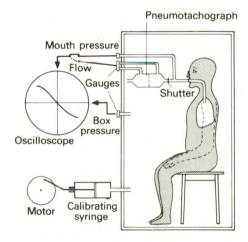

Fig. 15.10. A constant-volume box plethysmograph. To measure thoracic gas volume the patient pants against the closed shutter whilst changes in mouth pressure (= alveolar pressure) and box pressure (= change in gas volume) are recorded on the oscilloscope. The box pressure signal is then calibrated against the known volume injected by the calibrating syringe. Thus the relationship between the changes in alveolar pressure and thoracic gas volume can be established. To measure airway resistance the patient pants through the pneumotochograph whilst flow and box pressure are recorded, and then pants against the closed shutter to establish the relationship between changes in alveolar pressure and box pressure. From these two relationships it is possible to relate flow rate to the pressure drop across the airways and so to derive airway resistance.

By applying Boyle's law $(PV = k)$ the following equation can be derived:

$$PV = (P + \Delta P)(V - \Delta V).$$

Since P is barometric pressure minus water vapour pressure, and ΔP and ΔV are measured, V can be calculated. Thoracic gas volume measured by this technique equals that measured by inert gas dilution techniques in patients with normal lungs, but in patients with airways obstruction the dilution methods yield lower values because of the volume of trapped gas which does not equilibrate with the inert gas (DuBois et al. 1956).

The body plethysmograph can also be used to measure airway resistance by causing the patient to pant through a pneumotachograph which is situated within the box. During panting the alveolar pressure rises and falls during expiration and inspiration because of the resistance to airflow within the airways. There is a simple inverse relationship between the changes in alveolar pressure and the changes in volume recorded by the plethysmograph which can be determined by panting against the closed shutter. When this has been determined the resistance of the airways (R_A) can be calculated from the equation:

$$R_A = \frac{\Delta P}{\Delta V} \times \frac{\Delta V}{\dot{v}}$$

where $\dot{v}$ is the instantaneous flowrate recorded by the pneumotachograph. The advantage of this technique is that it yields a measure of airway resistance which is unaffected by tissue resistance. It also obviates the need to swallow an oesophageal balloon for measurement of oesophageal pressure (DuBois, Botelho & Comroe 1956).

In practice the change in box volume is displayed on the x-axis of an oscilloscope screen and mouth pressure or flow on the y-axis (Fig. 15.10) so that the inter-relationships can be derived directly from the slope of the resulting trace.

IMPEDANCE PNEUMOGRAPHY

Changes in the volume of the thorax can also be detected by measuring the impedance between electrodes situated on opposite sides of the chest wall. A high frequency alternating current (in the kilohertz range) is used to avoid tissue stimulation, pain and the danger of cardiac arrest and the change in impedance is then displayed on a chart recorder.

It is possible to obtain a reasonably linear relationship between the change in impedance and tidal volume for any given individual but the signal has to be calibrated against a spirometer before use. Furthermore, the relationship may be altered by changes in body position and electrode movement. The method is chiefly of value for monitoring purposes (Geddes & Baker 1975; Juett 1977).

CAPACITANCE SPIROMETRY

Respiratory activity has also been detected by placing one plate of a capacitor above the patient and the other behind the back. Changes in tidal volume change the capacitance so that respiratory movements can be detected. However, the method has not been used in clinical practice.

WASHOUT AND DILUTION METHODS

These techniques are most frequently used for measurements of functional residual capacity (FRC) but can also be used to measure other gas volumes which cannot be derived by water displacement. The principle can be illustrated by the nitrogen washout method of determining FRC. The patient breathes air through a non-breathing valve. At the end of a normal expiration two valves are turned so that the inspired gas is abruptly changed to pure oxygen, whilst the expired gas is directed into an empty Douglas bag. The patient continues to expire into the bag until the nitrogen has been washed out of the lungs (about 7 minutes in those with normal lungs) and the volume of the expired gas and its nitrogen concentration are measured. Since the gas in the lungs initially contained approximately 80% nitrogen the FRC must have been 100/80 times the volume of nitrogen collected in the bag. In practice corrections must be applied for the volume of nitrogen eliminated into the lungs from the tissues during the washout period, and for the small quantity remaining in the alveoli at the end of the washout.

The other common technique for determining FRC is the closed-circuit helium method. A measured volume of an insoluble gas such as helium is added to a spirometer containing oxygen. The gases are mixed by recirculating around the closed circuit of the spirometer and the volume of the spirometer circuit derived from the volume of helium added and its final concentration. The spirometer is then connected to the patient at the end of expiration and rebreathing continued until the gases in the lung and spirometer are thoroughly mixed. If He_1 and V_1 represent the initial concentration of He and the volume of gas in the spirometer, and He_2 is the final concentration of helium after dilution by the volume of gas in the lung (FRC), then

$$He_1 \times V_1 = He_2 \times (V_1 + FRC).$$

Thus FRC can be calculated.

Measurement of steady gas flow rate

Two basic principles are employed. In the first, flow rate is calculated from the volume of gas collected in unit time. This principle is of limited application but is widely used to standardize other methods. The second, which is the basis of most clinical methods of measuring flow, depends on the relationship between the pressure drop and flow rate across a resistance. In one application the pressure drop is maintained constant and flow is assessed by measuring the size of the orifice required to transmit the flow (variable orifice flowmeter). In the second method the size of the orifice is kept constant and the flow rate is determined by measuring the pressure drop across the orifice (fixed orifice flow meter).

Volume/time methods

The volume of gas is determined by collecting it in a container of known size or by measuring it with a gas meter, spirometer or some other volume measuring device. The simplest clinical application of this method is the measurement of rotameter or oxygen by-pass flow on an anaesthetic machine by measuring the time taken to fill the 2 litre reservoir bag. If this takes 5 seconds the flow rate is $2/5 = 0.4$ litres per second or 24 litres per minute. More accurate measurements are obtained by passing a large volume of the gas through a wet or dry gas meter for a known time, but if the volume is small, the greatest accuracy is obtained by using a carefully-calibrated spirometer. Most accurate flowmeters are calibrated by spirometers, appropriate corrections being made for any changes in pressure and temperature between the flowmeter and spirometer. The wet spirometer has the additional advantage that changes in flow rate during the measurement can be identified from changes in the slope of the record of volume against time.

Pressure drop/orifice methods

VARIABLE ORIFICE FLOWMETERS

Rotameter

This type of flowmeter has now displaced most of the other types of flowmeter previously used in anaesthesia. Although it was patented in Aachen in 1908 and first used in anaesthesia in 1910, it was not fitted to the Boyle's machine until 1937.

A rotameter consists of a vertical glass tube inside which rotates a light metal alloy bobbin. The flow of gas is controlled by the fine-adjustment flow control valve at the bottom of the rotameter and when this is opened the pressure of the gas forces the bobbin up the tube. The inside of the tube is shaped like an inverted cone, so that the cross-sectional area of the annular space around the bobbin is greater at the top end of the tube than it is at the bottom. Since the weight of the bobbin is constant, the bobbin will rise until the cross-sectional area of the annular space yields a pressure drop which exactly opposes the downward pressure resulting from the weight of the bobbin. The pressure drop therefore remains constant throughout the range of flows for which the tube is designed, and the bobbin floats freely in the stream of gas. Friction between the bobbin and tube wall is avoided by adding vanes to the bobbin so that it rotates in the stream of gas, and additional stability at low flow rates is achieved by modifying the shape of the bobbin (Fig. 15.11).

Each rotameter has to be calibrated for a specific gas. The reason for this becomes apparent when the physical principles are considered (Fig. 15.12). At the bottom of the rotameter the length of the bobbin is much greater than the distance between the bobbin and glass. The channel therefore approximates to a tube and, providing flow is laminar, Poiseuille's formula is applicable. In this situation viscosity is an important determinant of pressure drop:

pressure difference

$$\propto \frac{\text{viscosity} \times \text{length} \times \text{flow rate}}{(\text{radius})^4}$$

As the bobbin rises, the distance between bobbin and tube increases, so that the space around the bobbin approximates more to an orifice than to a tube. For flow through an orifice the density becomes an important factor: pressure drop $\propto$ density $\times$ (velocity)^2. Since the transition from a tubular space to an orifice is not clearly defined, and since a certain amount of turbulence must occur even at low flow rates, it is apparent that each rotameter must be calibrated

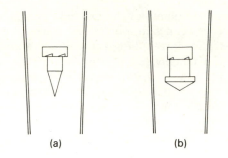

Fig. 15.11. Rotameter tubes showing a. original shaped bobbin and b. bobbin modified to increase stability at low flow rates.

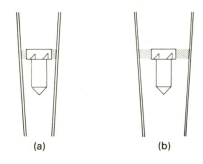

Fig. 15.12. Physical principles underlying measurement of flow by rotameter. a. At the bottom of the tube the length of the annular space is greater than the distance between tube and bobbin. b. At the top of the tube the annular space approximates to an orifice.

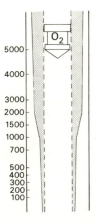

Fig. 15.13. Non-linear scale on rotameter. The shaded area illustrates how the annular space between bobbin and tube increases as the bobbin moves up the tube.

specifically for one gas. Furthermore, since viscosity and density vary with temperature and pressure, the calibration must be carried out under the appropriate conditions.

The flow rate is indicated by the position of the top of the bobbin. Under ideal conditions the indicated flow rate should be within $\pm 2\%$ of the true flow rate. However, as indicated later (p. 195) this accuracy is rarely retained under clinical conditions (Waaben, Stokke & Brinkløv 1978).

Further complexities in calibration have resulted from the introduction of rotameters in which portions of the scale are expanded so that increased accuracy of reading is available over specific ranges of flow. This feature is made possible by varying the taper of the cone in different parts of the tube. However, if the scale is read carelessly or the marking is not clear, serious errors can result from incorrect gas flow settings. It is essential therefore to observe where the deviations from linearity occur, before using the flowmeter (Fig. 15.13).

Other variable orifice flowmeters

A number of other types of variable orifice flowmeters have been used in the past but are now only of historical interest. The main types are illustrated in Fig. 15.14.

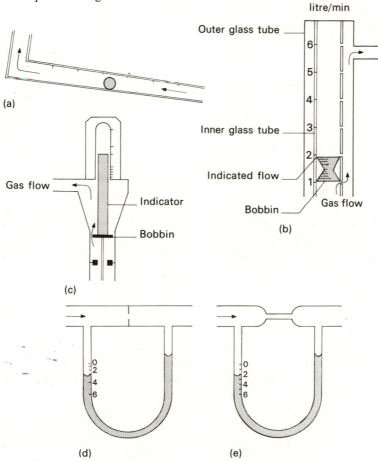

Fig. 15.14. Other forms of variable orifice constant pressure drop flowmeters used in the past. a. Ewing (two balls were used for stability in the inclined tube flowmeter on the Connell 'stratosphere' anaesthetic machine), b. Coxeter, c. Heidbrink, d. Orifice type water depression flowmeter with non-linear scale, e. laminar flow type with linear scale.

VARIABLE-PRESSURE FLOWMETERS

Water-depression flowmeter

This type of flowmeter was widely used in the United States on Foregger anaesthetic machines. There were two basic designs (Fig. 15.14). In one the gas was caused to flow through an orifice and the pressure drop across the orifice was measured with a water manometer. Since the pressure drop across an orifice is proportional to the square of the flow rate, the scale was non-linear, being crowded at the lower readings and expanded at the higher readings. This was obviously undesirable for anaesthesia, and so parallel-sided tubes were substituted for the orifice. This ensured that flow was laminar, and consequently the pressure drop was proportional to flow rate: a linear scale could therefore be obtained. It was, however, necessary to provide a number of flow-meters in parallel to obtain accuracy over a wide range of flow rates, and there was always the danger of blowing water into the patient circuit when the cylinders were suddenly opened.

Bourdon gauge flowmeter

In this instrument a Bourdon gauge is used to sense the pressure drop across an orifice so that the scale is nonlinear (Fig. 15.15). The meter is rugged, not affected by changes in position, and useful for metering the flow from gas cylinders when transporting patients from one place to another. It is, however, affected by back pressure, and complete occlusion of the outlet will cause the meter to record maximum flow. In some types of meter an aneroid system is used

instead of the Bourdon gauge to detect the pressure difference.

VARIABLE ORIFICE AND VARIABLE PRESSURE DROP FLOWMETERS

Water-sight flowmeter

This type of flowmeter was used in the earlier models of the Boyle's machine (Fig. 15.16). Both the pressure drop and the cross-sectional area of the orifices increased as flow increased. The gas was passed through

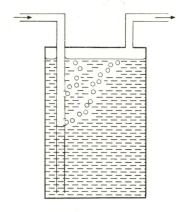

Fig. 15.16. Water-sight flowmeter.

a tube which was immersed in water and escaped through one or more holes bored in the side of the tube. The pressure drop across the hole was balanced by the hydro-static pressure of the external water column. If flow rate was increased the pressure drop across the hole was increased and the water in the flowmeter was forced down until the gas could escape through a lower hole. Observation of the lowest hole through which the gas was bubbling yielded a

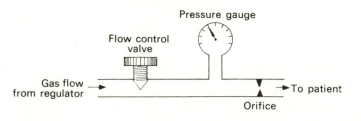

Fig. 15.15. Bourdon gauge flowmeter.

measure of flow rate. The height of water in the reservoir had to be kept constant and high flows of gas could not be used since the resultant excessive bubbling prevented proper observation of the tubes.

SOURCES OF ERROR WHEN USING FLOWMETERS

Errors most commonly occur as the result of sticking of the rotameter bobbin. This may be caused by the tube not being vertical, by the presence of dirt in the tube or by the attraction between bobbin and tube produced by electrostatic charges. Errors from the latter source are particularly common when the bobbin is being regularly depressed by the use of intermittent positive pressure ventilation and at low flow rates may result in an inaccuracy of up to 35% of the reading (Hagelsten & Larsen 1965; Greenbaum & Hesse 1978).

Sticking of the bobbin was at one time very common in cyclopropane flowmeters. The trouble developed when manufacturers started to fit flowmeter control valves which isolated cyclopropane under pressure in the tube connecting the cylinder to the flowmeter control valve. When the ambient temperature fell at night the gas liquified and dissolved small quantities of grease and debris from the connecting tube. These impurities were carried into the flowmeter when flow was next restored (Russell 1961). This problem was overcome by changing the type of grease used in the flowmeter control valve and by connecting the cylinder to the rotameter with metal instead of rubber tubing.

Errors in delivered gas concentration may be caused by factors other than flowmeter inaccuracy. The most common causes are a leak from a cracked rotameter tube, a deficient sealing washer between the tube and the rotameter block or a leak from the tube connecting the top of the flowmeters (Thompson 1976). To reduce the risk of hypoxia caused by a leak between the oxygen and nitrous oxide flowmeters Eger et al. (1963) suggested that the oxygen

flowmeter should be situated nearest the outlet from the flowmeter bank. This suggestion has not been taken up because of the possible confusion which might occur during any transition period. Finally, it is important to remember that the position of the bobbin may not be noticed if it is driven to the top of the rotameter tube by a high gas flow. This complication can only be prevented by checking that all flowmeter control valves are at the 'off' position before the flowmeters are put into service.

EFFECT OF PRESSURE ON FLOWMETERS

The pressure within a flowmeter may be altered by a variation in ambient pressure or by a change in the resistance to outflow. The effects of changes in ambient pressure are seen at altitude or when the flowmeter is used in a hyperbaric chamber. Alterations in outflow resistance are more commonly encountered and may be caused by the attachment of anaesthetic vaporizers, nebulizers or gas-driven ventilators (e.g. the Manley).

Under hyperbaric conditions the density of the gas is increased so that at a given flow rate a larger orifice will be necessary to maintain the same pressure difference. In other words a rotameter will read high in a pressure chamber. McDowall (1964) has found that the actual flow (F_A) is given by the equation:

$$F_A = F_I \times \sqrt{\frac{\rho_0}{\rho_1}}$$

where F_I is the indicated flow under hyperbaric conditions whilst ρ_0 and ρ_1 are the densities of the gas at atmospheric and hyperbaric pressures respectively. Thus, if pressure is increased to two atmospheres absolute, density is doubled and

$$\sqrt{\frac{\rho_0}{\rho_1}} = \sqrt{\frac{1}{2}}$$

so that F_A is 71% of F_I. It should be noted that F_A is the volume flow rate which is actually occurring under the hyperbaric conditions existing in the chamber. Similar reasoning indicates that with a constant orifice meter (e.g. Bourdon gauge meter) the pressure difference for a given flow rate will be greater under hyperbaric conditions so that this too will read high.

When back pressure is exerted on a rotameter by attaching a nebulizer or ventilator to the outlet the circumstances are different, for the gas issuing from the nebulizer or expired by the patient on a ventilator is at atmospheric pressure. It is necessary therefore to consider both the effect of the back pressure on the rotameter reading and the change in gas volume resulting from the transition to atmospheric pressure. As has already been shown, increasing the pressure in the rotameter increases the density so that the actual flow is less than the indicated flow. However the density of a gas is proportional to its absolute pressure so that if P_F represents the pressure in the flowmeter and P_B represents atmospheric pressure

$$F_A = F_I \sqrt{\frac{P_B}{P_F}}.$$

But F_A represents the actual flow measured under the pressurized conditions in the flowmeter. When the pressure of this gas becomes atmospheric its volume will increase in the ratio P_F/P_B so that the flow measured at atmospheric pressure (F_B) will be:

$$F_B = F_I \sqrt{\frac{P_B}{P_F} \times \frac{P_F}{P_B}} = F_I \sqrt{\frac{P_F}{P_B}}.$$

Thus, the flow at atmospheric pressure will be larger than the flow indicated on the flowmeters. If the back pressure is of the order of 13 kPa (100 mmHg or 860 mmHg absolute), the actual flow is about 7% greater than indicated flow (Conway 1974).

There is a further error in the flow measurement arising from the effect of increased outlet pressure on flow through the flow control valve. This also depends on the pressure drop across it, normally about 4 bars (400 kPa). If the outlet pressure rises by 13 kPa, there is a 3.25% fall in the pressure drop across the orifice of the fine-adjustment needle valve and a corresponding real drop in the flow. Thus, a seven litre flow of N_2O will fall by about a quarter of a litre.

The problems introduced by back pressure on rotameters can be easily overcome by placing the fine-adjustment flow control valve on the outlet side of the rotameter instead of the inlet side. The gas in the tube is thus constantly pressurized to regulator-outlet pressure, and back pressure effects are reduced to the effect on the flow through the flow control valve. Special precautions have to be taken to prevent leaks from the rotameter, and the flowmeter must be calibrated under the correct pressure conditions, but such pressure-compensated flowmeters are now being widely used.

Measurement of unsteady gas flow rates

The instruments so far described possess marked inertia so that they respond relatively sluggishly to rapid changes in flow rate. Furthermore, they are essentially direct reading instruments which cannot be connected easily to a recording system. More sophisticated instruments are therefore required to record flow rates which vary rapidly with time.

VARIABLE PRESSURE DROP (FIXED ORIFICE) FLOWMETERS

Pneumotachograph

This instrument measures flow rate by sensing the pressure drop across a laminar resistance. The pressure difference across the resistance is kept small (usually less than 0.1 kPa or 10 mmH$_2$O) so that the flow of gas is minimally affected by the resistance, and the pressure tappings are carefully designed to ensure that the differential manometer senses the true lateral pressure exerted by the gas on each side of the resistance element.

Two types of pneumotachograph head are in common use (Finucane, Egan & Dawson 1972). In the Fleisch head (Fig. 15.17a) the resistance consists of a bundle of parallel-sided tubes each tube having a diameter of 1–2 mm. Since reducing the diameter of a tube increases both the pressure drop and the critical velocity, this arrangement yields the biggest possible pressure drop whilst conserving laminar flow. The number of tubes is matched to the desired range of flow rates. The resistance unit is made by rolling strips of corrugated and plain foil into a cylinder and then enclosing the unit within an electric coil. The coil is heated to prevent condensation when the instrument is being used with moist gases. The pressure tappings consist of a series of holes in the casing at each end of the resistance unit. These lead into two annular chambers ('piezometer rings') which are connected to the differential manometer by flexible tubes.

In the Lilly type of head (Fig. 15.16b) the resistance unit consists of a layer of metal or plastic gauze, the pressure tappings being taken from each side of the gauze. When metal gauze is used it may be heated to prevent condensation. A plastic mesh causes less condensation and does not require heating if used for short periods. Recently, it has been suggested that the problem of condensation can be overcome by using a resistance unit which consists of a diaphragm with a V-shaped incision in it. The resulting flap opens progressively as flow is increased and so maintains a direct relationship between pressure and flow. This type of head may be very useful for long-term monitoring (Osborn 1978). When using both types of head it is important to ensure that the gas flow is spread evenly across the resistance unit. It is also essential to adjust the size of head to the expected flow rates, for turbulence causes non-linearity if the specified flow is exceeded. On the other hand the use of too large a head results in a very small pressure signal and an unnecessarily large dead space. A Fleisch No. 2 head, for example, has a dead space of 16 ml, is linear to within $\pm 5\%$ from 0–60 l/min, and gives a pressure of about 0.1 kPa (10 mmH$_2$O) at the maximum rated flow rate. The size of the pressure drop depends not only on the characteristics of the resistance but also on the viscosity of the gas. This in turn, is temperature and, to a small extent, pressure dependent (Hobbs 1967). Thus, whilst it is relatively easy to achieve an output signal which does not deviate by more than $\pm 5\%$ of the actual flow when a single gas is being measured at atmospheric temperature and pressure, it is much more difficult to compensate for the differences in pressure, temperature, humidity and composition between the inspired and expired gas of a patient on a ventilator. (Humidity is a particular problem since water vapour has a markedly lower viscosity than dry air.)

The differential manometer needs to be very sensitive to record the small changes

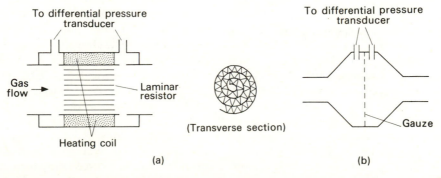

(a)

(b)

Fig. 15.17. Pneumotachograph. a. Longitudinal section and transverse sections of Fleisch head showing corrugated foil wound into a spiral. b. Longitudinal section of Lilly type of head.

in pressure across the resistance. Furthermore, since this signal may be integrated to give volume, the manometer must have very good zero and gain stability. It is important to ensure that the geometry of the gas path from each side of the transducer diaphragm to the head is similar so that abrupt changes of pressure within the head (e.g. from intermittent positive pressure ventilation) do not produce transient pressure artefacts from the transducer (Kafer 1973; Churches *et al.* 1977). Pneumotachographs have been widely used in both respiratory and anaesthetic research. Although their principles are easy to understand their practical application is very much more difficult.

Two other types of variable-pressure flowmeter must be mentioned, although they have not been widely used clinically.

Venturi tube flowmeter

When gas passes through a narrowed portion of tube it accelerates. Some potential energy is thus converted to kinetic

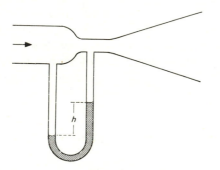

Fig. 15.18. Venturi tube flowmeter. The difference in pressure *h* is related to the flow rate.

energy and the pressure recorded from a side arm in the constricted part of the tube is less than the pressure in the wider part of the tube (Fig. 15.18). Because the pressure difference is roughly proportional to the square of the flow rate, the scale is nonlinear, sensitivity being least at low flow rates. Furthermore, the instrument is very sensitive to changes in the density of the gas.

Pitot tube flowmeter

This again utilizes the difference between the amount of potential and kinetic energy possessed by the gas. The potential energy is proportional to its pressure, and the kinetic energy is proportional to its velocity. In the pitot tube flowmeter (Fig. 15.19) the kinetic energy is sensed by the difference

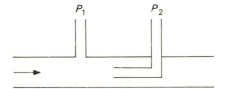

Fig. 15.19. Pitot tube flowmeter.

in pressure between a tube facing into the stream of gas and a tube measuring the lateral pressure exerted by the gas. This pressure difference is proportional to the square of flow rate, so that the scale is again nonlinear. Furthermore the range of flow which can be accommodated by any particular instrument is somewhat limited. These disadvantages have discouraged its use in clinical practice.

VARIABLE ORIFICE (FIXED PRESSURE DROP) FLOWMETERS

The peak flowmeter

The peak expiratory flow rate which can be achieved by normal adults often exceeds 500 litres/min. Peak flow can be measured by a pneumotachograph or dry spirometer, but a more useful clinical instrument is the peak flowmeter (Wright & McKerrow 1959). This is basically a variable orifice meter and is capable of measuring flows up to 1000 litres/min with the imposition of only a small resistance to gas flow.

The meter consists of a metal cylinder about 12 cm in diameter and 6 cm deep. The cylinder contains three compartments (Fig. 15.20). The first is shallow and contains the dial and pointer. The middle compartment

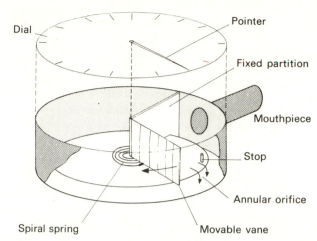

Fig. 15.20. Peak expiratory flowmeter.

contains the measuring apparatus and communicates with the third compartment via an annular orifice around the circumference of a metal partition. A mouthpiece is attached to the wall of the middle chamber and a fixed partition deflects the expired air onto a movable vane. The vane fits the inside of the cylinder closely and is free to rotate around a central axle. The air flow causes the vane to rotate against the force exerted by a light spiral spring. The movement of the vane opens up a section of the annular orifice which thus permits the air to escape through holes in the outer casing of the third compartment to the atmosphere. As the force exerted by the spiral spring is essentially constant throughout the range of movement of the vane, the position adopted by the vane depends primarily on the flow rate and on the area of the annular orifice which must be exposed to the air flow to maintain a constant pressure difference. The vane is very light and rapidly attains a maximum position in response to the peak expiratory flow. It is then retained in this position by a ratchet, which can be released after the reading has been taken. The reading is obtained from a pointer which is attached at an angle of 180° to the vane, and so balances it. The meter tends to under-read when compared with the peak expiratory flow rate recorded by a pneumotachograph, but there is a consistent relationship between the two measurements.

The patient must be encouraged to expire as rapidly as possible but the total volume expired is much less than that of an FVC manoeuvre, since only peak flow rate is being measured. It is essential that the meter should be held with the axis of the mouthpiece horizontal and with the dial pointing to the right of the patient. This minimizes the effect of gravity on the position of the vane. The peak flowmeter is now tending to be replaced by various types of peak flow gauge which are cheaper and yet yield similar results (Campbell *et al.* 1974; Wright 1974; Wright 1978). These work on a similar principle, a light piston being displaced down a cylinder to open up a linear orifice running down the length of the cylinder (Fig. 15.21). The piston is again opposed by a very light spring and is either held in the position of maximal displacement by a ratchet or displaces a sliding pointer which indicates the peak flow rate. The instrument must also be held horizontal when making the measurement and the breath expelled as rapidly as possible. With all these instruments the measurement is re-

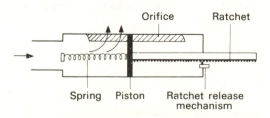

Fig. 15.21. Peak flow gauge.

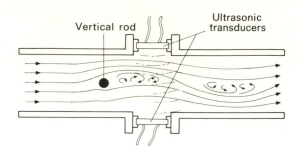

Fig. 15.22. Ultrasonic flowmeter.

peated 3–5 times and the maximum reading recorded. This is compared with normal values derived from a nomogram (e.g. Cotes 1975).

OTHER DEVICES FOR MEASURING GAS FLOW

Thermistor flowmeter

This consists of a small thermistor mounted in a tube. The change in temperature between inspired and expired air produces cyclical changes in temperature, which can be displayed on a meter or used as a ventilator failure alarm. Whilst this device is useful as a qualitative monitor of respiration, quantification is almost impossible since the composition of expired gas varies throughout expiration. However, when the temperature and composition of the flowing gas can be kept constant, the cooling effect on a heated wire or heated thermistor can be used to measure flowrate. Such a device has been incorporated into a venturi system. The expired gas is passed through a venturi which in turn sucks air through a thermistor probe unit attached to the narrow part of the venturi. Since the gas passing over the thermistor has a constant composition (air) it is possible to produce a quantitative result.

Ultrasonic flowmeter

Although a system utilizing the Doppler technique has been used for respiratory function testing the most successful technique appears to be that employed in the Ohio ventilation monitor. In this system the gas is passed through a tube containing a rod which is placed at right angles to the direction of gas flow (Fig. 15.22). The eddies created by this rod set up a series of oscillations in the flowing gas which are sensed by an ultrasonic detector working on the Doppler principle. Since the frequency of the oscillations is related to flow rate, a flow signal can be derived which can be electronically integrated to give volume. It is claimed that the system is little affected by temperature, humidity or changes in the composition of respired gas.

References

ADAMS A.P., VICKERS M.D.A., MUNROE J.P. & PARKER C.W. (1967) Dry displacement gas meters. *British Journal of Anaesthesia*, **39**, 174.

BERNSTEIN L., D'SILVA J.L. & MENDEL D. (1952). The effect of the rate of breathing on the maximum breathing capacity determined with a new spirometer. *Thorax*, **7**, 255.

BYLES P. (1960). Observations on some continuously acting spirometers. *British Journal of Anaesthesia*, **32**, 470.

CAMPBELL I.A., PRESCOTT R.J., SMITH I., ANDERSON C., JOHNSON A. & CAMPBELL J. (1974) Peak-flow meter versus peak-flow gauge. *Lancet*, **ii**, 199.

CHURCHES A.E., LOUGHMAN J., FISK G.C., ABRAHAMS N. & VONWILLER J.B. (1977) Measurement errors in pneumotachography due to pressure transducer design. *Anaesthesia and Intensive Care*, **5**, 19.

COLLINS M.M., McDERMOTT M. & McDERMOTT J.T. (1964) Bellows spirometer and transistor timer for the measurement of forced expiratory volume and vital capacity. *Journal of Physiology (London)*, **172**, 39P.

CONWAY C.M. (1974) Anaesthesia and Measurement. *Proceedings of the Royal Society of Medicine*, **67**, 1087.

CONWAY C.M., LEIGH J.M., PRESTON T.D., WALTERS F.J.M. & WEBB D.A. (1974) An assessment of three electronic respirometers. *British Journal of Anaesthesia*, **46**, 885.

COTES J.E. (1975) *Lung Function: Assessment and Application in Medicine*. 3rd Ed. Oxford: Blackwell Scientific Publications.

COX L.A., ALMEIDA A.P., ROBINSON J.S. & HORSLEY J.K. (1974) An electronic respirometer. *British Journal of Anaesthesia*, **46**, 302.

DREW C.D.M. & HUGHES D.T.D. (1969) Characteristics of the Vitalograph spirometer. *Thorax*, **24**, 703.

DuBois A.B., BOTELHO S.Y., BEDELL G.N., MARSHALL R. & COMROE J.H. (1956) A rapid plethysmographic method of measuring thoracic gas volume. A comparison with a nitrogen washout method for measuring FRC in normal subjects. *Journal of Clinical Investigation*, **35**, 323.

DuBois A.B., BOTELHO S.Y. & COMROE J.H. (1956) A new method of measuring airway resistance in man using a body plethysmograph. Values in normal subjects and in patients with respiratory disease. *Journal of Clinical Investigation*, **35**, 327.

EGER E.I., HYLTON R.R., IRWIN R.H. & GUADAGNI N. (1963) Anesthetic flowmeter sequence—a cause for hypoxia. *Anesthesiology*, **24**, 396.

FINUCANE K.E., EGAN B.A. & DAWSON S.V. (1972) Linearity and frequency response of pneumotachographs. *Journal of Applied Physiology*, **32**, 121.

GEDDES L.A. & BAKER L.E. (1975) *Applied biomedical instrumentation*. 2nd Ed. New York: John Wiley & Sons.

GREENBAUM R. & HESSE G.E. (1978) Electrical conductivity of flowmeter tubes. *British Journal of Anaesthesia*, **50**, 408.

HAGELSTEN J.O. & LARSEN O.S. (1965) Inaccuracy of anaesthetic flowmeters caused by static electricity. *British Journal of Anaesthesia*, **37**, 637.

HOBBS A.F.T. (1967) A comparison of methods of calibrating the pneumotachograph. *British Journal of Anaesthesia*, **39**, 899.

JUETT D.A. (1977) Impedance pneumography and plethysmography. *British Journal of Clinical Equipment*, **2**, 69.

KAFER E.R. (1973) Errors in pneumotachography as a result of transducer design and function. *Anesthesiology*, **38**, 275.

McDOWALL D.G. (1964) Anaesthesia in a pressure chamber. *Anaesthesia*, **19**, 321.

NUNN J.F. & EZI-ASHI T.I. (1962) The accuracy of the respirometer and ventigrator. *British Journal of Anaesthesia*, **34**, 422.

OSBORN J.J. (1978) A flowmeter for respiratory monitoring. *Critical Care Medicine*, **6**, 349.

RUSSELL F.R. (1961) Deposits in the cyclopropane flowmeter. *British Journal of Anaesthesia*, **33**, 323.

THOMPSON P.W. (1976) Safety of anaesthetic apparatus. Chapter 9 in *Recent advances in anaesthesia and analgesia*. Number 12. Eds C.L. Hewer & R.S. Atkinson. London: Churchill-Livingstone.

WAABEN J., STOKKE D.B. & BRINKLØV M.M. (1978) Accuracy of gas flowmeters determined by the bubble meter method. *British Journal of Anaesthesia*, **50**, 1251.

WRIGHT B.M. & McKERROW C.B. (1959) Maximum forced expiratory flow rate as a measure of ventilatory capacity. *British Medical Journal*, **2**, 1041.

WRIGHT B.M. (1974) Peak-flow meter and peak-flow gauge. *Lancet*, **2**, 1151.

WRIGHT B.M. (1978) A miniature Wright peak-flow meter. *British Medical Journal*, **2**, 1627.

Chapter 16
Measurement of Blood Flow

The principles of flow measurement described in the last chapter can also be applied to the measurement of blood flow. However, the much greater density and viscosity of blood necessitate a number of modifications to the apparatus. Furthermore blood has some properties, such as electrical conductivity, which permit other measurement techniques to be used. In all these applications it is particularly important to differentiate between the measurement of flow rate and flow velocity (p. 182). For further details of the methodology see Roberts (1972) and McDonald (1974).

Direct measurement of steady flow in blood vessels

VOLUME/TIME METHODS

A number of relatively simple instruments have been used in physiological research to measure mean flow. The simplest method is to divert the flow into a graduated vessel for a known time. To prevent physiological alterations due to loss of blood from the circulation the Ludwig stromuhr can be utilized (Fig. 16.1).

ROTAMETERS

Rotameters have found a wide application both in industry and medicine. The basic principle is similar to the gas rotameter but the movement of the bobbin is sensed by recording the change in inductance in a coil when a soft-iron core attached to the rotameter rises within the coil (Fig. 16.2). By careful design the effect of viscosity changes

in the blood can be minimized so that calibration does not change appreciably with changing haematocrit.

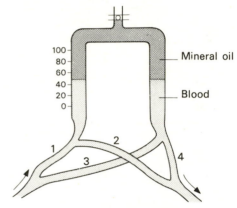

Fig. 16.1. Ludwig stromuhr. Blood normally flows in the direction shown by arrows. When tubes 2 and 3 are clamped blood flows into one chamber and out of the other. By using a stop watch it is possible to calculate the flow rate. On the next occasion tubes 1 and 4 are clamped to reverse the flow.

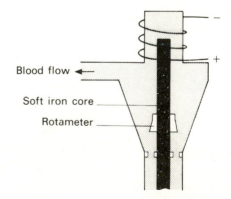

Fig. 16.2. Liquid rotameter. An increase in flow causes the rotameter to move upwards. This is sensed by the change of inductance in the coil produced by the movement of the soft iron core attached to the rotameter.

Another instrument utilizing a rotating vane is the Potter electroturbinometer. In this instrument the vane is built around a permanent magnet which is free to rotate in a tube inserted between the cut ends of a blood vessel. The speed of rotation of the rotor is sensed by a pick-up coil situated in the wall of the instrument. This instrument is remarkably stable and is capable of an accuracy of $\pm 5\%$. However, the resistance to flow is greater than with a good rotameter and it ceases to rotate at very low flows.

Heat-dissipation methods

The thermostromuhr is an example of an instrument which has been widely used. In one of the more recent modifications two thermistors are placed in close apposition to the blood vessel. The thermistors are separated by a heating coil and it is arranged that their electrical outputs oppose each other. When the heating coil is switched on the downstream thermistor will record a higher temperature than the upstream thermistor. The difference in temperature between the two thermistors is inversely related to blood flow. This instrument is reasonably accurate if flow is nonpulsatile, but may become very inaccurate when pulsatile flow is present.

Other heat-dissipation methods have been used. One of the simplest was a length of resistance wire passed down the length of the blood vessel. An electrical current was passed down the wire to heat it and the loss of heat, which was proportional to blood flow, was detected by measuring the change in resistance of the wire. A similar catheter tip flowmeter utilizing thermistors has been used more recently to measure pulsatile flow (p. 208).

LIMB PLETHYSMOGRAPHY

A simple clinical technique for measuring limb blood flow is that known as plethysmography. The venous return is intermittently occluded by abruptly pressurizing

a proximal cuff to a pressure of about 6–7 kPa (50 mmHg). After allowance for an initial occlusion artefact, the rate of increase of volume of the limb during the first few seconds after occlusion is directly related to the arterial flow. A number of techniques are available for measuring the rate of change of limb volume. In air or water plethysmographs the limb is sealed into a box and surrounded with air or water at a constant temperature close to that of the skin, the increase in limb volume being transmitted directly to a small recording spirometer. Some air-filled plethysmographs have a fixed volume, and measure

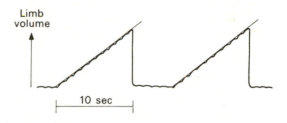

Fig. 16.3. Limb plethysmography. Recorded changes in limb volume following two occlusions of 10 s each. In this recording there was no initial occlusion artefact.

instead the small changes in pressure (Greenfield, Whitney & Mowbray 1963). Another simple form of plethysmograph is based on the demonstration by Whitney (1953) that the change in limb girth bears a direct relation to the change in limb volume. This change in girth is recorded with a mercury-in-rubber strain gauge which surrounds the limb. When the rubber tube containing the mercury is stretched it becomes longer and narrower. The electrical resistance of the column of mercury therefore increases. This change in resistance can be detected, amplified and recorded (Fig. 16.3).

The change in limb volume can also be recorded by measuring the change of electrical impedance of the limb (Nyboer 1970; Geddes & Baker 1975).

Direct measurement of oscillatory flow in blood vessels

METHODS BASED ON PRESSURE MEASUREMENT

In one method the difference in pressure between two points situated proximally and distally in the vessel is sensed with a double-lumen catheter and a differential electro-manometer. If the diameter of the vessel can be measured by angiographic techniques and if the velocity profile is reasonably laminar, it is possible to apply Poiseuille's equation to derive instantaneous flow. Unfortunately the mathematical analysis of the pressure curves is extremely complex and very high fidelity recordings are essential. The method has therefore not been widely applied in clinical practice.

Other methods are based on the analysis of the pulse wave contour recorded by intra-arterial pressure measurement (Wesseling et al. 1974). The analysis of the wave form is performed by a small bedside computer which can display beat-to-beat values for stroke volume, heart rate and cardiac output. However a preliminary calibration against some other standard technique (e.g. dye-dilution) is required to establish correction factors for each patient. Although preliminary observations appear promising, methods using this principle have not found wide favour.

ELECTROMAGNETIC FLOWMETERS.

These are the most widely-used instruments for the direct measurement of blood flow in both the experimental and clinical situation. The measurement technique is based on the laws of electromagnetic induction described by Faraday. If blood or other electrolyte flows at right angles to a magnetic field, then an electromotive force (e.m.f.) will be induced in a plane which is mutually perpendicular to the magnetic field and to the direction of fluid flow. The induced voltage can be measured by two electrodes situated in the appropriate plane and connected to a suitable detector circuit (Fig. 16.4). The induced voltage is proportional to the strength of the magnetic field and to the velocity of blood flow within the blood vessel. Since the flowmeter wraps around the blood vessel and forms a snug fit, the diameter of the vessel is held constant. By the application of a suitable calibration factor the velocity signal can therefore be read in terms of flow.

Although many of the earlier electromagnetic flow meters employed a constant magnetic field the method proved unsatisfactory, for the constant field generated a steady current round the detector circuit which caused polarization of the detector electrodes (p. 49). To overcome this, most modern instruments utilize an alternating magnetic field produced by an electromagnet supplied with either a sinusoidal, square wave or trapezoidal alternating

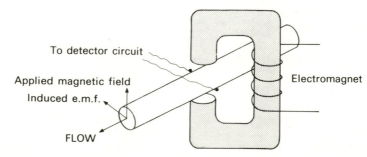

Fig. 16.4. Principle of electromagnetic flowmeter.

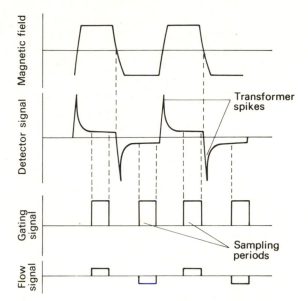

Fig. 16.5. Processing of signal from square wave electromagnetic flowmeter. The gating system causes the detector signal to be sampled when interference from the 'transformer spikes' is minimal. The flow signal is then rectified and displayed.

current (Geddes & Baker 1975). The use of an alternating field creates large artefactual signals in the detector circuit which result from the inductive forces generated by the rising and falling of the a.c. current. With a sine wave current the error signals are also sinusoidal, but out of phase with the flow signal and so can be eliminated by suitable electronic processing. In the case of the square-wave flowmeter, the error signals appear as spikes each time the curve reverses. These can be eliminated by using a simple gating technique (Fig. 16.5).

Although sine wave flowmeters are more complex than square wave instruments they are more efficient. This is an important consideration for it means that a smaller excitation current and magnet are required to produce any given output signal. However, many other factors must be considered when choosing an instrument for a given application.

One important factor is zero stability. In the experimental situation the zero reading can be checked by occluding the vessel with a clamp or pneumatic occluder. However, this is often impossible in the clinical situation or when flowmeters are used on the aorta or pulmonary artery. The problem has now been minimized by

using a pulsed energizing current as shown in Fig. 16.6. With this waveform there is a period of zero current flow; this can be used to automatically re-zero the instrument.

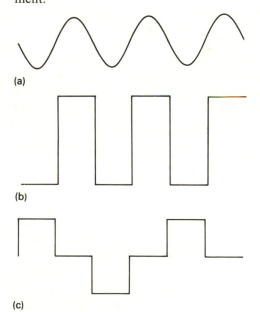

Fig. 16.6. Energising waveforms for electromagnetic flowmeters. a. Sinusoidal, b. square wave, c. pulsed-square wave with 'no-flow' interval which permits automatic zeroing of instrument.

A second factor is the type of probe which can be used. In some types of flow-meter the probe is an integral part of a cannula which is inserted between the cut ends of a blood vessel or, more commonly. incorporated into an extracorporeal per-fusion circuit. For most clinical and experi-mental applications the probe is C-shaped so that it can be slipped around the vessel. The probe must be carefully chosen so that it fits snugly round the vessel but does not compress it. This type of probe can be designed to produce a very even magnetic field, so that accurate measurements can be obtained, but it is important to ensure that changes in blood pressure or vessel tone do not impair the signal by creating a disparity between vessel and probe diameters. This not only alters the calibration but also impairs the detection of the very small voltages which are generated by the flow. A reduction in signal will also occur if the direction of the magnetic field deviates significantly from the perpendicular plane. With very small vessels an I-type probe is used. In this the electromagnet is placed to one side of the vessel. Although the resulting magnetic field is not as even as with the C-type, the resulting errors are usually acceptable providing the vessel is small. A recent introduction is a probe which is shaped like a strap and which can be wrapped round the aorta after cardiac surgery and used to monitor left ventricular output during the postoperative period. When measurements have been completed the probe is withdrawn through the chest incision with little more difficulty than withdrawing a chest drain.

The electromagnetic principle has also been used in a catheter-tip flow probe which can be passed into the heart or large vessels. In this probe both the detectors and electromagnet are within the catheter. Since the resulting magnetic field is very uneven the instrument yields measurements of the velocity of blood flow in close proximity to the catheter tip (Fig. 16.7). In the aorta where the velocity profile is relatively flat the positional error is not

great. However, absolute flow rates can only be measured if the aortic diameter can be determined by some other method.

Flow probes can be calibrated *in vitro* or *in vivo*. *In vitro* calibration is accom-plished by collecting the blood in a measur-ing cylinder for a given time and comparing this with the integrated signal from the flowmeter. *In vivo* calibration can be per-formed by placing a clamp distal to the flow

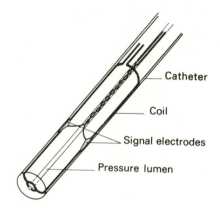

Fig. 16.7. Catheter tip flow probe (after Mills 1968).

probe and by withdrawing a measured quantity of blood through a needle placed between the probe and clamp. Alternatively the measurement can be calibrated against some indirect method of measuring flow, e.g. the indicator-dilution technique. The calibration factor of each probe remains reasonably constant with time so that once this has been established the machine can be set to match the flow probe in use. However the probe must be recalibrated if haematocrit changes. Flow probes are relatively robust and have been implanted for long term experiments in animals. How-ever, regular checks of their performance are desirable.

ULTRASONIC FLOWMETERS

These instruments detect the velocity of flow so that the actual flow rate can only be determined if the vessel diameter has been determined by an independent technique.

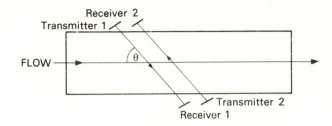

Fig. 16.8. Ultrasonic flow meter using transit time difference.

The fundamental requirement when using ultrasound is that the wavelength must be short compared with the dimension of the system being measured. Two different principles are used (see Chapter 9). In the first, two transmitter-receiver crystals are placed on opposite sides of the vessel so that one lies downstream from the other (Fig. 16.8). The upstream crystal transmits a pulse of ultrasound to the downstream crystal and the process is then reversed about 800 times a second. The transit time of the pulses between the two crystals depends on the speed of transmission of ultrasound in blood and the distance between the two crystals. However, the transit time of the pulses moving downstream will be shorter than that of the pulses moving upstream because the transmitting medium is also moving downstream. This difference in transit time will depend on the angle between the transmitter-receiver axis and the direction of blood flow, and on the velocity of blood flow. Since the position of the crystals is fixed by the flowmeter the difference in transit time between the two directions can be related directly to blood velocity. An extremely sensitive and stable detecting device is required to measure the very small difference between the transit times, but the method has the advantage that the direc-tion, as well as the velocity, of flow is indicated.

The second type of ultrasonic flowmeter utilizes the Doppler principle. In this instrument a combined transmitter-receiver crystal is directed at an angle to the flowing stream (Fig. 16.9). The ultrasound beam is reflected from the moving corpuscles, the frequency of the reflected sound depending upon the direction and velocity of blood flow. Ultrasound reflected from corpuscles moving away from the transmitter will have a lower frequency than that transmitted, while that reflected from corpuscles moving towards the transmitter will have a higher frequency. The difference between transmitted and received frequencies is the *Doppler* frequency (see Chapter 9) which is directly proportional to the velocity of the reflecting surface with respect to the transmitter. Since the difference is small, the Doppler frequency is usually within the audible range, so can be monitored using a loudspeaker or headphones. The Doppler flowmeter generates a signal whose amplitude is proportional to the frequency of the Doppler signal, and therefore to mean corpuscular velocity. Simple instruments cannot discriminate between blood flowing towards or away from the transmitter. If flow reversal is possible in the vessel under study, a more sophisticated device must be

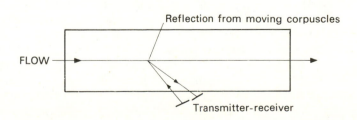

Fig. 16.9. Ultrasonic flow meter utilizing Doppler principle.

used, which by detecting whether the reflected signals are higher or lower in
frequency than the transmitter, can be made
fully directional.

Doppler instruments have proved useful
in many clinical situations for the transducer can be situated some distance away
from the vessel. Ultrasound is reflected by
an air-tissue interface so that the transducer
must be coupled to the vessel or skin with
a liquid or gel acoustic coupling medium.
Ultrasound is also reflected strongly by
bone so that blood-flow measurements
within the skull are impracticable. Some
attenuation of the ultrasound beam by body
tissues also occurs. Since the attenuation
increases with frequency, and the best
resolution is only obtained at high frequencies, some compromise in respect of
frequency must be made. Another problem
is that the recorded velocity depends on the
angle between the ultrasound beam and the
direction of flow. Despite these problems
the instrument has proved useful in detecting the presence of flow in peripheral
arteries or in peripheral veins. Thus it has
been used to detect flow in the radial
artery after prolonged arterial cannulation
(Bedford & Wollman 1973), to detect
peripheral venous thrombosis in the legs,
to measure flow in the aorta (see p. 116 &
217) and to localize the placenta (Brown
1967, 1971).

THIN-FILM FLOWMETERS

Considerable advances in thermal techniques of measuring flow have been made
by Bellhouse *et al.* (1968). The probe consists
of a small glass bead on the end of a catheter.
Three thin metallic rings about 1 μm in
thickness are deposited on the bead. The
central ring acts both as a resistance
thermometer (page 266) and as a heating
element. It is incorporated in a Wheatstone
bridge which is in turn connected to a high
gain amplifier so that any fall in temperature
of the resistance causes an increased heating
current to flow through the element. Thus
the temperature is maintained constant

slightly above the surrounding blood
temperature whatever the prevailing flow
conditions. Changes in flow velocity are
then detected by measuring the fluctuations
in power necessary to balance the bridge.
The two end rings are used to detect the
direction of flow by sensing the difference
in temperature of blood which has passed
over the central, heated ring. The instrument
has minimal thermal inertia and a remarkably fast response time. However, its
use has been mainly restricted to research
applications.

Indicator techniques for measuring blood flow

THE FICK PRINCIPLE

The Fick principle was enunciated in 1870
and has since formed the basis of many
techniques for measuring liquid flow. The

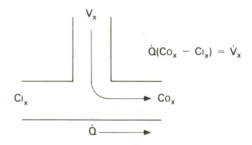

Fig. 16.10. The Fick principle. The quantity of
indicator exchanged per minute ($\dot{V}_x$) equals the
product of the flow per minute ($\dot{Q}$) multiplied
by the difference between the output and input
concentrations (C_O, C_I).

principle applies to any flowing stream of
liquid when a substance either enters or
leaves the stream. The principle states that
the flow of liquid in a given period of time
is equal to the amount of substance entering
or leaving the stream in the same period of
time, divided by the difference between the
concentrations of the substance before and
after the point of entry or exit (Fig. 16.10).

Use of O_2 and CO_2

When measuring cardiac output the uptake of oxygen or elimination of carbon dioxide from the blood is utilized. If the arterio-venous content difference is known then the flow can be calculated from the O_2 or CO_2 exchange in the lung. For example, if the arterio-venous O_2 difference is 50 ml/litre, then 50 ml of O_2 must be exchanged for every litre of blood flowing through the lungs. If the oxygen consumption is 300 ml/min then the cardiac output must be

$$\frac{300}{50} = 6 \text{ litres/min}$$

or cardiac output (litres/min)

$$= \frac{O_2 \text{ consumption (ml/min)}}{\text{arterio-venous } O_2 \text{ content difference (ml/litre)}}$$

Similar calculations can be applied to CO_2. One of the main problems in this *direct* Fick method is the difficulty of obtaining a sample of mixed venous blood. Mixed venous P_{CO_2} (but not P_{O_2}) can be estimated by the rebreathing technique (page 246) and CO_2 content calculated from the CO_2 dissociation curve, but the accuracy of such an *indirect* Fick method is inadequate for most clinical work. Furthermore, large errors result from the use of CO_2 as an indicator gas if changes in alveolar and arterial P_{CO_2} occur during the course of the measurements. The Fick technique can only be applied in steady-state conditions, the limiting factor being the accuracy of measurement of O_2 consumption or CO_2 output (usually $\pm 10\%$). Despite the technical difficulties and other objections to the method (Visscher & Johnson 1953; Chamberlain 1975) this still remains the standard by which other methods are judged.

Foreign gases

The Fick principle can also be applied to the absorption of a foreign gas by the blood during its passage through the lungs. If the concentration of the inert gas in mixed-venous blood is zero the rate of uptake from the lungs will be equal to the product of pulmonary capillary blood flow and the quantity contained in unit volume of end-pulmonary capillary blood. The latter can be calculated from the alveolar tension (P_{A_x}) and the blood solubility of the gas (λ_x). Then if $\dot{V}_x$ is the rate of uptake of the gas from the alveoli, the blood flow ($\dot{Q}$) is given by:

$$\dot{Q} = \frac{\dot{V}_x}{P_{A_x} \lambda_x}.$$

This fundamental principle forms the basis of three groups of techniques for measuring pulmonary blood flow. In the first group, the gas mixture containing a known concentration of a soluble gas is inhaled, the breath is held for a fixed period and the alveolar gas concentration then determined by analysis of an end-tidal sample. The procedure is repeated several times using different breath-holding periods and the rate of uptake at zero time obtained by extrapolating the semilog plot of gas concentration against time back to the ordinate. The pulmonary blood flow is then calculated from a knowledge of the solubility coefficient of the gas in the blood and from the alveolar volume at zero time. The latter is obtained by recording the change in concentration of an inert, insoluble gas, such as helium. This is included in the gas mixture to provide an indication of the dilution of inspired gas which occurs in the absence of absorption.

In the second group of methods the mixture of inert and soluble gases is rebreathed from a bag and the end-tidal concentrations are measured by continuously aspirating a small sample of gas from the mouthpiece into a mass-spectrometer. This technique overcomes many of the objections to the breath-hold methods but introduces other errors which are associated with the rebreathing procedure. However, the method is rapid, noninvasive and appears to give a reasonably accurate measurement of pulmonary capillary blood flow and lung tissue volume. Since the latter includes lung water, the technique has attractions for those working in the intensive care situation (Petrini, Peterson and Hyde 1978: Peterson *et al.* 1978).

The third technique enables instantaneous capillary flow to be measured continuously. The patient is seated in a body plethysmograph (page 189) and inhales a gas mixture containing about 15% of nitrous oxide (a moderately soluble gas). The uptake of the gas is measured continuously by recording the change in volume of the gas in the plethysmograph and the arterial concentration of the gas is obtained from the breath-holding or rebreathing technique as in the other two methods. The duration of the breath-hold or rebreathing period in all these techniques must, of course, be less than the recirculation time (20 s) otherwise the uptake of the soluble gas will be modified by the presence of this gas in mixed venous blood (Lee & DuBois 1955).

These three methods and the indirect Fick method measure pulmonary capillary flow through ventilated alveoli and therefore exclude flow through intrapulmonary shunts. This contrasts with the Fick and indicator dilution techniques which measure total blood flow. The three soluble gas methods also become inaccurate in the presence of ventilation/perfusion inequalities.

Kety–Schmidt technique

This technique was used to measure cerebral blood flow and represented another modification of the Fick principle (Kety & Schmidt 1945). The subject inhaled 10% nitrous oxide in air over a period of 10 minutes. During this period blood samples were taken at intervals from an artery and from the main venous drainage of the organ under study (e.g. internal jugular bulb). The blood samples were analysed for N_2O and the results plotted on a graph (Fig. 16.11). The arterial concentration rose quickly and

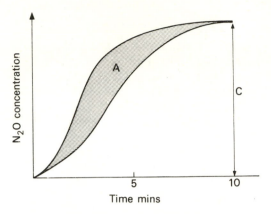

Fig. 16.11. Principle of Kety–Schmidt technique for measuring cerebral blood flow. The area (A) between the arterial and venous N_2O concentration time curves represents the quantity of N_2O taken up by the brain. At the end of 10 min inhalation the brain is fully saturated and the arterial and venous concentrations are almost equal (C).

the venous more slowly, but at the end of 10 minutes, both arterial and venous concentrations were almost equal. At this time venous concentration presumably equalled brain concentration. The quantity of nitrous oxide taken up by unit weight of brain must equal the final concentration (C) multiplied by the solubility coefficient of nitrous oxide in brain (λ). The quantity of nitrous oxide must be represented by the area between the arterial and venous curves (A) i.e. it is the sum of all the arterio-venous differences throughout the period of inhalation multiplied by the cerebral blood flow. Hence cerebral blood flow ($\dot{Q}$) can be calculated from the equation

$$\lambda C = \dot{Q} \cdot A \quad \text{or} \quad \dot{Q} = \frac{\lambda C}{A}.$$

Other indicators

Yet another application of the Fick principle is seen in the measurement of splanchnic blood flow. In this situation the indicator (generally bromsulphalein or indocyanine green) is injected at a constant rate into a peripheral vein but is almost completely cleared from the arterial blood during its passage through the liver. The difference in concentration is obtained by sampling arterial and hepatic venous blood after equilibrium conditions have been established. At this time the quantity of indicator being cleared by the liver must equal the infusion rate (R) so that.

$$\dot{Q} = \frac{R}{C_A - C_V}$$

where C_A and C_V are the arterial and venous concentrations respectively.

INDICATOR-DILUTION TECHNIQUES

Constant infusion

A substance is injected in known concentration (C_1) at known flow rate (F_1) into the upstream segment of a large vessel and thoroughly mixed with the blood passing the injection point. The blood is then sampled downstream. If the flow of blood in the vessel is F_2 and the downstream concentration of the indicator is C_2 then

$$F_1 \times C_1 = F_2 \times C_2 \quad \text{or} \quad F_2 = F_1 \times \frac{C_1}{C_2}.$$

The technique can also be used to measure limb or organ blood flow provided that there are single input and output channels, that the indicator is not altered during its passage through the region and that recirculation does not occur. These restrictions greatly limit its application.

Single-injection indicator dilution

In this technique an indicator is injected as a 'slug' into the vena cava, the right heart or, preferably, the pulmonary artery. The concentration of the indicator reaching the systemic side of the circulation is then plotted against time. The flow is worked out in the following manner. Suppose that 5 mg of indicator was injected, that the duration of the curve was 30 s and that the mean concentration of the indicator on the systemic side was 2 mg/litre (the latter is calculated from the area under the curve

divided by the duration of the curve). Then the 5 mg of indicator must have been diluted by $5/2 = 2.5$ litres of blood during the 30 s. Hence, the cardiac output must have been $60/30 \times 2.5 = 5$ litres/min.

The general formula is:

cardiac output

$$= \frac{60 \times \text{indicator dose (in mg)}}{\text{average concentration} \times \text{time (s)}}$$

in litres/min.

One of the problems with this method is that recirculation of indicator occurs before the downslope of the curve is complete (Fig. 16.12a). A number of techniques have been proposed to overcome the difficulty, but the most commonly-used method utilizes the exponential character of the downslope. If such a curve is replotted on a semilogarithmic scale a straight line results (Fig. 16.12b). The slope of the semilogarithmic plot is established from the top portion of the recorded dye curve. Points from the lower portion of this slope are then replotted back onto the original curve to define the tail of the curve which would have been recorded if recirculation had not occurred (Fig. 16.12a). The area may be measured by counting squares, weighing the paper enclosed by the curve or by planimetry.* Other methods of calculating the area of the curve have been devised but all involve a variable degree of approximation.

A number of indicators have been used for this technique. Of the dyes used indocyanine green (Cardio-green or Fox-green) is the most popular. It is non-toxic and has a relatively short half-life, so that repeated measurements can be made. It has a peak spectral absorption at 800 nm, which is the wavelength at which the absorption of

---

* A planimeter is an instrument for manual measurement of the area of a curve. One end of the instrument is fixed whilst the small wheel on the other end is moved round the area to be measured. The instrument mechanically integrates the movements of the wheel in the x and y axes and so gives a direct reading of the area of the curve.

oxygenated and reduced haemoglobin is identical. The measurement is therefore not affected by changes in arterial saturation. Indicator dilution curves have also been inscribed using radioactive tracers such as radioactive human serum albumin or chromium-labelled red cells (see page 130).

In the original Stewart–Hamilton method the concentration of dye or isotope in the systemic circulation was obtained by allowing a continuous stream of blood from a peripheral artery to flow into a series of small tubes which were supported at the periphery of a rotating disc and sequentially moved under the open end of the sampling catheter. Each of the thirty or so blood samples was then analysed separately and the curve plotted by hand. Nowadays the dye concentration is recorded by spectro-

photometric means, the arterial blood being sampled at a continuous rate of about $30\,ml \cdot min^{-1}$ through a cuvette densitometer by means of a motorized syringe. For radioactive measurements the arterial blood is drawn through a small coil situated within a scintillation detector. Baseline adjustments for both dye and radioactivity detectors are made by passing the patient's blood through the detector and calibration is then performed with blood samples containing known amounts of the indicator. A dynamic calibration may also be used. This is achieved by drawing a sample of the patient's blood through a mixing unit consisting of a small glass tube filled with glass beads. A known amount of the indicator is injected proximal to this tube so that an indicator–dilution curve appears down-

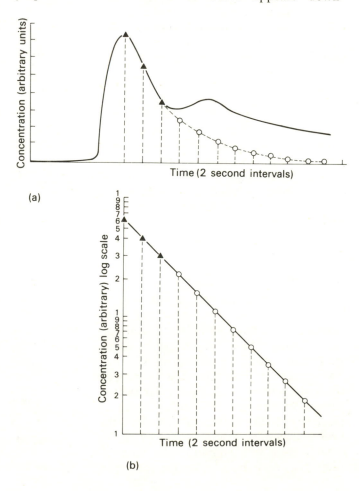

Fig. 16.12. a. Single injection indicator dilution curve showing distortion of downslope produced by recirculation. b. Replot on semilogarithmic paper.
▲ = points taken from the downslope in (a) to establish the slope of the replot in (b).
○ = points taken from (b) to plot tail of curve in (a).

stream to the mixing unit. The blood is then drawn through the densitometer or scintillation detector and the curve recorded in the usual way. The cardiac output may be calculated from the sampling flow rate, the doses of indicator injected into patient and mixing unit, and the areas under the two indicator dilution curves (Emmanuel *et al.* 1966).

Many attempts have been made to sense the changes in indicator concentration non-invasively. Earpiece densitometers have been extensively studied and have proved adequate for monitoring the direction of change in cardiac output but have not proved reliable for absolute measurements. A similar level of success has been achieved with radioactive indicators and external counting over the heart.

Thermal dilution methods have now become popular, particularly in the intensive care situation where pulmonary artery catheterization is frequently required for the monitoring of left-sided filling pressures. The principle of the method is similar to other indicator dilution methods but the injection and sampling are performed on the right side of the heart. Typically a slug of 10 ml normal saline or 5% dextrose solution at room temperature is injected into the right atrium and the temperature change is recorded by a thermistor in the pulmonary artery. The dilution curve which results is similar in shape to a dye dilution curve but there is no recirculation. The calculation is also similar but must naturally be worked out in terms of the 'heat dose'. Thus the numerator is the product of the difference in temperature between the injectate and blood multiplied by the density, specific heat and volume of the injectate. The denominator is the area under the temperature-time graph multiplied by the density and specific heat of blood.

Thermal dilution methods have a number of advantages (Wilson *et al.* 1972; Weisel, Berger & Hechtman 1975; Buchbinder & Ganz 1976). The indicator is cheap, non-toxic and repeated measurements may be made without much alteration in the 'base-line'. (With dyes or isotopes the background

level builds up progressively so limiting the number of estimations which can be performed.) Arterial puncture and blood withdrawal is not necessary and the absence of a recirculation curve greatly facilitates measurement of the area under the curve, particularly in low output, high central blood volume states where the recirculation curve may make dye dilution estimates of output grossly inaccurate. There are however a number of disadvantages to the thermal dilution technique. Firstly, it requires the passage and correct placement of a special catheter with a thermistor probe which is carefully matched to the processor. Such probes are expensive, particularly if combined with triple lumen catheters which permit injection of indicator and the recording of pulmonary artery and wedge pressures. A second disadvantage is that the bolus is large and mixing with the venous blood may be incomplete. The third disadvantage is that pulmonary arterial flow varies much more with intermittent positive pressure ventilation than does systemic flow: furthermore there are respiratory fluctuations in temperature in the pulmonary artery. Injection during inspiration may then give very different results from those obtained with injection during expiration. Finally, there is always the problem of correcting for the change of temperature of the injectate as it passes along the catheter.

Both dye and thermal dilution methods may now be used in association with mini-computers (Equipment review 1976). With the dye technique the initial part of the downslope is sampled automatically by the computer and all the computations are then carried out in a similar manner to those already described. The computer rejects the curve if the section sampled is not exponential or if the quality of the curve is unsatisfactory for some other reason. The dye calibration is also incorporated in the processing so that a direct digital or printed display is available within a few seconds of the curve being inscribed. The thermal dilution computer similarly utilizes the volume and temperature of the injectate, the patient's blood temperature and the dilution curve to produce the result. The use of such on-line techniques has greatly improved the understanding of acute circulatory problems.

Radioisotope techniques for measuring blood flow

The great advantage of radioisotopes over other indicators is that their radioactivity can often be detected by external counting as well as by blood sampling and counting *in vitro*. This greatly extends their possible range of use. There are, however, a number of difficulties which have to be overcome if they are to be used successfully. First, radioactive decay is a random process, so that accurate count rates can only be achieved by accumulating relatively large numbers of counts. Since the dose of radioactivity which can be administered is limited by possible radiation hazards it may be necessary to use prolonged counting periods or to use wide-angle collimators so that counts are collected from a wide area. As a result definition may be lost. A second problem is that radioactive counts may emanate from a number of tissues which lie within the field of view of the collimator. Thus radioactivity in the lung may be affected by radioactivity in the chest wall whilst count rates accumulated over the head may arise from brain, muscle and skin. Since the overlying tissues are closer to the counter they may unduly influence the total count rate. A third problem is that beta-particles are absorbed by a very small thickness of tissue so that external counting can usually only be carried out with gamma-emitting isotopes. Gamma-radiation with a low energy also tends to be easily absorbed whilst high energy radiation may penetrate the relatively thin layers of lead used in gamma camera collimators thus impairing definition. These considerations limit the choice of isotopes for a particular application.

Basically isotope techniques for measuring blood flow can be divided into those using nondiffusible indicators which remain within the bloodstream and those using diffusible indicators which diffuse throughout the body tissues.

NON-DIFFUSIBLE INDICATORS

Constant infusion

This technique is only suitable for measurements within large blood vessels or for measurements of flow through limbs or organs where all the flow enters and leaves the tissue through a single artery and vein. In the case of large blood vessels such as the inferior vena cava or aorta the radio-isotope is injected at a constant rate through one lumen of a double lumen catheter which is so designed that the indicator is caused to mix rapidly with the flowing blood. A sample is then withdrawn through the second lumen of the catheter, the tip of which is situated downstream from the injection site. In the organ or limb the injection is made into the artery and the sample withdrawn from the vein. Then, if A_1 and A_2 represent the concentration of the radioactivity in the injectate and sampled blood, and F_1 and F_2 represent the flow of injectate and blood flow respectively then:

$$F_1 \times A_1 = F_2 \times A_2 \quad \text{or} \quad F_2 = F_1 \times \frac{A_1}{A_2}.$$

Suitable indicators are albumin labelled with ^{125}I, ^{131}I or ^{113}In^m. Obviously recirculation of indicator will occur, thus altering the input of indicator to the system. Measurements must thus either be confined to a period of about 10–15 s after starting the injection or a correction must be applied for recirculation. Since the indicator does not diffuse into the tissues this can be achieved by sampling proximal to the site of injection. In most applications the sample can be obtained from a peripheral artery when equilibrium conditions have been achieved. Then if the arterial concentration of radioactivity is B:

$$(F_1 \times A_1) + (F_2 \times B) = (F_2 \times A_2)$$

or $$(F_1 \times A_1) = F_2(A_2 - B)$$

or $$F_2 = \frac{(F_1 \times A_1)}{(A_2 - B)}.$$

Bolus injection

A bolus of radioactivity can be injected into a central vein or the pulmonary artery and the radioactivity in a peripheral artery determined by drawing the sample at a constant rate through a coil situated in a well counter. The dose injected is obtained by measuring the radioactivity in the syringe before and after injection, and the sensitivity of the well counter is determined by aspirating a known dilution of the injected radioisotope through the coil. The technique is thus exactly analogous to that using a dye as the indicator.

Many attempts have been made to achieve noninvasive measurements by external counting over the heart. Although reasonable correlations with other methods of measuring cardiac output have been obtained by a number of authors it is difficult to obtain good curves and the method has therefore not become popular.

DIFFUSIBLE INDICATORS

Many diffusible indicators have been employed for measurement of blood flow. Probably the most popular is ^{133}Xe dissolved in saline. This radioisotope has a half-life of 5.3 days and emits gamma radiation, mainly in the two ranges of 30 keV and 81 keV, the latter energy being suitable for use with a gamma camera. Other radionuclides which have been used are ^{85}Kr, ^{13}N$_2$ and ^{81}Kr^m. ^{13}N$_2$ has the advantage that it is less soluble in blood than either xenon or krypton and is therefore almost completely cleared from the blood during its first passage through the lungs. However it has a short half-life (10 min) and is only available where there

is a cyclotron. ^{81}Kr^m is an isotope with a very short half-life (13 s) but is produced continuously by a portable generator utilizing a radioactive rubidium column. The generator is activated by irradiating the column in a cyclotron and produces a continuous supply of ^{81}Kr^m, the half-life of the generator being about $4\frac{1}{2}$ hours.

Diffusible indicators can be used to measure pulmonary blood flow by the Fick technique or to measure cerebral blood flow by the Kety–Schmidt method. Their use in the latter application obviates the time-consuming analyses of N$_2$O required for the performance of the original method (Lassen & Klee 1965) but the technique has now been dropped in favour of the clearance technique because of the general disadvantages of the Kety–Schmidt technique already mentioned.

Clearance methods

These are based on the two properties of diffusibility and relative insolubility. Thus after intra-arterial injection or absorption from the lungs the gas is distributed freely throughout the organ of interest. When the inflow of the gas is suddenly stopped the arterial blood will wash the isotope out of the tissue, the rate of clearance being exponential in character and dependent on the blood flow to the tissue. Good examples of clearance methods are those used to measure brain or muscle blood flow.

One technique for cerebral blood flow measurement employs a bolus of radioactive tracer which is injected into a carotid artery and detected by an array of scintillation detectors placed over the appropriate side of the head. The curve which is obtained (Fig. 16.13a) rises to a peak and then declines as the xenon is washed out by the subsequent blood flow. When this curve is analysed by replotting on semilog paper it is usually found to have an initial steep decline followed by a prolonged straight section (Fig. 16.13b). This indicates that the curve is probably representative of two tissue components, one having a relatively

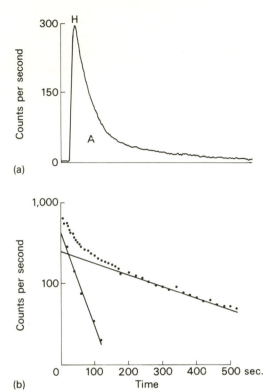

(a)

(b)

Fig. 16.13. a. ^{133}Xe clearance curve from brain after bolus injection into carotid artery. Blood flow can be calculated from the peak height (H) and the area under the curve (A) or from the initial slope. b. Semilogarithmic replot of a clearance curve showing fast and slow components.

fast washout and the other a much slower washout. These may correspond with the flows through white and grey matter. If the line drawn through the tail of the curve on the semilog plot is now projected back to cut the y-axis it is possible to subtract he values on this line from the values of the original curve to define the rate constant of the fast curve. This process is termed 'exponential stripping' and is now usually performed by a digital computer program.

However, it appears that for most practical purposes it is the fast component of the washout curve which is important so that it is usual to compare regional washouts by determining the initial slope. This is obtained by measuring the $T\frac{1}{2}$, the time taken for the curve to decline to half its initial value (McDowall 1969; Harper 1970). Then

$$\text{initial slope} = \frac{0.693}{T\frac{1}{2}}.$$

Attempts have been made to render the method noninvasive by giving the patient radioactive xenon to breathe until the brain tissue is saturated and then suddenly switching the breathing circuit to room air. Unfortunately the extracerebral tissues contribute significantly to the activity recorded and it is impossible to obtain a step change in arterial radioactivity because the lung radioactivity takes some time to washout. The analysis is therefore more complicated (McDowall 1976).

Another example of the use of this technique is the assessment of renal function. The isotope is injected intravenously and the radioactivity over the kidney is monitored. A curve is obtained which shows three, or sometimes, four phases (Fig. 16.14). There is an initial rapid rise in activity as the bolus of activity is transported to the kidney by the blood. This is followed by a slower rise in activity as the isotope is extracted from the blood and concentrated in the renal tubules. There is then a slow decline in activity as the radioisotope is carried away by the urine. Variations in the shape of the resultant renogram yield diagnostic information concerning the nature of the disturbance in renal function.

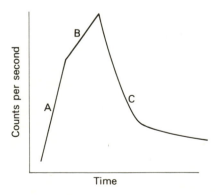

Fig. 16.14. A normal renogram. A = blood flow. B = tubular reabsorption. C = excretion.

A variation on this clearance technique can be used to measure muscle blood flow. In this case radioactive sodium or ^{133}Xe solution is injected directly into the muscle and the subsequent clearance followed with an external counter mounted above the site of injection.

Indirect techniques for estimation of cardiac stroke volume

Numerous methods have been devised, but none have become clinically established, due to difficulty of calibration and/or inherent inaccuracy.

Doppler ultrasonography

A beam of ultrasound is directed from the suprasternal notch towards the transverse arch of the aorta and is reflected from the blood cells as they move away from the transducer in the axis of the ultrasound beam. A geometrically-valid estimate of blood *velocity* can therefore be obtained from the Doppler signal (Cross & Light 1974). To derive a value for stroke volume, the velocity signal is multiplied by the cross-sectional area of the aorta and then integrated with respect to time during the ejection phase of the cycle. This calculation is based on the assumption that flow is turbulent and the velocity profile therefore uniform, and that the aortic dimensions remain constant. The cross-sectional area must be estimated from either aortography or more indirectly, from the result of simultaneous dye-dilution or thermal-dilution studies. The technique can yield reliable estimates of changes in stroke volume (Hanson & Bilton 1978) but absolute values are more difficult to obtain.

Ballistocardiography

In this technique, the patient is placed on an 'inertial table' which enables movements in the horizontal plane to be measured by sensitive accelerometers. The stroke volume can be deduced from the forces transmitted to the table during the course of systole. The method is complex, expensive, and does not readily lend itself to clinical practice (Smith 1969).

Impedance plethysmography

Since the electrical impedance of a block of tissue fluctuates according to the blood volume contained therein, it follows that a study of thoracic impedance changes should yield a signal from which stroke volume might be derived. Two circumferential electrodes are placed around the neck and two around the upper abdomen. A small (< 1 mA), constant, high frequency (> 1 kHz) alternating current is passed between the outer electrodes and the resulting potential difference detected by the inner pair. This potential is rectified, smoothed, and 'backed off' to yield a zero value. Changes in impedance due to respiration and cardiac activity are now seen as voltage fluctuations about this zero value. The respiratory signals are appreciably larger than those due to cardiac activity, so that measurements must be made either with the subject breath holding, or by utilizing an averaging technique. This is accomplished by using the ECG 'R' wave as a synchronizing signal, and averaging the impedance cardiogram over several cardiac cycles, so that the respiratory artefact, being asynchronous, is eliminated (Hull & Flanagan, 1969). The signal thus obtained represents changes in thoracic blood volume, and clearly resembles the pulse waveform. Since aortic flow carries blood out of the thorax in the later stages of systole, the stroke volume cannot be inferred directly from the signal, but must be computed indirectly. The initial rise in impedance represents the initial ejection of blood from the heart, and its first derivative the initial ejection flow rate. If the initial flow value is multiplied by the ejection period, a rough index of ejection volume is obtained. The ejection period can be derived from the impedance waveform, but is perhaps better defined by a simultaneous phonocardiogram. This index of stroke volume can be translated into absolute volume terms by comparison with simultaneous dye or thermal dilution studies. Comparing impedance and dye-dilution measurements in man, Baker (1969) showed that although a change in the impedance cardiogram correlated well with the direction of a change in stroke volume, it did not correlate well with the magnitude of change.

For a further discussion of the use of impedance measurements see Nyboer (1970); Geddes & Baker (1975); Juett (1977).

High-speed cine-ventriculography followed by planimetry and computation of serial ventricular volumes has also been used for estimation of stroke volume, as has *analysis of the aortic pressure waveform*. These techniques have not found any clinical usefulness.

References

BAKER L.E. (1969) Biomedical applications of electronic impedance measurements. In: *Progress in medical electronics*. Editors D.W. Hill and B. Watson. Cambridge: Cambridge University Press.

BEDFORD R.F. & WOLLMAN H. (1973) Complications of percutaneous radial-artery cannulation. *Anesthesiology*, **38**, 228.

BELLHOUSE B.J., SCHULTZ D.L., KARATZAS N.B. & LEE G. DE J. (1968) A catheter tip method for the measurement of pulsatile blood flow velocity in arteries. In *Blood flow through organs and tissues* Editors W.H. Bain and A.M. Harper. Edinburgh: Churchill Livingstone.

BROWN R.E. (1967) Ultrasonic localisation of the placenta. *Radiology*, **89**, 828.

BROWN R.E. (1971) Doppler ultrasound in obstetrics. *Journal of the American Medical Association*, **218**, 1395.

BUCHBINDER N. & GANZ W. (1976) Hemodynamic monitoring: invasive techniques. *Anesthesiology*, **45**, 146.

CHAMBERLAIN J.H. (1975) Cardiac output measurement by indicator dilution. *Biomedical Engineering*, **10**, 92.

CROSS G. & LIGHT L.H. (1974) Non-invasive intrathoracic blood velocity measurements in the assessment of cardiovascular function. *Biomedical Engineering*, **9**, 464.

EMMANUEL R., HAMER J., CHING B., NORMAN J. & MANDERS, J. (1966) A dynamic method for the calibration of dye dilution curves in a physiological system. *British Heart Journal*, **28**, 143.

Equipment review (1976) Cardiac output computers. *Biomedical Engineering*, **11**, 421.

GEDDES L.A. & BAKER L.E. (1975) *Principles of applied biomedical instrumentation. 2nd Ed.* New York: John Wiley and Sons.

GREENFIELD A.D.M., WHITNEY R.J. & MOWBRAY J.F. (1963) Methods for the investigation of peripheral blood flow. *British Medical Bulletin*, **19**, 101.

HANSON G.C. & BILTON A.H. (1978) Clinical experience with transcutaneous aortovelography: preliminary communication. *Journal of the Royal Society of Medicine*, **71**, 501.

HARPER A.M. (1969) Measurement of cerebral blood flow. In: *Cerebral Circulation*, Editor D.G. McDowall. Boston: Little Brown.

HULL C.J. & FLANAGAN G.J. (1969) The impedance cardiograph: development and application. *British Journal of Anaesthesia*, **41**, 791.

JUETT D.A. (1977) Impedance pneumography and plethysmography. *British Journal of Clinical Equipment*, **2**, 69.

KETY S.S. and SCHMIDT C.F. (1945) Determinations of cerebral blood flow in man by use of nitrous oxide in low concentrations. *American Journal of Physiology*, **143**, 53.

LASSEN N.A. & KLEE A. (1965) Cerebral blood flow determined by saturation and desaturation with Krypton 85. *Circulation Research*, **16**, 26.

LEE G. & DuBOIS A.B. (1955) Pulmonary capillary blood flow in man. *Journal of Clinical Investigation*, **34**, 1380.

McDONALD D.A. (1974) *Blood flow in arteries. 2nd Edition.* London: Edward Arnold.

McDOWALL D.G. (1969) Regional blood flow measurement in clinical practice. *British Journal of Anaesthesia*, **41**, 761.

McDOWALL D.G. (1976) Monitoring the brain. *Anesthesiology*, **45**, 117.

MILLS C.J. (1968) A catheter tip electromagnetic velocity probe for use in man. *In blood flow through organs and tissues*, p. 38. Editors W.H. Bain and A.M. Harper. Edinburgh: Churchill Livingstone.

NYBOER J. (1970) *Electrical impedance plethysmography. 2nd Edition.* Springfield, Illinois: Thomas.

PETERSON B.T., PETRINI M.F., HYDE R.W. & SCHREINER B.F. (1978) Pulmonary tissue volume in dogs during pulmonary edema. *Journal of Applied Physiology: Respiratory, Environmental and Exercise Physiology*, **44**, 798.

PETRINI M.F., PETERSON B.T. & HYDE R.W. (1978) Lung tissue volume and blood flow by rebreathing: theory. *Journal of Applied Physiology: Respiratory, Environmental and Exercise Physiology*, **44**, 782.

ROBERTS C. (ed.) (1972) *Blood flow measurements.* London: Sector Publishing.

SMITH N.T. (1969) Cardiac function evaluation. In *Techniques in clinical physiology.* Editors J.W. Bellville and C.S. Weaver. London: Collier-Macmillan.

VISSCHER M.B. & JOHNSON J.A. (1953) The Fick principle: analysis of potential errors in its conventional application. *Journal of Applied Physiology*, **5**, 635.

WEISEL R.D., BERGER R.L. & HECHTMAN H.B. (1975) Current concepts: measurement of cardiac output by thermodilution. *New England Journal of Medicine*, **292**, 682.

WHITNEY R.J. (1953) The measurement of volume changes in human limb. *Journal of Physiology (London)*, **121**, 1.

WILSON E.M., RANIERI A.J., UPDIKE O.L. & DAMMAN J.F. (1972) An evaluation of thermal dilution for obtaining serial measurements of cardiac output. *Medical Biological Engineering*, **10**, 179.

WESSELING K.H., SMITH K.T., NICHOLS W.W., WEBER H., DE WIT B. & BENEKEN J.E.W. (1974) Beat to beat cardiac output from the arterial pressure contour. In *Measurement in Anaesthesia*, Editors S.A. Feldman, J. Leigh & J. Spierdijk. London: University Press.

Further reading

PRYS-ROBERTS C. (1980) Measurement of cardiac output and regional blood flow. p. 531 in *The circulation in anaesthesia.* Ed. C. Prys-Roberts. Oxford: Blackwell Scientific Publications.

SMITH N.T. (1980) Non-invasive assessment of the cardiovascular system. p. 561 in *The circulation in anaesthesia.* Ed. C. Prys-Roberts. Oxford: Blackwell Scientific Publications.

Chapter 17
Gas and Vapour Analysis

There are four main applications of gas and vapour analysis to clinical practice. They are:

1 To establish the identity and concentrations of gases and vapours delivered to the patient by an anaesthetic circuit, incubator, oxygen tent or pipe-line installation.

2 To detect the presence of atmospheric pollution.

3 To assess metabolic or cardiorespiratory function either by the analysis of the respired gases (O_2, CO_2 and N_2) or by the use of inert tracer gases such as He, CO or Ar.

4 To detect the presence of abnormal concentrations of gases such as H_2 or CH_4 in expired air as an indication of abnormal bacterial colonization of the gut.

Chemical methods

Chemical methods of gas analysis are most commonly used for the estimation of oxygen and carbon dioxide. They involve the removal of fractional volumes from the gas phase by the production of nongaseous compounds, the fractional concentration being determined by the reduction in volume which occurs.

CARBON DIOXIDE

The concentration of CO_2 in gas mixtures can be determined by measuring the reduction in volume after absorption of the gas in 10–20% potassium hydroxide solution. This method cannot be used without modification if another gas soluble in potassium hydroxide (e.g. N_2O) is present. The difficulty can be overcome by allowing for the absorption of nitrous oxide during analysis (Glossop 1963) or by using

saturated sodium hydroxide, in which N_2O is relatively insoluble, to absorb the CO_2 (Nunn 1958a). The latter technique is difficult since the solution is extremely viscous and forms a precipitate of sodium carbonate which obscures the meniscus. A better method is to saturate the absorbent solution with N_2O before use (Owen–Thomas & Meade 1975). Many types of apparatus have been described for carrying out this analysis, the best known being the Haldane, Lloyd–Haldane (Lloyd 1958) and the Scholander (Scholander 1947). A simple modification of the Haldane apparatus described by Campbell (1960) illustrates the principle of the method.

This apparatus consists of a burette, absorption chamber and reservoir for the absorbent solution (Fig. 17.1). The burette has a volume of 10 ml and the stem is graduated from 8.5 to 10 ml in 0.1 ml increments. A mercury column driven by a syringe is used to transfer gas from one chamber to another.

Before starting the analysis the absorption chamber is opened to atmosphere and the height of the absorbent reservoir is adjusted until the meniscus is aligned with the hair line. This ensures that the volumes of absorbent in the reservoir and absorption chamber are exactly balanced when at atmospheric pressure. The gas sample to be analysed is attached to the side limb of tap A. A preliminary sample is aspirated into the burette by raising the syringe plunger, and discharged to atmosphere through tap B. Another sample is then aspirated into the burette and the excess gas is discharged through tap B, approximately 10 ml being retained in the burette for analysis. (The 10-ml volume shown on

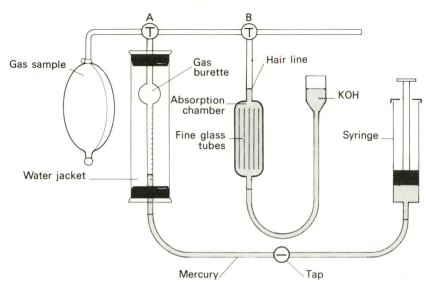

Fig. 17.1. Simplified CO_2 analyser (Campbell 1960).

the scale of this apparatus includes the volume in the tube joining taps A and B.) The burette and absorption chamber are then interconnected by the appropriate adjustment of taps A and B and the gas is driven to and fro between the gas burette and the absorption burette, between ten and fifteen times. The absorbent meniscus is again adjusted to the level of the hair line by manipulating the syringe plunger, and the reduction in volume of the gas in the burette is read from the level of the mercury meniscus in the stem of the burette. The absorption process is repeated and the gas volume checked to ensure that absorption is complete. Thus

concentration of CO_2

$$= \frac{\text{reduction in gas volume}}{\text{original volume}}.$$

If the original volume is adjusted exactly to 10 ml the concentration may be read directly from a second scale on the opposite side of the burette.

Care should be taken to ensure that the taps are well lubricated and that the apparatus is free from leaks. The burette must be kept acidified with a few drops of dilute sulphuric acid and the tube between the taps must be cleaned with a pipe-cleaner soaked in dilute H_2SO_4 if the KOH is accidentally drawn into it. The KOH should be replaced whenever absorption takes longer than twelve to fifteen swings. After a little practice operators should be able to achieve duplicates within $\pm 0.1\%$ CO_2 (approximately 1 mmHg). A number of simpler, but less accurate, analysers have also been developed (Nunn 1958b; Essex & Pask 1964; Brey & Holloway 1971).

OXYGEN

The concentration of oxygen in a gas mixture can be determined by absorbing the gas in alkaline pyrogallol or sodium anthraquinone. Since these solutions also absorb CO_2, the CO_2 analysis must be completed first. A standard Haldane apparatus with two absorption chambers is necessary (Haldane & Graham 1935). This apparatus has an additional burette which automatically compensates for changes in temperature during the analysis. The accuracy is therefore somewhat greater than the simplified apparatus ($CO_2 \pm 0.05\%$; $O_2 \pm 0.1\%$). Again, a number of simpler but less accurate methods have been proposed (Pask 1959; Smith & Pask 1959).

Physical methods

The main advantage of the physical methods of gas analysis is their speed. Indeed, they can often be adapted for continuous operation.

When a machine is designed to follow rapid changes in gas concentration it is essential to know the speed of response of the complete system. This may be divided into two components—the time required for the sample to flow along the sampling catheter, and the time required for the instrument to react to the change in gas concentration (Fig. 17.2). The former is often called the transit, or delay, time, whilst the latter is usually called the response, or rise, time.

The transit time usually accounts for the greater part of the total delay. It is reduced by using a narrow and short sampling catheter with a rapid sampling rate. The response time of the instrument is chiefly a function of the time required to wash out the analysis cell, but additional delays may be imposed by the mechanism used to detect the change in gas concentration. Commonly, the instrumental response to a square wave change in gas concentration is sigmoid in shape: it is therefore usual to express the instrumental response time as the time required to obtain a 90 or 95% response to the change in gas concentration.

Most gas analysers are subject to drift and variations in sensitivity and have to be calibrated frequently, either with a known input signal or with known gas mixtures. Such mixtures can now be produced with reasonable accuracy by special gas-mixing pumps. Alternatively, mixtures of the approximate concentration required may be made by decanting from other cylinders and then subjected to chemical analysis (Hill 1961). Known concentrations of a vapour may be prepared by using a highly-accurate vaporizer such as the Dräger 'Vapor' (Hill 1963), by preparing saturated vapours at a known temperature and then diluting them (Herchl 1970; Nunn, Gill & Hulands 1970), or by vaporizing known weights of a liquid in known volumes of a diluent gas. For example 1 gram-molecule of halothane vapour (molecular weight 197 g) occupies 22.4 litres at S.T.P.D. Therefore, 1 litre of halothane vapour weighs $197/22.4 = 8.8$ g. To make a 2% v/v concentration 8.8 g of halothane must be vaporized in 50 litres of air.

Physical methods of analysis may be classified into specific and nonspecific methods according to the property of the gas which is used for analysis.

Non-specific methods

These methods use a property of the gas which is common to all gases but possessed by each gas to a differing degree. Examples of the properties used are density, viscosity, thermal conductivity, refractive index, velocity of sound in the gas and magnetic

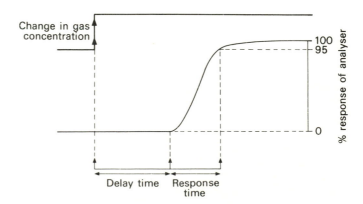

Fig. 17.2. Transit (or delay) time and rise (or response) time after square wave change in sampled gas concentration.

Table 17.1. Physical properties of some common gases and vapours.

	Refractive index*† (sodium D line) STP	Relative‡ magnetic susceptibility (change in zero reading with 100% gas)	Thermal* conductivity (mW·m⁻¹·K⁻¹)	Velocity of* sound (m·s⁻¹ STP)	Viscosity* (Pa·s)	Density* (kg·m⁻³ STP)
Air	1.000 29	–	24.283	331	17.1	1.29
Argon	1.002 81	−0.22	16.621	319	21.0	1.78
Carbon dioxide	1.000 45	−0.27	14.235	259	13.9	1.98
Carbon monoxide	1.000 33	+0.01	23.404	338	16.7	1.25
Chloroform	1.001 45	NS	12.099 (16°C)	171	9.9	5.34§
Diethylether	1.001 55	NS	137.452 (30°C)	206	7.2	3.31§
Enflurane	1.001 44	NS	–	–	–	8.25§
Halothane	1.001 58	NS	–	–	–	8.78§
Helium	1.000 04	+0.30	147.375	965	18.9	0.18
Hydrogen	1.000 14	+0.24	174.170	1284	8.5	0.09
Krypton	1.000 43	−0.51	8.876	–	23.3	3.71
Methane	1.000 44	−0.20	30.186	430	10.3	0.72
Methoxyflurane	1.000 47§	NS	–	–	–	7.36§
Nitrogen	1.000 30	0.00	24.283	334	16.7	1.25
Nitric oxide	1.000 30	+43.00	23.864	324	18.8	1.34
Nitrous oxide	1.000 52	−0.2	15.407	263	13.5	1.98
Oxygen	1.000 27	100.00	24.492	316	19.5	1.43
Trichloroethylene	1.001 78	NS	116.184 (20°C)	–	21.0	5.86§
Xenon	–	−0.95	5.191	–	–	5.85

NS = no significant effect with concentrations used in clinical practice.
* Data from *Handbook of Respiration* (1964).
† Data from *Handbook of Chemistry and Physics* (1971).
‡ Data from Tayler Instrument Analytics Ltd. Instrument calibrated with $N_2 = 0\%$, and $O_2 = 100\%$.
§ Data from Lowe, H. J. (1972) *Dose-regulated Penthrane anesthesia.* Abbott.

susceptibility (Table 17.1). Nonspecific methods are most useful when the particular physical property of the gas to be analysed differs markedly from the background gas. Normally, nonspecific methods are only suitable for use with binary gas mixtures but they can be used for the analysis of more complex mixtures if the background gas mixture is constant (e.g. CO_2 in air), or if the relevant physical properties of the gas to be analysed differ widely from the background gases whilst the properties of the background gases differ little from each other.

Specific methods

By using some property of the gas which is unique to that gas, it can be identified in a gas mixture. Such methods may therefore be used when there are a number of background gases whose identity and concentration are unknown. Examples of the specific properties used are the absorption and emission of radiation of a particular wavelength, the detection of atomic nuclear properties or the conduction of electricity in response to an applied voltage (polarography).

Non-specific methods

DENSITY

This is one of the oldest methods and was employed by Waller (1908) in his chloroform balance. The principle of the balance is

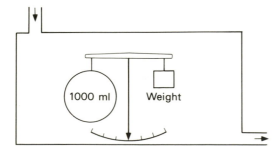

Fig. 17.3. Waller's chloroform balance.

shown in Fig. 17.3. A sealed glass bulb filled with air and of about 1000 ml capacity is exactly counterbalanced by a small weight within a gas-tight chamber. When a heavier than air vapour is admitted to the chamber there is an apparent decrease in weight of the glass bulb due to the difference in weight between the vapour/air mixture and the air which it displaces. One thousand millilitres of air weighs 1.3 g and 1000 ml of chloroform vapour weighs 5.3 g. Hence the apparent reduction in weight when pure chloroform vapour is passed through the chamber is $5.3 - 1.3 = 4.0$ g. If the reduction in weight is 0.04 g the vapour concentration must be 1%.

VISCOSITY

Viscosity is an important determinant of flow down a parallel-sided tube when flow is laminar. Use has been made of a pneumatic Wheatstone bridge to measure the difference in pressure across a capillary tube but the method has not found wide application because of the relatively small differences in viscosity between the common gases.

THERMAL CONDUCTIVITY

A gas with a high thermal conductivity conducts heat more readily than one with a low conductivity. This property is utilized in instruments known as katharometers. In these instruments the gas is passed over a heated wire. The degree of cooling of the wire depends on the temperature of the gas, the rate of gas flow and the thermal conductivity of the gas. The reduction in temperature of the wire reduces its resistance, and so provides a signal which can be related to the concentration. The change in resistance is detected with a Wheatstone bridge circuit and the output displayed on a meter (Fig. 17.4).

Katharometers can be made to detect changes in helium concentration of $\pm 0.1\%$ and, by situating the resistors out of the main gas stream, they can be made relatively

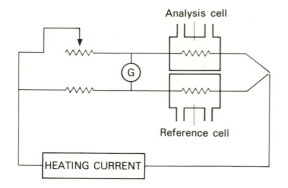

Fig. 17.4. Wheatstone bridge circuit used in a thermal conductivity analyser (katharometer). The resistances are heated by passing an electric current through them and the imbalance of the bridge produced by the analysis gas is showed by the galvanometer (G).

insensitive to changes of sample flow rate. The response time is then slow. If flow rate is rigidly controlled and the gas samples are passed through small analysis chambers at a very low pressure a katharometer can be made to respond quickly to changes in gas concentration. Indeed, the response of some instruments is sufficiently rapid to permit breath-by-breath analysis of CO_2.

The use of this type of instrument is obviously dependent on the difference in thermal conductivity between analysis and background gas (Table 17.1). For example the thermal conductivities of N_2 and O_2 are very similar and therefore analysis for one of these gases in the presence of the other is difficult. Helium however, has a high thermal conductivity. Since a complete change of background gas from N_2 to O_2 would only produce a small change in indicated helium concentration, the apparatus can easily be used for the analysis of helium in nitrogen/oxygen mixtures. In clinical practice katharometers are usually used for the measurement of CO_2 and He; they are also used as detectors in gas chromatography systems (see p. 237).

REFRACTIVE INDEX

Light travels at a speed of about 3×10^8 $m \cdot s^{-1}$ (186 282 miles per second) through a vacuum but at a slower speed through transparent materials. The relationship between the velocity of light through a vacuum and the velocity through a transparent substance determines the refractive index of that substance. Thus the speed of light through water is approximately 2.3×10^8 $m \cdot s^{-1}$ (143 000 miles per second) and the refractive index of water is therefore $3.0 \div 2.3 = 1.3$ approximately. The delay caused by the passage of light through a gas is less than that produced by an equal length of water so that the refractive indices of gases are smaller than the refractive index of water (Table 17.1). Since the delay depends on the number of gas molecules present, the refractive index varies with both the pressure and the temperature of the gas.

The only practicable way of measuring the extremely small delay resulting from the

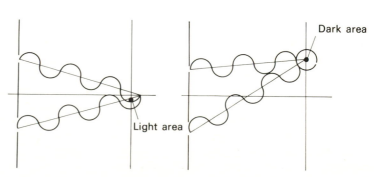

Fig. 17.5. Formation of interference bands. Left: light waves arriving in phase augment each other producing bright areas. Right: light waves arriving 180° out of phase cancel each other producing dark bands.

passage of light through a gas is to measure the phase lag by the principle of interference. This is illustrated in Fig. 17.5. Light consists of transverse waves, the colour being determined by the wavelength and the brightness by the amplitude of the wave. When light waves from a common source (and hence in the same phase) are passed through two linear slits in an opaque sheet and focussed onto a screen an interference pattern is produced. Waves which reach the screen at a point equidistant from the two slits will be in phase and so will reinforce each other and produce a central bright area. On each side there will be two dark bands. These are situated at a point where one light path is exactly half a wavelength longer than the other so that the waves reaching the screen are out of phase and thus cancel each other. Outside the dark bands there will be two light bands where the waves arriving at the screen are exactly in phase because one light path is exactly one wavelength longer than the other, and outside these there will be two more dark bands and so on. The pattern is only observed when the light source is monochromatic, i.e. emits light of only one wavelength. In many commercial interferometers white light is used; this consists of a mixture of wavelengths each of which produces an interference band at a different distance from the axis. In such instruments only the two innermost dark bands are clearly defined, the remainder of the field tailing off into spectral colours.

When a gas is introduced into one light path it delays the transmission of the light waves. Since the frequency of the waves is unchanged this must lead to a reduction in the wavelength and an alteration in the position of the dark bands. If the refractive index of the gas is known, the change in position can be related to the number of gas molecules in the light path and hence to the partial pressure of the gas.

Two types of refractometers are in common use. The Rayleigh refractometer is a large instrument (about 2 m long) which is used in the laboratory. Small and robust portable instruments, originally developed for the measurement of methane gas concentrations in mines, are used in clinical surroundings.

Rayleigh refractometer

Light from a tungsten bulb is focussed into a parallel beam and passed through two vertical slits and then through two chambers closed at each end with optically flat glass plates (Fig. 17.6a). One chamber (A) contains the gas to be analysed whilst the other (B) contains the background gas. The two beams of light then pass through two glass plates (X, Y) which are inclined at an angle to the optical axis. Plate X is fixed but plate Y can be rotated so that the length of the light path through the glass can be varied. Both light paths are then focussed onto a lens at the eye-piece of the instrument which magnifies the image in the horizontal plane. When the two tubes are filled with the same gas and X and Y are inclined at the same angle to optical path an interference pattern is produced. This appears at the eyepiece as a spectrum with a series of dark bands at its centre (Fig. 17.6b). If the gas in tube A is changed, the position of the interference bands is shifted. However, the shift can be counteracted by varying the thickness of glass in the light path by rotating Y so that the interference bands once again appear in their original position. The degree of rotation of plate Y can be measured with a Vernier scale and calibrated to indicate gas concentration in tube A.

In order to ensure that the interference pattern is correctly returned to the original position a duplicate pattern is reproduced below this movable pattern (Fig. 17.6b). This duplicate pattern is produced by the bottom half of the two beams of light issuing from the vertical slits. These beams pass beneath the two tubes and are diverted by the prism Z, so that their interference pattern appears immediately below the other.

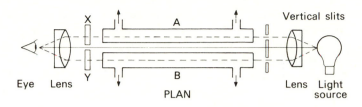

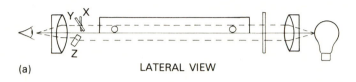

(a) LATERAL VIEW

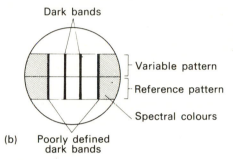

(b)

Fig. 17.6. a. plan and lateral view of the Rayleigh refractometer. b. the interference pattern viewed at the eye piece. For description see text.

Portable interference refractometers

The detailed arrangement of the optical pathways varies with the instrument but the basic principle is illustrated in Fig. 17.7. Light from a common source is split into two beams, one of which travels through a cell containing the gas to be analysed whilst the other forms the reference pathway. The beams form an interference pattern on a translucent scale which is viewed through the eyepiece. The zero is initially set with

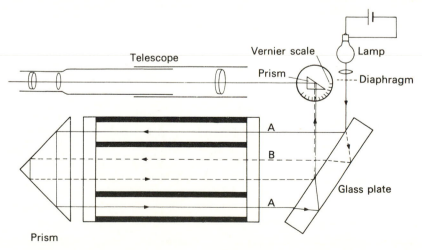

Fig. 17.7. Light path in a portable interference refractometer. A = reference cell. B = analysis cell.

the background gas in both the analysis and reference cells and the gas to be analysed is then aspirated through the analysis cell. The dark bands are shifted across the scale and the concentration is read directly from a previously prepared calibration graph (Hulands & Nunn 1970).

Both types of refractometer are usually calibrated by passing known concentrations of the gas or vapour through the instrument and plotting these against the reading on the instrument. The calibration lines are linear and once the calibration has been performed it remains stable. Although it is possible to encompass a range of sensitivities by adjusting the cell length, most instruments do not incorporate this facility. The main use for this method of analysis is in checking the output from anaesthetic machines and vaporizers, for one analyser can cover a range of gases and vapours, the readings may be made quickly, and the calibration is only likely to change if the machine is damaged.

VELOCITY OF SOUND

This property has been utilized in two ways, both now of only historic interest. In one type of instrument (Faulconer & Ridley 1950; Stott 1959), the gas was resonated in a small chamber by an electronic circuit. The frequency of oscillation which caused the gas to resonate depended on the velocity of sound in the gas mixture, and hence on the gas composition. In another instrument (Molyneux & Pask 1959) a pulse of sound was emitted at the end of a pair of one metre tubes. One tube contained the gas mixture and the other the background gas. The difference in time taken by the sound to travel down the tubes gave a measure of the gas concentration.

SOLUBILITY

A number of gases and vapours are soluble in other substances and alter their physical characteristics. An example of an analyser using this principle is the Dräger 'Narkotest' (Fig. 17.8). Four bands of silicone rubber are linked to a pointer and maintained under slight tension by a counterweight. The strips elongate as they absorb vapour and so move the pointer across the scale. The length of the strips is also affected by humidity and temperature so that compensation devices have to be included. The 'Narkotest' gives a linear response to cyclopropane, fluroxene, ethrane, diethyl ether, halothane and methoxyflurane but it is also affected by nitrous oxide, a 70% mixture of N_2O in O_2 yielding a reading of about 0.3%. When this gas is used with an anaesthetic vapour the zero should be adjusted with the N_2O/O_2 mixture (Lowe & Hagler 1971; White & Wardley-Smith 1972). Normal concentrations of O_2 have little effect on the instrument.

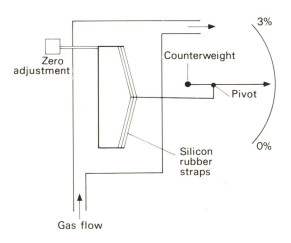

Fig. 17.8. Drager 'Narkotest' halothane analyser.

MAGNETIC SUSCEPTIBILITY

Because of their molecular structure gases may be influenced by a magnetic field. Most gases are repelled from the field and are called diamagnetic. Only two common gases, oxygen and nitric oxide, are strongly paramagnetic (i.e. attracted into a magnetic field). The paramagnetism displayed by oxygen is so characteristic that the use of this property could almost be called a specific method of analysis.

The analyser consists of a cell containing the pole pieces of a permanent magnet. Suspended within the nonhomogeneous magnetic field are two small glass spheres connected by a short bridge to a taut wire suspension. The spheres are filled with a weakly-diamagnetic gas such as nitrogen and are free to rotate though the suspension tends to return the spheres to a position in the strongest part of the magnetic field. When the molecules of a paramagnetic gas such as oxygen enter the cell they are attracted to the centre of the magnetic field and so displace the glass spheres to a zone where the magnetic field is weaker. Since the spheres are fixed by the vertical suspension the only movement open to them is rotation against the torsion of the vertical wire. The displacing force exerted by the oxygen molecules is related to the number of molecules present so that the new position of the glass spheres is determined by the concentration of oxygen present in the cell.

In the simplest instrument, such as that described by Pauling, Wood & Sturdivant (1946), the rotation of the glass dumb-bell is detected by shining a light onto a small

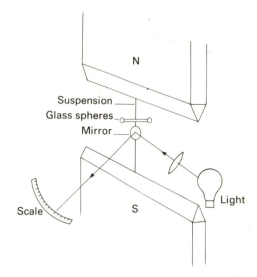

Fig. 17.9. Pauling type of paramagnetic oxygen analyser.

mirror attached to the bridge joining the spheres to the suspension (Fig. 17.9). The resulting light spot is directed onto a translucent scale calibrated from 0 to 100% O_2. This instrument is relatively delicate and the accuracy is limited by the nonlinearities introduced by variations in the strength of the magnetic field and by the mechanical suspension. More accurate readings are obtained by returning the glass 'dumb-bell' to its zero position by an electrical method. In one instrument an electrical current from a constant voltage source is fed into a small coil of wire attached to the dumb-bell (Fig. 17.10). The current passing through this coil is gradually increased by a helical potentiometer until the turning moment produced by the coil in the magnetic field exactly opposes the turning moment produced by

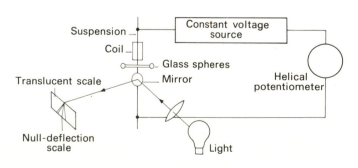

Fig. 17.10. Null-deflection type of paramagnetic oxygen analyser (Servomex 101).

the gas. The zero position is detected by a beam of light shining onto a small mirror attached to the dumb-bell and reflected onto a translucent screen with zero marking. The helipot is calibrated in terms of oxygen percentage and can be read to an accuracy of 0.1% O_2 (Nunn *et al.* 1964). In a more recent instrument the movement of the light beam reflected from the mirror is detected by two photocells (Fig. 17.11). Displacement of the mirror causes an imbalance between the amount of light received by the photocells and this alters their electrical outputs. The difference in output from the two cells is amplified and fed back to the coil, so returning the dumb-bell to its zero position. The current passing through the coil is directly related to the turning moment produced by the paramagnetic gas and can be displayed on a meter which can be calibrated in terms of oxygen concentration. Two scales are provided: 0–25% O_2 and 0–100% O_2, the discrimination between readings being 0·25% O_2 and 1% O_2 respectively.

In fact, the accuracy of the analyser is much greater than that displayed by the meter and by recording the electrical output on a digital voltmeter it is possible to achieve a degree of accuracy which is probably far in excess of that obtainable on a standard Haldane apparatus (Ellis & Nunn 1968).

Paramagnetic analysers are affected by the presence of high concentrations of a diamagnetic background gas. For accurate work it is therefore necessary to set the zero point with 100% background gas (e.g. N_2 or N_2O) and then to set the span with 100% O_2. However, small concentrations of a diamagnetic gas (such as carbon dioxide in expired air) have an insignificant effect on the reading. Another source of error is the presence of water vapour in the gas to be analysed. It has been recommended that all gases should be dried by passage through a tube of silica gel before entering the cell. However, when nitrous oxide is present in the gas mixture it appears to be adsorbed onto the drying medium so that a variable reading is obtained. When working with respired gas it is better to saturate both the calibration gases and the gases to be analysed by passing them over water. The cell is then dried by flushing with dry gas when the analyses have been completed.

Specific methods

EMISSION OF ELECTROMAGNETIC RADIATION

If suitably excited, all gases will emit electromagnetic radiation in some part of the ultraviolet, visible or infrared portions of the spectrum, the 'neon sign' being a common example of this phenomenon. This principle has been used in a number of gas analysers, but the only instrument available commercially is the nitrogen meter (Daniels, Couvillon & Lebrizzi 1975). This is used in such tests of respiratory function as the single-breath method of measuring anat-

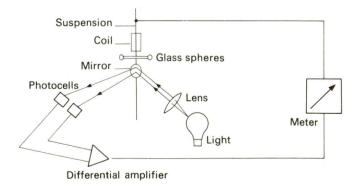

Fig. 17.11. Direct reading type of paramagnetic oxygen analyser utilising photocells to detect deviations from the zero position of the glass dumb-bell.

omical dead space and closing volume, and the nitrogen washout test for assessing the distribution of ventilation.

A powerful suction pump draws the gas sample through a fine needle valve (placed close to the patient) to a gas discharge tube (Fig. 17.12). Two electrodes are sealed into the ends of this tube and a potential of about 1500–2000 V is applied. This ionizes the gas, which glows, the wavelengths of the radiation emitted being characteristic of the gas. A reflector placed behind the tube directs the light through a filter onto a photoelectric cell. This cell produces a current which is proportional to the intensity of the radiation falling on it, and this current is then amplified and displayed on a meter.

The great advantage of the N_2 meter is its specificity and rapid response. The transit time from needle valve to discharge tube and the time required to wash out the tube are minimized by the reduction in pressure in the system, and the delay time and response time are accordingly very short, the total delay being in the order of 20–40 ms.

Unfortunately, the light output from the gas discharge tube is not directly pro-portional to the concentration of the gas and linearizing circuits have to be added This makes the machine expensive.

ABSORPTION OF RADIATION

All gases absorb electromagnetic radiation, in either the infrared or ultraviolet regions of the spectrum. The wavelengths are specific for each gas and depend on the molecular configuration (see Chapter 8).

Infrared gas analysers

Infrared radiation in the range 1–15 μm is absorbed by all gases with more than two atoms in the molecule provided those atoms are dissimilar. Thus O_2 does not absorb infrared radiation but CO does.

The instruments utilizing this analytical principle may be classified as *dispersive or nondispersive.*

The infrared spectrophotometer is an example of the dispersive type of analyser. In this instrument radiation from an infrared source passes through a prism or diffraction grating and is so dispersed that the radiations of different wavelengths are arranged in sequence. If now the gas to be

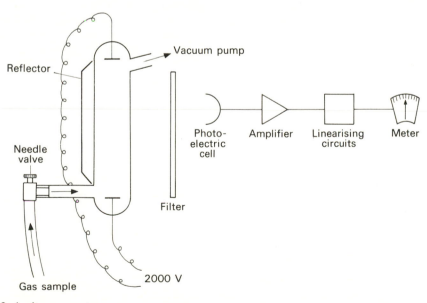

Fig. 17.12. A nitrogen meter.

analysed is placed in the path of the radiation it will absorb maximally in one or more regions of the spectrum. By scanning the whole spectrum a graph of absorption against wavelength can be plotted. Alternatively, the absorption at a particular wavelength can be studied. This type of instrument is versatile and can readily be adjusted for measurements on different gases which have different absorption spectra (see Chapter 8).

If interest is centred on only one gas the nondispersive type of analyser is usually employed (Hill & Powell 1968). In this instrument (Fig. 17.13) light from an infrared source (yielding a wide range of wavelengths) is directed down two tubes whose ends are sealed with a substance which transmits infrared radiation. The gas sample to be analysed is aspirated through the analysis cell, whilst the remainder of the tube on this side, and the reference tube, is flushed with air or other background gas. The gas in the analysis cell absorbs a small proportion of the infrared radiation and the strength of the radiation reaching the detector is therefore less than that impinging on the detector on the reference side.

The Luft type of detector (so-named after the originator) is now commonly used. This consists of two chambers containing the gas or vapour to be analysed. The gas in the chamber also absorbs the infrared radiation, and is therefore heated. This causes the gas to expand. The detector on the reference side receives more radiation than that on the analysis side and the difference in pressure in the two chambers is measured by recording the deflection of the elastic membrane separating them. This part of the detector is therefore a pressure transducer, the capacitance principle being most commonly used. To prevent drift due to slow heating of the detector cells the light from the infrared source is 'chopped' by a rotating shutter so that it cycles on and off at a frequency of 25–100 Hz. This produces an alternating output from the transducer which is then amplified and displayed. The accuracy is about $\pm 0.1\%$ in the range 0–10% CO_2 although the accuracy of an analyser can be improved tenfold with appropriate modifications (Cormack & Powell 1972).

Unfortunately, there are several sources of error in this technique. In the first place there is often some overlap in the absorption wavebands of different gases. For instance, the fundamental absorption bands for carbon dioxide, nitrous oxide, and carbon monoxide are at 4.3, 4.5 and 4.7 μm respectively. The absorption spectrum of each gas is in fact quite complex, centred about the fundamental wavelength, so that overlap is inevitable. As a result, a CO_2 analyser given a sample containing both CO_2 and N_2O will read high, since the N_2O will absorb some infrared energy *within* the absorption band-

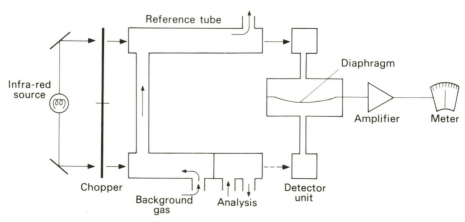

Fig. 17.13. Infrared analyser using Luft-type detector unit.

width for CO_2. This error can be overcome by narrowing the absorption band by special optical filters, or by filling the analyser (except the cuvette) with N_2O, so that no energy within the N_2O absorption band reaches the Luft detector.

A second error arises from the phenomenon of 'collision broadening' (also called 'pressure broadening') in which the absorption spectrum of one gas (i.e. CO_2) is actually *widened* by the physical presence of certain other gases such as N_2, N_2O or C_3H_6, so that absorption is increased. Collision broadening is not altogether prevented by the 'background gas filter' method. Correction factors for different concentrations of N_2O and CO_2 have been published (Cooper 1957; Severinghaus, Larson & Eger 1961; Kennell, Andrews & Wollman 1973), but the simplest method of eliminating this error is to calibrate the instrument with gas mixtures which contain the same background gas concentration as that to be analysed.

Since this type of analyser detects the *number* of molecules of absorbent gas in the cuvette, it is really a partial pressure detector, so that changes in atmospheric pressure will alter the reading for a given gas. Frequent calibration checks are therefore necessary to minimize errors from this source. Alternatively, the analyser can be calibrated in partial pressure terms by calculating the P_{CO_2} of the calibrating gas. Errors due to changes in atmospheric pressure will then be minimal.

By a combination of small cell-size ($<0.5\,ml$) and a suitable sampling rate ($500\,ml\cdot min^{-1}$), a 95% response time of $100\,ms$ with an overall error of $<0.1\%\,CO_2$ can be achieved, thus permitting detailed analysis of individual expiratory capnograms.

In addition to CO_2 analysis, infrared analysers have been used for the estimation of N_2O, ether, halothane, alcohol, and many other vapours. Very high resolution analysers are now available for measuring gas concentrations in the parts-per-million range, as are required for monitoring gas pollution in operating theatres.

Laser analysers

A number of organic compounds absorb strongly at $3.39\,\mu m$ which is the wavelength omitted by a helium–neon gas laser. By utilizing the intense, narrow beam generated by the laser it is possible to make the sample cell long and narrow, so that very high sensitivity is easily achieved. A reference beam and the 'sample' beam are chopped alternately by a rotating shutter, and directed onto a photocell so that the intensity of the two beams can be compared. The method has been used for the analysis of trace quantities of ethyl alcohol in expired air and is fast enough to follow breath-by-breath variations in end-tidal CO_2.

Ultraviolet gas analysers

A number of gases such as hydrogen, oxygen and nitrogen do not absorb in the infrared region of the spectrum but have characteristic absorption patterns in the

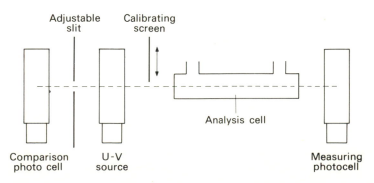

Fig. 17.14. Ultraviolet gas analyser.

ultraviolet region. However the greatest use for this method has been in the analysis of halothane which has a useful absorption band in the region of 200 nm. Ultraviolet light from a mercury lamp is filtered and passed through the analysis chamber to a photocell (Fig. 17.14). The output from this cell is compared with a similar reference photocell (to minimize errors due to changes in the output from the lamp) and is then amplified and displayed on a meter. The accuracy obtainable is about $\pm 0.2\%$ in the range 0–5% halothane (Robinson, Denson & Summers 1962). Halothane decomposes to a certain extent when exposed to the intense radiation from the mercury lamp so it must not be returned to the circuit. Similar considerations apply to trichloroethylene which can also be analysed by this technique. Recently a rapid response halothane analyser suitable for use with small sample flow rates has been described (Tatnall, West & Morris 1978).

MASS SPECTROMETRY

Mass spectrometers are capable of separating the components of complex gas mixtures according to their mass and charge by deflecting the charged ions in a magnetic field. There are basically two types of mass spectrometer, the magnetic sector type and the quadrupole.

Magnetic sector mass spectrometer

The earliest mass spectrometers built for medical purposes were of this type (Fowler & Hugh-Jones 1957). A gas sample of about 25 ml $\cdot$ min^{-1} is aspirated continuously through the sampling catheter and a small proportion of this sample is drawn into an evacuated ionization chamber through a molecular leak. In this chamber the molecules are bombarded by a transverse beam of electrons. The charged ions then diffuse out of a slit in the chamber wall and are accelerated by a plate to which a negative voltage is applied. The stream of ions passes out through a hole in this plate and comes under the influence of a magnetic field whose lines of force run at right angles to the stream of ions. The magnetic field deflects the ions according to their mass: charge ratio. Since most ions carry a single charge the separation is effectively governed by the mass of the ions, the lightest ions being deflected most and the heaviest least. This results in a fan-like series of beams of ions of different molecular weight (Fig. 17.15).

The position of the deflected beams may be altered by changing the velocity of the ions entering the magnetic field; this is achieved by varying the accelerating voltage on the plate. It is thus possible to direct each beam of ions across the detector unit in turn. The detector measures the rate at which ions impinge on it so that a measure of gas partial pressure is obtained. By relating the detector output on the *y*-axis to the accelerating voltage on the *x*-axis it is possible to display a mass spectrum on an oscilloscope screen (Fig. 17.16). The height of the peaks then represents the concentra-

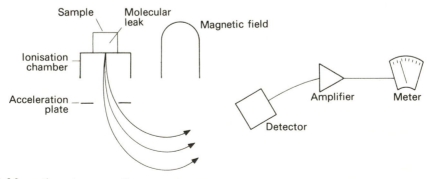

Fig. 17.15. Magnetic sector type of mass spectrometer.

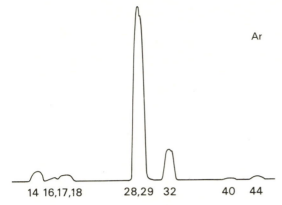

Fig. 17.16. Mass spectrum of room air. Concentration is in the vertical axis and mass/charge ratio along the abcissa. The large N_2 and O_2 peaks occur at 28 and 32. The other peaks are due to doubly charged O_2 at 16, water vapour at 18, Ar at 40 and CO_2 at 44.

tion of each gas whilst the position of the peak on the *x*-axis identifies the mass number of each peak.

Quadrupole mass spectrometer

In general the magnetic sector instrument is now being replaced by the quadrupole analyser, which is smaller and lighter. Furthermore, the balance between sensitivity and resolving power (ability to differentiate different masses) can be adjusted easily to suit a particular application.

As in the magnetic sector instrument a beam of ions is accelerated out of an ionization chamber. The ions then pass through the quadrupole mass filter. This consists of four parallel cylindrical rods (each about 0.5 cm in diameter and 5 cm long), the opposite pairs being electrically connected. A standing d.c. voltage is applied to the rods and a radio-frequency a.c. component is then applied to the opposite pairs (Fig. 17.17).

By adjusting this frequency it is possible to filter out all the ions except those with a particular mass:charge ratio and these then pass down the filter to the detector at the opposite end of the filter. All the other ions undergo increasing oscillations and eventually hit the rods and lose their charge. By varying the voltage applied to the plate it is possible to scan the mass spectrum and so determine the proportions of various masses present in the gas mixture.

Mass spectrometers are relatively bulky and expensive, although the introduction of specialized quadrupole machines for particular applications has greatly reduced both their size and cost. They have a very short response time (about 100 ms for a 95% response) and they require very small sample flow rates (about 20 ml·min^{-1} for normal respiratory work). The sample flow rates can be greatly reduced if a rapid response is not required; indeed the instrument can be used to measure blood-gases by sampling the gases which diffuse into the interior of a thin teflon catheter inserted into a blood vessel. However there are still

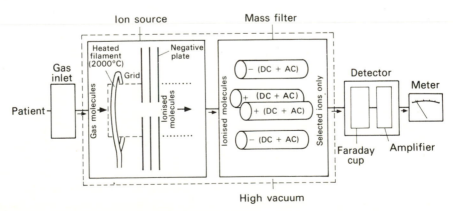

Fig. 17.17. Quadrupole type of mass spectrometer.

many practical problems in the application of this technique. All mass spectrometers operate under conditions of very high vacuum and it takes some time for the various pumping systems to achieve the required working pressures. When these have been achieved the pumps must run continuously. Water-vapour condensation in the sampling tube is prevented by heating the tube but the response time for water vapour is often longer than that for other gases and vapours. Another problem is that some molecules may lose two electrons without disintegrating and so become doubly charged. They then behave like ions with half the mass. Some fragmentation of molecules also occurs in the ionization process resulting in the production of a mass spectrum rather than a single peak for each molecule. These secondary peaks can usually be recognized easily and can often be used to advantage. For example in anaesthesia it would be impossible to separate CO_2 from N_2O since the parent peak of each occurs at 44 amu (atomic mass units). However, nitrous oxide produces a strong secondary peak which is about 30% of the parent peak height at 30 amu and carbon dioxide produces a secondary peak at 12 amu. Since the ratio of secondary peaks to parent peaks remains reasonably constant these can be used to determine the concentrations of the two gases in a mixture. In most instruments the spectrum is scanned 25 times per second so that it is possible to produce a continuous record of the changing concentration of any gas. Commonly a mass spectrometer can provide a continuous record of the changing concentrations of up to eight separate gases. These are selected by tuning the analyser to the appropriate peaks on the mass spectrum and then setting the zero and gain controls on each channel of the recorder to provide the appropriate scale on the recording.

GAS CHROMATOGRAPHY

This is a contraction for the term gas–liquid chromatography. The use of the word chromatography to describe the process of separating colourless gas or vapour mixtures into their constituents is derived from the older technique of liquid–liquid chromatography, in which the separated components were identified by their natural colours, or by colours produced by chemical treatment.

The principle used to achieve separation of the components of a mixture is that of partition chromatography: this is based on the fact that molecules of a solute partition between two solvents in a way that reflects the balance of attractive and repulsive forces between solute and solvent. In the gas–liquid chromatograph one solvent is adsorbed onto an inert material such as firebrick granules or a diatomaceous earth. This constitutes the stationary phase and is packed into a narrow, stainless steel or glass tube (up to 2 m long) to form the chromatographic column. The second solvent is a stream of gas, such as helium, nitrogen or argon, which flows through the column at a rate of about 50 ml $\cdot$ min^{-1}. The mixture to be analysed is injected as a bolus into this stream of carrier gas and its constituents then partition between the two solvents as the mixture is carried down the column. Components which have a high volatility or low solubility in the stationary phase are eluted before the less volatile or more soluble compounds and so are the first to appear at the outlet of the column. The various components of the mixture thus emerge at varying time intervals after the injection and pass to a nonspecific detector unit which yields an electronic signal proportional to the quantity of each substance present.

When the substance is a gas or vapour at room temperature it is injected directly into the stream of carrier gas. In order to ensure that an accurately known volume of gas is delivered into the system it is a common practice to use a special gas sampling valve to isolate a known volume of gas before injection. When the substance is a liquid it is necessary to heat part or all of the column to volatilize the components of the mixture. It is also often necessary to heat the column to ensure that the stationary phase is a liquid when the column is in use. For this reason the column is usually enclosed in a thermostatically controlled oven.

Columns are of two main types: the packed columns already mentioned, and open tubular columns in which the liquid phase is deposited on the wall of the tube. The latter have a high resolving power (i.e. produce good separation of the components of the mixture), but the packed columns are cheaper and easier to work with and have a much greater sample capacity, i.e. permit more samples to be analysed before the column has to be changed. The liquid phase is usually a wax or gum with a carbon or silicon base. The column filling must be free from absorptive or catalytic sites and is usually acid-washed and treated with a special blocking agent to prevent such action.

The temperature of the column is of great importance. As the temperature is increased beyond the melting point of the stationary phase, the partition is pushed towards the gaseous phase. This shortens the retention time of the compound (the interval between the injection and the peak of the signal on the detector). It is quite common for two components of a mixture to have widely-different retention times, so increasing the duration of each analysis. To overcome this problem most modern instruments have facilities for temperature programming. The temperature is maintained at a constant level for a preset period after injection and then programmed to rise at a finite rate to a maximum value. This method may also be used to separate two substances which have a similar solubility in the liquid phase, but different volatility.

Unfortunately, temperature programming may give rise to the troublesome phenomenon of 'column bleed', in which small amounts of the liquid phase volatilize and pass to the detector. At constant temperature and carrier gas flow rate this effect gives rise to a constant background current which can be offset electronically.

However, when the temperature is increased the effect is more pronounced and leads to a constantly shifting baseline.

The first essential, then, is to choose the most appropriate column for the mixture to be analysed and to arrange the temperature programming so that each constituent in the mixture arrives at the end of the column over a narrow time interval which is clearly separated from each of the other constituents. It is then necessary to record the quantity and identity of each component present. These are the functions of the detector. Many different types of detector are used for this purpose but all are non-specific; that is they produce a signal proportional to the quantity of the substance present but they are incapable of identifying the substance. The choice of detector is governed by the nature of the substances being analysed.

Perhaps the simplest detector is the *thermal conductivity* or katharometer detector (page 224). The detector consists of a heated resistance wire which forms part of a Wheatstone bridge. When a gas with a thermal conductivity different from that of the carrier gas passes the detector there will be a difference in the amount of heat conducted away from the wire. As a result its temperature will change and so will its resistance. This change in resistance unbalances the bridge and produces a signal which can be amplified and displayed on a chart recorder. This type of detector is chiefly used when inorganic gases such as oxygen, nitrogen, carbon dioxide and nitrous oxide are being analysed. Since the thermal conductivity of helium differs widely from the other inorganic gases (Table 17.1) it is often used as a carrier gas in such situations.

The *flame ionization detector* is commonly employed when trace amounts of organic vapours have to be analysed. The detector contains a small flame produced by hydrogen burning in air and the carrier gas emerging from the column is fed into this flame. The presence of an organic component results in the production of positive ions which are then attracted to a charged collecting electrode. The resulting ionization current is detected and fed to a suitable amplifier and recorder. This type of detector is widely used, gives a linear response over a wide range of concentrations, is very sensitive and has a small background current. The detector responds to all compounds containing carbon and has the added advantage of not being affected by water vapour.

The electron-capture detector is used for the selective analysis of organic compounds containing an electron-capturing atom such as a halogen. The detector consists of a small chamber containing a radioisotope which emits beta-radiation, i.e. negatively charged electrons. A small voltage is applied to the collector electrode (anode) and the resulting current (carried by the electron stream) detected and amplified. When an electron-capturing molecule passes through the detector, some of the electrons are 'captured', and so fail to reach the anode. The reduction in current can then be recorded. The detector is very sensitive but the output is only linear over a narrow range of concentrations. It is particularly useful when measuring anaesthetic agents in blood, for these are commonly extracted into heptane before being injected into the chromatograph. Heptane tends to produce a wide peak which masks the smaller halothane peak when the flame ionization detector is used, but this problem does not arise with the electron capture detector.

Many other forms of detector have been used for specific purposes but perhaps one of the most powerful analytical tools is provided by the combination of a gas chromatograph with a mass spectrometer. The latter instrument can identify the molecular fragments present in any component eluted from a chromatograph column and so greatly aid identification of an unusual compound.

However, in normal practice it is still necessary to identify the source of the deflection produced by the nonspecific detector. When analysing known mixtures identification can usually be performed by determining the retention time for each constituent of the mixture and identifying the peaks on this basis. It is then necessary to quantify the amount of each substance present, for the response of the detector varies with the substance. One way of calibrating the deflection is to inject a known quantity of each of the substances being analysed and to relate these to the deflections produced. However the injection of small quantities (often in the microlitre range) is not very accurate and it is therefore wise to incorporate an internal standard into each sample. This standard must have characteristics similar to those of the constituents of the sample but must be readily identifiable and must not interfere with the other components of the mixture. The inclusion of such a standard obviates errors due to changes in column conditions, gas flow or amplifier gain and greatly improves the accuracy of the technique. If the column has once been calibrated for this internal standard and the test substance, the concentration of the latter can be derived.

The electrical output of a detector is proportional to the mass of the substance passing through the detector at that instant. If the sample size is fixed, concentrations can be derived. The output appears as a deflection from the base line, and if this is drawn on paper moving at constant speed, the area between the curve and the base line is proportional to the total mass of that compound in the sample. If the chromatographic separation is good, the deflection has an abrupt onset, short duration, and abrupt termination, and appears as a peak. Under these conditions, the peak bears a close approximation to a triangle, and the area can be found as

$$\frac{\text{half height}}{\text{base}}$$

or more commonly, height times width at half height (since the base may be distorted by contaminants). If the base is always the same, then the peak height alone is proportional to area, and is an acceptable simplification. However, where peaks are broad, area must be measured. This can be done mechanically or electronically.

The gas–liquid chromatograph may be used for purposes other than gas analysis. Thus, it can be used to analyse blood samples containing volatile or local anaesthetic agents (Wortley et al. 1968; Douglas, Hill & Wood 1970; Jones, Molloy & Rosen 1972). It is also widely used to measure the concentrations of other drugs such as the anticonvulsants, barbiturates and tranquillizers. For further references to the use of this technique readers are referred to Hill (1973) and Moore & McVittie (1978).

CHEMICALLY-SENSITIVE ELECTRODES

Polarography

If two electrodes are connected by a buffered electrolyte and a potential of about 0.6 volts is maintained between them it is found that the current which flows is proportional to the concentration of oxygen present in the electrolyte. By imprisoning a thin layer of electrolyte under a membrane the electrode can be made to respond to changes in oxygen concentration in a gas on the other side of the membrane (Wilson & Laver 1972). This is the basis of the oxygen electrode (see Chapter 18). By using a gold cathode with a large polarizing voltage it is possible to measure N_2O concentration (Albery et al. 1978).

CO_2 electrode

The concentration of CO_2 in a gas may be measured by determining the change in pH of a thin layer of bicarbonate solution surrounding a pH-sensitive electrode (Chapter 18).

THE FUEL CELL

Various forms of fuel cell have been used to sense oxygen concentration (Wilson & Laver 1972). A fuel cell is a device which converts energy from an oxidation–reduc-

tion chemical process into electrical energy. It is thus analogous to a primary cell in a battery though it differs from a battery in that the output is dependent on the oxygen concentration present. The chemical reaction uses up the components of the fuel cell so that its life depends on the concentration of oxygen to which it is exposed and on the duration of exposure. Modern fuel cell analysers for oxygen are compact and are reasonably accurate though the response is relatively slow (Torda & Grant 1972).

RADIOACTIVE ISOTOPES

Respired gases can be 'labelled' by incorporating radioactive isotopes in the mixture. This enables their fate in the body to be followed with great accuracy. There are many technical difficulties associated with this type of work, but the principle has now been widely used in respiratory physiology and has contributed greatly to our knowledge of the distribution of pulmonary ventilation and blood flow (see Chapter 10).

References

ALBERY, W.J., BROOKS W.N., GIBSON S.P. & HAHN C.E.W. (1978) An electrode for P_{N_2O} and P_{O_2} analysis in blood and gas. *Journal of Applied Physiology: Respiratory, Exercise & Environmental Physiology*, **45**, 637.

BREY O. & HOLLOWAY R. (1971) Dry method for estimation of mixed venous CO_2 concentration. *British Medical Journal*, **4**, 292.

CAMPBELL E.J.M. (1960) Simplification of Haldane's apparatus for measuring CO_2 concentration in respired gases in clinical practice. *British Medical Journal*, **1**, 457.

COOPER E.A. (1957) Infrared analysis for the estimation of carbon dioxide in the presence of nitrous oxide. *British Journal of Anaesthesia*, **29**, 486.

CORMACK R.S. & POWELL J.N. (1972) Improving the performance of the infra-red carbon dioxide meter. *British Journal of Anaesthesia*, **44**, 131.

DANIELS A.U., COUVILLON L.A. & LEBRIZZI J.M. (1975) Evaluation of nitrogen analyzers. *American Review of Respiratory Disease*, **712**, 571.

DOUGLAS R., HILL D.W. & WOOD D.G.L. (1970) Methods for the estimation of blood halothane concentration by gas chromatography. *British Journal of Anaesthesia*, **42**, 119.

ELLIS F.R. & NUNN J.F. (1968) The measurement of gaseous oxygen tension utilizing paramagnetism: an evaluation of the "Servomex" OA 150 analyser. *British Journal of Anaesthesia*, **40**, 569.

ESSEX L. & PASK E.A. (1964) A simple CO_2 gas analyzer. *Lancet*, **i**, 311.

FAULCONER A. & RIDLEY R.W. (1950) Continuous quantitative analysis of mixtures of oxygen, nitrous oxide and ether with or without nitrogen. *Anesthesiology*, **11**, 265.

FOWLER K.T. & HUGH-JONES P. (1957) Mass spectrometry applied to clinical practice and research. *British Medical Journal*, **1**, 1205.

GLOSSOP M.W. (1963) A simple method for the estimation of carbon dioxide concentration in the presence of nitrous oxide. *British Journal of Anaesthesia*, **35**, 17.

HALDANE J.S. & GRAHAM J.I. (1935) *Methods of air analysis, 4th Edition*, London: Griffin.

HERCHL R. (1970) The preparation of accurate standard mixtures of inhalation anaesthetic agents. *Canadian Anaesthetists' Society Journal*, **17**, 624.

HILL D.W. (1961) The production of accurate gas and vapour mixtures. *British Journal of Applied Physics*, **12**, 410.

HILL D.W. (1963) Halothane concentrations obtained from a Dräger "Vapor" Vaporizer. *British Journal of Anaesthesia*, **35**, 285.

HILL D.W. & POWELL T. (1968) *Non-dispersive Infra Red Gas Analysis in Science, Medicine and Industry*. London: Adam Hilger.

HILL D.W. (1973) *Electronic techniques in anaesthesia and surgery, 2nd Edition*. London: Butterworth.

HULANDS G.H. & NUNN J.F. (1970) Portable interference refractometers in anaesthesia. *British Journal of Anaesthesia*, **42**, 1051.

JONES P.L., MOLLOY M.J. & ROSEN M. (1972) A technique for the analysis of methoxyflurane in blood by gas chromatography. *British Journal of Anaesthesia*, **44**, 124.

KENNELL E.M., ANDREWS R.W. & WOLLMAN H. (1973) Correction factors for nitrous oxide in the infrared analysis of carbon dioxide. *Anesthesiology*, **39**, 441.

LLOYD B.B. (1958) A development of Haldane's gas analysis apparatus. *Journal of Physiology, London*, **143**, 5P.

LOWE H.J. & HAGLER K. (1971) Clinical and laboratory evaluation of an expired anesthetic gas monitor (Narkotest). *Anesthesiology*, **34**, 378.

MOLYNEUX L. & PASK E.A. (1959) A sonic analyser for anaesthetic vapours. *Anaesthesia*, **14**, 191.

MOORE R.A. & MCVITTIE J.D. (1978) Gas–liquid chromatography. *British Journal of Clinical Equipment*, **3**, 25.

NUNN J.F. (1958a) Respiratory measurements in the presence of nitrous oxide. *British Journal of Anaesthesia*, **30**, 254.

NUNN J.F. (1958b) The Dräger carbon dioxide analyser. *British Journal of Anaesthesia*, **30**, 264.

NUNN J.F., BERGMAN N.A., COLEMAN A.J. & CASSELLE D.C. (1964) Evaluation of the Servomex paramagnetic oxygen analyser. *British Journal of Anaesthesia*, **36**, 666.

NUNN J.F., GILL D. & HULANDS G.H. (1970) Apparatus for preparing saturated vapour concentrations of liquid anaesthetic agents. *Journal of Physics E*, **3**, 331.

OWEN-THOMAS J.B. & MEADE F. (1975) The estimation of carbon dioxide concentration in the presence of nitrous oxide, using a Lloyd–Haldane apparatus. *British Journal of Anaesthesia*, **47**, 22.

PASK E.A. (1959) An oxygen analyser. *Lancet*, **i**, 273.

PAULING L., WOOD R.E. & STURDIVANT J.H. (1946) An instrument for determining the partial pressure of oxygen in a gas. *Journal of the American Chemical Society*, **63**, 795.

ROBINSON A., DENSON J.S. & SUMMERS F.W. (1962) Halothane analyzer. *Anesthesiology*, **23**, 391.

SCHOLANDER P.F. (1947) Analyzer for accurate estimation of respiratory gases in one-half cubic centimetre samples. *Journal of Biological Chemistry*, **167**, 235.

SEVERINGHAUS J.W., LARSON C.P. & EGER E.I. (1961) Correction factors for infrared carbon dioxide pressure broadening by nitrogen, nitrous oxide and cyclopropane. *Anesthesiology*, **22**, 429.

SMITH H. & PASK E.A. (1959) Method for the estimation of oxygen in gas mixtures containing nitrous oxide. *British Journal of Anaesthesia*, **31**, 440.

STOTT F.D. (1959) Sonic gas analyzer for measurement of CO_2 in expired air. *Review of Scientific Instruments*, **28**, 914.

TATNALL M.L., WEST P.G. & MORRIS P. (1978) A rapid response u.v. halothane meter. *British Journal of Anaesthesia*, **50**, 617.

TORDA T.A. & GRANT G.C. (1972) Test of a fuel cell oxygen analyzer. *British Journal of Anaesthesia*, **44**, 1108.

WALLER A.D. (1908) The chloroform balance. A new form of apparatus for the measured delivery of chloroform vapour. *Journal of Physiology, London*, **37**, 6P.

WHITE D.C. & WARDLEY-SMITH B. (1972) The "Narkotest" anaesthetic gas meter. *British Journal of Anaesthesia*, **44**, 1100.

WILSON R.F. & LAVER M.B. (1972) Oxygen analysis: advances in methodology. *Anesthesiology*, **37**, 112.

WORTLEY D.J., HERBERT P., THORNTON J.A. & WHELPTON D. (1968) The use of gas chromatography in the measurement of anaesthetic agents in gas and blood. *British Journal of Anaesthesia*, **40**, 624.

Chapter 18
pH and Blood–Gas Analysis

pH measurement

The SI unit defining the acidity or alkalinity of the blood is the hydrogen-ion concentration $[H^+]$. This is expressed in nanomoles per litre ($nmol \cdot l^{-1}$). However, it is not possible to measure $[H^+]$ directly in aqueous solutions so that the acid–base state is usually defined by measuring the pH with a glass electrode. This electrode produces a voltage which is related to the tendency for the hydrogen ions to escape from the solution: it thus measures the effective concentration or 'activity' of the hydrogen ions. The activity is only equal to the true concentration in infinitely dilute solutions where interactions between the various ions are negligible. In blood the concentration of hydrogen ions is greater than the activity seen by the electrode, but the difference between the two measurements is variable and difficult to define.

There are other reasons why pH remains a useful measurement. The pH electrode produces an electrical output of about 60 mV per pH unit so that the scale is linear and adjustments for drift and electrode scale length are easily made. Furthermore $[H^+]$ changes act biologically in a logarithmic way so that a unit alteration of pH provides a better indication of the magnitude of a biological effect than a unit change in $[H^+]$. For these reasons most workers continue to express results in pH units. The conversion of one measurement to another is detailed in Table 18.1.

pH can be measured by the use of indicators or electrodes, and can also be calculated from a knowledge of P_{CO_2} and bicarbonate or total CO_2 content using the Henderson–Hasselbalch equation. How-

ever, inaccuracies are introduced by the assumption of a fixed pK′ so that the use of the Henderson–Hasselbalch equation is limited to clinical situations where there are fairly gross acid–base changes and where accuracy is less important than speed of

Table 18.1. Conversions between pH and hydrogen ion activity ($nmol \cdot l^{-1}$).

pH	$[H^+]$ $nmol \cdot l^{-1}$	pH	$[H^+]$ $nmol \cdot l^{-1}$
6.80	158.3	7.35	44.6
6.90	125.7	7.40	39.8
7.00	100.0	7.45	35.5
7.10	79.4	7.50	31.6
7.20	63.1	7.55	28.2
7.25	56.2	7.60	25.1
7.30	50.1	7.70	20.0

Example 1. Convert pH 7.80 to $[H^+]$. Since the negative logarithm of $[H^+]$ is 7.80 the logarithm is -7.80. This can be written $+0.20-8.00$. The antilogarithm of 0.20 is 159 and the antilogarithm of -8 is 10^{-8}. The product of 159 and 10^{-8} is 15.9×10^{-9} moles per litre = 15.9 $nmol \cdot l^{-1}$.
Example 2. Convert 12.6 $nmol \cdot l^{-1}$ to pH. This $[H^+]$ is equivalent to 12.6×10^{-9} $mol \cdot l^{-1}$. The logarithm of the product of two numbers is equal to the sum of the logarithms of the numbers. Therefore $\log (12.6 \times 10^{-9}) = \log 12.6 + \log 10^{-9}$ The logarithm of 12.6 is 1.1 and the logarithm of 10^{-9} is -9. Consequently $\log [H^+] = \log (12.6 \times 10^{-9}) = 1.1 -9 = -7.9$ or pH = 7.9.

$[H^+]$ may also be calculated from the following versions of the Henderson–Hasselbalch equation:

$$[H^+] \, nmol \cdot l^{-1} = \frac{180 \, P_{CO_2} \, kPa}{[HCO_3^-] \, mmol \cdot l^{-1}}$$

or $$[H^+] \, nmol \cdot l^{-1} = \frac{24 \, P_{CO_2} \, mmHg}{[HCO_3^-] \, mmol \cdot l^{-1}}.$$

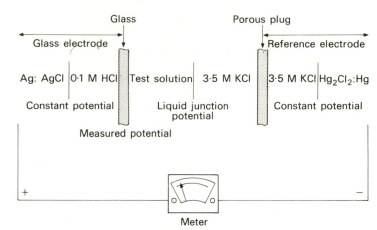

Glass electrode				Reference electrode
Ag: AgCl	0·1 M HCl	Test solution	3·5 M KCl	3·5 M KCl	Hg₂Cl₂:Hg
Constant potential		Liquid junction potential		Constant potential

Glass — Porous plug

Measured potential

Fig. 18.1. The measurement of pH: arrangement of electrodes and pH meter.

+ — Meter

diagnosis. Similarly, the accuracy of indicators is limited unless complex techniques of colour measurement are used. For this reason the description of the measurement of pH will be limited to the use of electrodes.

pH ELECTRODES

Although other electrodes have played an important part in research, pH measurements are now made with the glass electrode. This is versatile, unaffected by the solution to be measured and can be used with suspensions as well as solutions. The glass electrode assembly consists of two half-cells (just as a battery consists of two half-cells) each of which develop a potential when connected together. One, the reference half-cell (commonly called the reference electrode) maintains a constant potential, whilst the other, the glass half-cell (or glass electrode), develops a potential which is proportional to the concentration of hydrogen ions present. The complete cell is shown in Fig. 18.1, and a representative commercial example in Fig. 18.2.

The potential of the calomel reference electrode varies with temperature and takes several hours to stabilize at a new temperature. It is therefore important to maintain the electrodes at a constant temperature of 37°C. The calomel electrode is connected to the solution under test with a solution of potassium chloride. The junction between the KCl and test solution is sometimes made through a porous plug, which allows the KCl solution to flow very slowly into the test solution. In other electrodes the

Fig. 18.2. Glass electrode assembly (Radiometer). The test solution is aspirated into a glass capillary which is constructed of pH sensitive glass. The column of test solution is continued into a polyethylene capillary, the end of which can be dipped into a thermostatted glass cup containing the KCl. The KCl solution in the cup can be easily renewed when contaminated. Connection to the rest of the KCl bridge and the calomel electrode is accomplished through a porous plug.

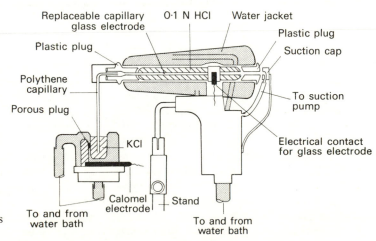

junction is made within a glass or plastic capillary tube, the porous plug in this arrangement usually preventing contamination of the calomel. What matters is that there should be a sharply-defined junction between the two liquids which can be formed accurately and reproducibly for each measurement, and which does not break up during the course of the measurement. The reason for this is that a potential (the liquid junction potential) is always developed at the junction between two salt solutions. Since this potential is part of the total e.m.f. of the cell, it is most important that it should remain constant during a measurement and should be reproducible with each measurement.

At 37°C the glass electrode assembly normally produces about 60 mV per pH unit change. The internal resistance of the cell is high so that if an appreciable current is drawn from the cell when the e.m.f. is measured, a low value will be obtained. It is therefore essential that the pH meter should have a very high input impedance.

Buffers

Although pH is defined as the negative logarithm of the hydrogen ion *concentration*, it is the *activity* of the hydrogen ions which affects the electrical output of the glass electrode. The activity of hydrogen ions only equals the concentration of hydrogen ions in infinite dilutions. For this reason, and also because of the unknown magnitude of the liquid junction potential, it is not possible to relate the measurement of pH directly to the actual concentration of hydrogen ions present. The measurement is therefore standardized against buffer solutions. These solutions usually consist of a weak acid and its salt with a strong base or a weak base and its salt with a strong acid. The characteristic of such a solution is that its pH remains stable despite the addition of relatively large quantities of acids or alkalis.

Unfortunately, a number of buffer scales have been used, the original Sørensen scale differing from some modern scales by as much as 0.4 pH unit. Most workers have now standardized on the National Bureau of Standards scale, since this bears the closest relation to theoretically defined values and also has a series of buffer solutions which are convenient for clinical use.

In practice, therefore, the span of the electrode is set with phosphate buffers of pH 6.835 and 7.386, and the latter buffer is used as a reference against which blood samples are read.

TECHNIQUE OF pH MEASUREMENT

The water bath temperature is first checked to ensure that the electrode is at $37°C \pm 0.1°C$. After setting up the electrode system so that the meter correctly spans the pH interval between the two buffers, a sample of the 7.386 buffer is placed in the electrode. The buffer adjustment is manipulated so that the needle reads exactly 7.386 on the meter, and a sample of blood is aspirated into the electrode. After a pause of 10–15 s (to allow diffusion of H^+ ions between the blood and the glass electrode) a second sample of blood is aspirated into the electrode. The reading is taken when the needle becomes steady, and the blood is then immediately washed out of the electrode with several aliquots of saline (water precipitates globulins which poison the glass of the electrode). Buffer is then reinserted into the electrode and the buffer reading again obtained. This should agree with the previous reading to within 0.005 pH units.

Certain points of technique are important. The electrodes must be kept scrupulously clean and the KCl in the glass cup must be changed whenever it becomes contaminated. The electrode should always be kept filled with water or buffer when not in use. The sample and buffer should be introduced in two increments and care should be taken to ensure an unbroken column of fluid from one end of the capillary to the other. If the electrode response is slow the glass electrode should be filled with 0.1% pepsin in 0.1 N HCl for about 30 min. This will dissolve the protein deposit which sometimes forms. Not infrequently the electrode responds normally with buffers but abnormally with blood samples. This error is difficult to detect unless the electrode is checked by reading the pH of the blood sample on a second electrode system. Alternatively, the electrode may be checked with a stabilized serum preparation (G. W. Burton: see Adams, Morgan-Hughes & Sykes 1967, 1968; Bird & Henderson 1971).

OTHER ION ELECTRODES

A number of other electrodes have now been developed for measuring cations such as K^+, Na^+ and Ca^{++} (Lambie 1980). The calcium electrode utilizes an ion exchange membrane and has proved especially useful for measurements of ionized calcium in blood.

Carbon dioxide

In conscious patients with normal lungs the P_{CO_2} of alveolar (end-tidal) gas approximates to the P_{CO_2} of the arterial blood. In anaesthetized patients and in patients with lung disease there is an increase in alveolar dead space which results in an arterial to end-tidal P_{CO_2} difference. In anaesthetized patients with normal lungs the end-tidal P_{CO_2} is usually about 0.7 kPa (5 mmHg) lower than the arterial P_{CO_2} so that an end-tidal sample can be used to provide a reasonable guide to the arterial P_{CO_2}. However, in patients with lung disease, the arterial to end-tidal P_{CO_2} difference may be increased to 2 or 3 kPa (15–20 mmHg), thus rendering the estimation of arterial P_{CO_2} by this method quite inaccurate. An increase in the arterial to end-tidal P_{CO_2} difference also occurs when cardiac output is markedly reduced so that end-tidal sampling cannot be used to estimate arterial P_{CO_2} in shock states. Conversely, if ventilation is being controlled at a fixed volume, end-tidal monitoring can be used to detect acute disturbances of the circulation. Under these circumstances a sudden reduction in end-tidal P_{CO_2} indicates an acute reduction of blood flow to the lung, whilst an end-tidal CO_2 of zero indicates a cardiac arrest.

The problem of an increased arterial to end-tidal P_{CO_2} difference is obviated by the use of rebreathing methods in which gas in a reservoir bag is rebreathed and caused to come into equilibrium with mixed venous blood. Such methods are simple and are very suitable for repeated measurements. However the arterial P_{CO_2} is calculated from oxygenated mixed venous P_{CO_2} by assuming a value of 0.8 kPa (6 mmHg) for the arterio-venous P_{CO_2} difference. Since this difference increases when cardiac output is reduced the use of rebreathing methods is restricted to patients with a normal cardiovascular status.

The calculation of P_{CO_2} from pH and bicarbonate concentration using the Henderson–Hasselbalch equation is now rarely used, since it has been found that pK' varies with pH and temperature. When this error is added to the known errors of pH measurement the method becomes too inaccurate for general use.

The indirect estimation of arterial P_{CO_2} by the Astrup interpolation technique is much more accurate than the use of the Henderson–Hasselbalch equation, since the slope of the buffer line is determined on each blood sample. It also has the advantage that the nonrespiratory component of acid–base balance is determined as well. It is, however, subject to the error resulting from the difference between the *in vitro* and *in vivo* buffer lines, and there are also a number of other possible errors in the technique which can summate.

The CO_2 electrode provides the most accurate method of determining blood P_{CO_2}; it is basically a glass electrode which measures the change in pH of a bicarbonate solution which has been equilibrated with the blood sample. The direct chemical analysis of a gas bubble which has been equilibrated with the blood sample (Riley technique) cannot be carried out in the presence of an anaesthetic gas, is technically very difficult and is now rarely used.

CO$_2$ tension

REBREATHING METHODS

There are many variations on the basic method, but the successful application of the technique depends more on a thorough understanding of the principles than on the actual technique employed.

The method is based on the discovery by Plesch (1909) that the rebreathing of a suitable gas mixture will lead to its equilibration with mixed venous blood (Fig. 18.3). Provided this equilibration is achieved before recirculation has occurred, subtraction of the normal arterio-venous difference of 0.8 kPa (6 mmHg) from the Pco$_2$ of the gas in the bag yields a reasonable approximation to arterial Pco$_2$. In fact a more accurate estimate is obtained by multiplying the oxygenated mixed venous Pco$_2$ by 0.8 (McEvoy, Jones & Campbell 1974).

The attainment of equilibrium between the gas in the bag, lungs and mixed venous blood within one circulation time (say 20 s) can only be achieved by ensuring that the initial Pco$_2$ of the gas in the bag is close to mixed venous Pco$_2$ and that thorough mixing between bag and lungs occurs during the rebreathing procedure. If a rapid response CO$_2$ analyser is available the correct gas mixture can be found by trial and error, the attainment of equilibrium being shown by a plateau on the trace of CO$_2$ concentration recorded at the mouth. This plateau must occur at least 10 s after the start of rebreathing and must last for at least 3 breaths. If a rapid analyser is not available the correct gas mixture must be generated by one or more preliminary periods of rebreathing. In one method, a 2-litre reservoir bag is filled with about 750 ml of oxygen and rebreathed for three separate periods of 15 s at one- to two-min intervals, the Pco$_2$ in the bag at the end of a fourth period of rebreathing being taken as the oxygenated mixed venous Pco$_2$. In another method a similar volume of oxygen is rebreathed for 1–1½ min. The bag is then

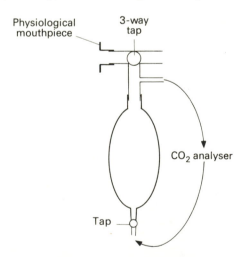

Fig. 18.3. Reservoir bag, 3-way tap and physiological mouthpiece used for rebreathing technique. Intermittent samples are normally removed through the tail of the bag. However, if a rapid analyser is employed the sample is continuously aspirated through a side arm on the tap and returned through the tail of the bag.

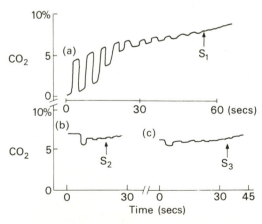

Fig. 18.4. CO$_2$ concentration as sampled at the mouth during the rebreathing method for determining mixed venous Pco$_2$. The three periods of rebreathing (a, b and c) are separated by intervals during which the patient eliminates the CO$_2$ retained during the rebreathing procedure. The arrows S_1, S_2, S_3 indicate the times of sampling when chemical analysis is used.

disconnected for 2–3 min to allow the patient to eliminate the CO_2 retained during rebreathing and the gas mixture is then rebreathed for 20 s to achieve the final equilibrium (Campbell & Howell 1962). Shallow breathing or gas leaks may delay the final equilibrium so that it is wise to repeat the final rebreathing for a period of 30–40 s (Fig. 18.4). The PCO_2 at the end of this period may be 0.1–0.5 kPa higher than the previous value due to recirculation, but a figure within this range confirms that equilibrium was attained in the previous 20-s rebreathing period.

Gas samples may be analysed on an infrared analyser, on a modified Haldane's apparatus (Chapter 17) or on a CO_2 electrode. The rebreathing technique should yield an accuracy of about ± 0.4 kPa (± 3 mmHg) and may be applied to the neonate and infant where arterial sampling may prove difficult (Sykes 1960; Heese & Freeseman 1964).

ASTRUP INTERPOLATION TECHNIQUE

Principle

This technique is based on the observation that there is an almost linear relationship between the pH and log PCO_2 of any particular blood sample over the physiological range, pH falling as PCO_2 is increased (Fig. 18.5). The line obtained by plotting the pH readings against the relevant PCO_2 values (plotted on a logarithmic scale) represents the buffer line of that particular blood sample. The slope of the line depends on the buffering power of the blood and hence on the concentration of plasma proteins and haemoglobin. The changes in plasma proteins encountered in clinical practice have little effect, so that the slope of the line depends predominantly on haemoglobin concentration, the slope being steepest when the haemoglobin concentration is high.

The position of the line in relation to

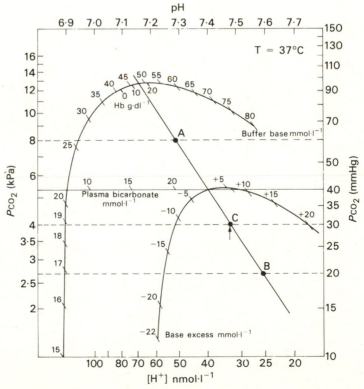

Fig. 18.5. Principle of Astrup interpolation technique plotted on a Siggaard–Andersen nomogram (1962). Points A and B are obtained by measuring the pH of two samples of the patient's blood which have been equilibrated with two $O_2 - CO_2$ gas mixtures of known PCO_2 (in this case 8 kPa and 2.7 kPa — 60 and 20 mmHg). Point C is interpolated from the measured pH of the patient's blood. The PCO_2 can then be read off the ordinate. The base excess (zero) is read from the lower curve. In a nonrespiratory alkalosis the buffer line A — B is shifted to the right and in a nonrespiratory acidosis it is shifted to the left.

the ordinate depends on the nonrespiratory state of the blood sample, the line being displaced to the left if there is a non-respiratory (or metabolic) acidosis and to the right if there is a nonrespiratory alkalosis. Three scales are provided on the nomogram to enable the nonrespiratory component to be quantified. The *base excess* curve indicates the change in pH which would occur if increments of acid or base were added to a normal sample of blood. Thus the addition of 5 mmol/litre of acid would result in a base deficit of 5 mmol/litre, or a base excess of −5 mmol/litre, whilst the addition of 5 mmol/litre of alkali would result in a base excess of 5 mmol/litre. This measure of the nonrespiratory component is independent of haemoglobin concentration since the curve defines the points at which the buffer lines of blood of different haemoglobin concentration, but equal base deficit or excess, intersect (Fig. 18.6). This measure of the nonrespiratory component

greatly simplifies the task of correcting any abnormality which is present, since it gives a direct indication of the quantity of acid or base which must be added to correct the deficit. The second scale commonly shown is the *standard bicarbonate*. This represents the bicarbonate concentration of the plasma of the blood sample when the latter has been equilibrated with a CO_2–O_2 gas mixture with a P_{CO_2} of 5.3 kPa (40 mmHg) at 37°C. Since this value refers to plasma bicarbonate, any deficit in base will only be made good if the dose of bicarbonate given is 1.1 to 1.2 times the deficit in standard bicarbonate. The third scale is that referring to buffer base. The normal buffer base depends on the haemoglobin concentration, since it represents the total quantity of buffer anions present in the sample. The normal buffer base value for each haemoglobin concentration is shown by reference to the haemoglobin scale situated on the buffer base curve. If the normal buffer base

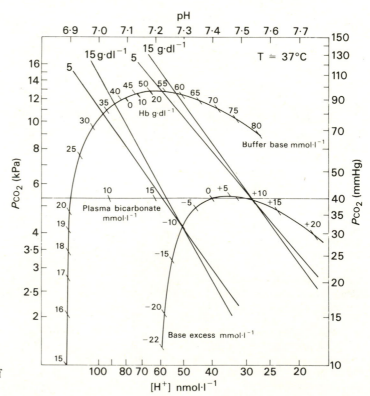

Fig. 18.6. Buffer lines for normal blood samples containing 5 and 15 g·dl⁻¹ of haemoglobin before and after the addition of 10 mmol·l⁻¹ of base.

is subtracted from the buffer base of the sample the true excess or deficit of base will be obtained. This is equivalent to the base excess.

Method

Two aliquots of the blood sample are equilibrated with humidified CO_2–O_2 gas mixtures of known composition (usually 4 % and 8 % CO_2) in a thermostatted micro-tonometer (Fig. 18.7). The microtonometer is oscillated rapidly by an electric motor and rocker arm so that the blood is spread into a thin film, equilibration of a 150 μl blood sample usually being complete in 3–5 min. The pH of each blood sample is then determined with a glass electrode system and the pH plotted against the known gas P_{CO_2} on a pH/log P_{CO_2} diagram. The pH of the original blood sample is interpolated in the buffer line and the P_{CO_2} read off the ordinate.

Sources of error

The first essential is to know the exact composition of the CO_2–O_2 gas mixtures used for equilibration since the actual concentration of CO_2 may differ from the nominal value. The composition may be determined by chemical analysis (p. 220) or by obtaining a certificate of analysis from the manufacturer. Since the gas is humidi-fied at 37°C the P_{CO_2} equals per cent CO_2 × (barometric pressure–water vapour pres-sure). At 37°C water vapour pressure is

6.27 kPa or 47 mmHg. A second source of error is incomplete equilibration with the CO_2–O_2 mixtures, the greatest error tend-ing to occur when the P_{CO_2} of the gas mixture differs markedly from that of the blood sample (Kelman, Coleman & Nunn 1966). Incomplete equilibration can usually be detected by inspecting the slope of the buffer line (Fig. 18.8) or by checking that the haemoglobin concentration indicated on the top scale is within ± 3 g · dl^{-1} of that determined by photometric means (Fig. 18.9). Other common sources of error are failure to ensure that the circulating water jacket is at 37°C at all points in the circuit, and the errors associated with the measure-ment of pH. With care an accuracy of ± 0.02 pH units, which is equivalent to an error of ± 0.25 kPa (2 mmHg) P_{CO_2} or ± 2.5 mmol · l^{-1} base excess, can be achieved.

In vitro and in vivo buffer lines

The buffer line plotted on the Siggaard–Andersen nomogram refers to *in vitro* con-ditions. *In vivo* a certain amount of the bicarbonate generated by the addition of CO_2 passes into the cells. The body as a whole, therefore, does not buffer a change in P_{CO_2} as well as blood alone, and the whole-body buffer line has a slope which is comparable with a dilute Hb solution of about 5 g · dl^{-1}, i.e. the slope is more hori-zontal than the *in vitro* buffer line. Conse-quently, if a blood sample is taken from a patient with a high P_{CO_2} and then equili-brated as described above, it will appear to

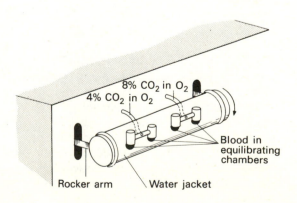

Fig. 18.7. Microtonometer on Astrup apparatus.

Fig. 18.8. Sources of error in the use of the Astrup technique. Line A − A represents a normal buffer line determined by the pH of the blood when equilibrated with gases of P_{CO_2} = 8kPa (60 mmHg) and 3.0kPa (22.5 mmHg). The base excess is zero. Points B − B represent the pH's recorded when equilibration with the gases is incomplete. If the pH of the original blood sample is now interpolated in this line (B′) the P_{CO_2} so determined is too low. The error can be detected by checking whether the patient's haemoglobin corresponds to that illustrated on the buffer base curve. (See Fig. 18.9.) Line C − C represents the effects of using inaccurate buffers or the presence of an abnormal electrode response to blood. Since all three blood pH readings are affected equally the P_{CO_2} is correct but the base estimate is in error. The error in C − C can only be detected by checking the electrode with a stabilized serum preparation with a known buffer line or by repeating the measurements on a second electrode system.

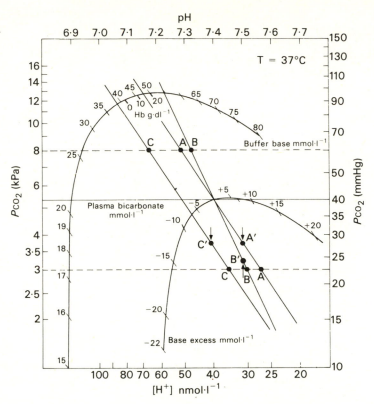

have a base content which is below the value which would have been obtained if the blood had been sampled when the P_{CO_2} was normal (Fig. 18.10). This error only exceeds 3–4 mmol·l^{-1} when the P_{CO_2} is above 12 kPa (90 mmHg) so it can usually be ignored.

The CO_2 *electrode*

The electrode consists of a glass pH electrode with a flattened tip which is in contact with a thin film of sodium bicarbonate solution trapped in a cellophane or nylon mesh (Fig. 18.11). The bicarbonate solution is separated from the CO_2 (in solution or in gaseous form) by a thin teflon or latex rubber membrane which is permeable to CO_2 but not to liquids or solids. CO_2

diffuses into the bicarbonate solution and the change in pH is recorded by the electrode (Fig. 18.12). To ensure a high degree of accuracy it is essential to use a stable pH meter which can discriminate changes in pH of 0.002 pH unit. Before use the electrode must be calibrated with two known concentrations of CO_2 (such as 4% and 8% in O_2). A standardizing gas with a P_{CO_2} close to that of the blood sample is then read before and after each determination. It takes about 3 min for the electrode to reach equilibrium with each sample of blood and gas, even if one or two increments of sample are added to speed up the response (Smith & Hahn 1975). The electrode is thermostatted to 37°C ± 0.1°C and must be maintained exactly at this temperature to ensure stability. The cuvette must be kept filled

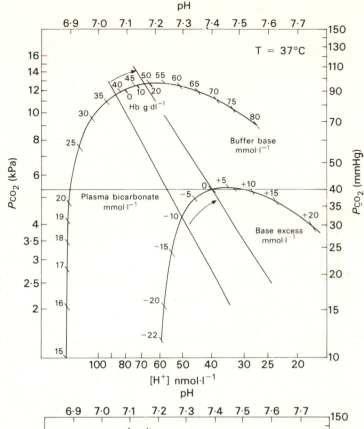

Fig. 18.9. Method of checking slope of buffer line when base excess is not zero. In this example base excess is -10 mmol·l^{-1} so that 10 mmol·l^{-1} must be added to the buffer base value to obtain the Hb concentration (see arrows).

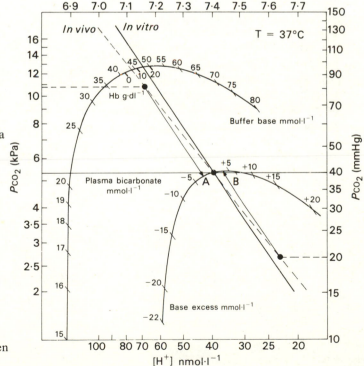

Fig. 18.10. Error in acid–base measurement due to the difference between *in vitro* and *in vivo* equilibration lines. It is assumed that the patient normally has a $P\text{CO}_2$ of 5.3 kPa (40 mmHg) and base excess of zero. An acute respiratory acidosis is then induced (*in vivo* curve) and the blood sampled at a $P\text{CO}_2 = 10.7$ kPa (80 mmHg). When this blood sample is equilibrated *in vitro* the equilibration line will be displaced to the left. The apparent base deficit is indicated by the arrow (A). The opposite effect occurs during a respiratory alkalosis (B).
A revised chart incorporating *in vivo* changes has been published by Siggaard–Andersen (1971).

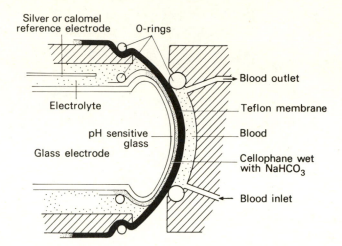

Fig. 18.11. The CO_2 electrode and cuvette.

with wash solution when not in use and the gases used for calibration must be humidified and flushed through very gently. With care and patience an accuracy $\pm 0.15\,kPa$ ($\pm 1\,mmHg$) is attainable (Hahn & Smith 1975). The electrode is not affected by O_2 or anaesthetic agents and is therefore most useful for gas or blood–gas measurements during anaesthesia.

CO_2 electrodes are relatively reliable, but a small hole in the membrane can produce aberrant results with liquids even though gases read correctly. This is due to the passage of H^+ ions from the liquid into the bicarbonate solution. The membrane can be checked electrically to obviate this source of error. An alternative test is to equilibrate a dilute solution of hydrochloric acid with gas of a known P_{CO_2} and then to read this in the electrode. If it reads correctly it is unlikely that there is a hole in the membrane.

TRANSCUTANEOUS AND INTRAVASCULAR CO_2 ELECTRODES

Transcutaneous electrodes are now at an advanced state of development and are subject to most of the problems encountered with transcutaneous oxygen electrodes. Intravascular electrodes which can be inserted through an arterial cannula are also available, though they are subject to changes in sensitivity due to the deposition of fibrin on the membrane.

CO_2 content

The total CO_2 contained in a blood sample consists of the dissolved CO_2 plus the com-

Fig. 18.12. The principle of the CO_2 electrode. CO_2 diffuses into the $NaHCO_3$ solution where it forms (H^+) and (HCO_3^-). The H^+ ions are detected by the glass electrode.

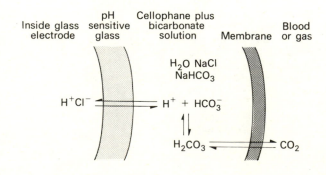

bined CO_2 (bicarbonate, carbonate and carbamino compounds). The CO_2 carried as carbamino compounds represents about 5% of the total and is customarily included in the bicarbonate measurement.

The standard method of measuring CO_2 content is based upon vacuum extraction and absorption by KOH in the manometric Van Slyke apparatus (Van Slyke & Neill 1924). However, this technique requires great technical skill and is time consuming. The micro-apparatus of Natelson (1951) may be used to measure plasma bicarbonate but although the apparatus is easier to handle, the results are less accurate. A convenient alternative is to measure the change in Pco_2 resulting from the addition of a large volume of acid to the blood (Severinghaus 1962; Horabin & Farhi 1978). The acid drives the CO_2 out of combination and the resulting increase in Pco_2 is related to the volumes of blood and acid and to the solubility of CO_2 in the final mixture. The Pco_2 is measured with a CO_2 electrode and the method is calibrated with standard bicarbonate solutions (Linden, Ledsome & Norman 1965).

In most chemical pathology laboratories plasma bicarbonate is measured by an autoanalyser technique or is derived from measurements of pH and Pco_2 as already described.

Oxygen

Arterial oxygenation may be assessed by measuring the tension, saturation or content, the relationship between these three measurements being determined by the shape and position of the O_2 dissociation curve (Fig. 18.13). Since there are many causes of variations in both the shape and position of the curve it is usually necessary to measure the variable of interest directly. Thus tension measurements are required for most respiratory problems, though saturation or content may be required if the percentage shunt is to be calculated. Saturation and tension are necessary to define the dissociation curve whilst content measurements are required when O_2 transport is being considered.

In the past, Po_2 was determined directly by the analysis of a gas bubble equilibrated with the blood sample. This was technically difficult, and nowadays Po_2 is usually measured directly by means of the oxygen electrode. Saturation is determined by photometric techniques involving the trans-

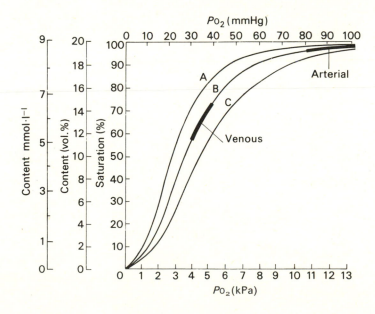

Fig. 18.13. O_2 dissociation curves for (A) $Pco_2 = 2.7$ kPa (20 mmHg); (B) $Pco_2 = 5.3$ kPa (40 mmHg); (C) $Pco_2 = 8$ kPa (60 mmHg). The normal arterial and mixed venous ranges are shown.

mission or reflection of light at certain wavelengths, or from measurements of oxygen content and capacity. O_2 content is measured by vacuum extraction and chemical absorption, by driving the O_2 into solution and measuring the increase in Po_2, or by a galvanic-cell analyser. O_2 capacity is determined by measuring the O_2 content of the blood sample after it has been fully saturated with oxygen. Then

$$\% \text{ saturation} = \frac{O_2 \text{ content}}{O_2 \text{ capacity}} \times 100$$

Oxygen tension

THE OXYGEN ELECTRODE

The modern electrode is based on a design originated by Clark (1956). The electrode assembly (Fig. 18.14) consists of a small cylinder with a plastic membrane, which is permeable to gases but not to liquids or solids, stretched over one end. The cylinder contains a buffered electrolyte solution (which minimizes the effects of CO_2 on the electrode), a silver–silver chloride anode and a platinum wire cathode. The cathode is about $20\,\mu m$ in diameter and is sealed into a glass rod so that only the tip is exposed. The tip of the glass rod is usually roughened so that a thin layer of electrolyte is trapped between the cathode and the plastic

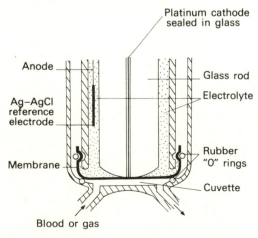

Platinum cathode
sealed in glass

Anode

Glass rod

Ag–AgCl
reference
electrode

Electrolyte

Membrane

Rubber
"O" rings

Cuvette

Blood or gas

Fig. 18.14. The O_2 electrode.

membrane. The electrode assembly is then inserted into a glass or metal cuvette which is maintained at 37°C by water circulated from a thermostatically-controlled water bath. A constant polarizing voltage of about 0.6 volts is applied between the anode and cathode. When the oxygen diffuses from the cuvette to the cathode it is reduced according to the reaction:

$$2H_2O + O_2 + 4e^- \rightarrow 4OH^-.$$

The resulting current flow, which is proportional to the number of oxygen molecules reaching the cathode, amounts to about $10^{-10}\,A\cdot kPa^{-1}$ ($10^{-11}\,A/mmHg$). This is amplified and displayed as a voltage drop across a high resistance by a voltmeter. The zero point is obtained either by injecting a reducing solution into the cuvette, or by flushing the cuvette with oxygen-free nitrogen. Since cylinders of this gas have a black shoulder marked with a white spot the gas is known as 'white spot' nitrogen. The span or gain control is set with either air or oxygen and the other gas is used to check the linearity of the instrument. Air is used as the calibrating gas for a Po_2 which is expected to be below $30\,kPa$ ($225\,mmHg$) and oxygen if the Po_2 is expected to be higher. The humidified calibrating gas is allowed to flow slowly through the cuvette before and after each measurement and the membrane is kept continually moist by frequent washings with an antiseptic-detergent wash solution. The electrode response should be brisk and should be complete within 30–60 s. As with the CO_2 electrode, strict temperature control at 37°C $\pm$ 0.1°C is necessary.

Sources of error

In most oxygen electrodes the Po_2 reading obtained with a blood or liquid sample is less than that obtained with gas of the same Po_2. This difference is believed to be caused by a distortion of the diffusion gradient close to the membrane due to the consumption of oxygen by the electrode. The blood-gas difference depends on the design of the electrode and on the membrane material and should be determined by measuring the Po_2 of liquid or blood which has been equilibrated with gas of a known Po_2 in a tonometer (Adams & Morgan-Hughes 1967; Chalmers, Bird & Whitwam 1974). In most of the modern electrodes the difference is less than 4% of the reading (Bird, Williams & Whitwam 1974) and is frequently much less.

At a polarizing voltage of about 0.6V the method is reasonably specific for oxygen though other substances, such as halothane, may also be reduced and so may interfere with the analysis (Severinghaus *et al.* 1971; Dent & Netter 1976). Other gases are reduced at higher polarizing voltages: for example the method has recently been utilized for determining the tensions of both nitrous oxide and oxygen (Albery *et al.* 1978). Interference by both halothane and nitrous oxide may produce marked errors in some commercial electrodes (Douglas *et al.* 1978; Evans & Cameron 1978).

In careful hands the accuracy of Po_2 measurement is ± 0.25 kPa (± 2 mmHg) at tensions up to 20 kPa (150 mmHg). At higher Po_2 levels the accuracy is less owing to the rapid fall in dissolved Po_2 due to metabolism by leucocytes, and to the inherent inaccuracy of the electrode and recording system (Hahn, Davis & Albery 1975). Other causes of inaccurate measurements are holes in the membrane, bubbles between the membrane and cathode, protein or clot on the membrane, poor temperature control and the presence of infected material in the cuvette.

Rapid response electrodes

Recently, pulsed electrodes have been introduced (Zick 1976). A bare gold cathode 75 μm in diameter is used with a silver–silver chloride anode and the polarizing voltage is applied in bursts of 5 ms duration. This electrode has a linear response, is not flow-sensitive and has an extremely short response time which permits breath-by-breath monitoring of Po_2.

INTRAVASCULAR MONITORING OF Po_2

Miniature, catheter-tip electrodes for intravascular monitoring are now available commercially and have been used successfully for periods of up to 1 or 2 days. The electrode system is subject to long-term electronic drift but this can be corrected by comparing the electrode reading with the Po_2 of blood samples which have been withdrawn through the catheter. The main problem with such electrodes is that fibrin deposition or thrombosis leads to changes in electrode sensitivity or to electrode failure. Intravascular electrodes have a fairly rapid response (between 5 and 60 s for a 95% response) and provide a useful record of acute changes in Po_2 resulting from nursing procedures such as opening an incubator, turning, endotracheal tube aspiration or temporary disconnection from the ventilator (Rolfe 1976a, b). They have also been used in adults to monitor changes in mixed venous Po_2 associated with rapid changes in circulatory status (e.g. after open-heart surgery). Recently, a catheter tip combined Po_2 and Pco_2 electrode has been described (Parker, Delphy & Lewis 1978). Intravascular measurements have also been performed by analysing the gases which diffuse from the blood into an intravascular silicone or Teflon catheter. Since the rate of diffusion is slow the sample flow rate is low. Analysis can therefore only be achieved by the use of a mass spectrometer. Difficulties in calibration and the occurrence or thrombosis round the catheter have limited the application of this technique.

TRANSCUTANEOUS MONITORING OF Po_2

Recent developments in electrode technology have led to the successful application of transcutaneous Po_2 monitoring devices (Huch *et al.* 1977; Skeates 1978; Blackburn 1978). There are two basic problems. Firstly, transcutaneous Po_2 is lower than arterial Po_2 because of the metabolic consumption of oxygen by the skin, so that a constant relationship between the two only develops when the skin vessels are maximally dilated. Secondly, diffusion of oxygen through the skin is slow. Full dilation of skin vessels can only be achieved by heating the skin to about 44°C by means of a thermo-statically-controlled heater around the electrode. Whilst such heating greatly improves the correlation between transcutaneous Po_2 and arterial Po_2 it is associated with a significant risk of injury to the skin, and superficial burns have occurred in long-term monitoring in neonates when temperatures of 44–45°C have been used. The relatively good correlation of transcutaneous Po_2 and arterial Po_2 is due to a fortunate balance between opposing factors. The heating of blood in the skin capillaries above 37°C shifts the O_2 dissociation curve to the right and decreases the solubility of oxygen in blood, so increasing the Po_2 in the capillary blood (Kelman & Nunn 1966). This increase offsets the diffusion gradient and the in-creased tissue metabolism resulting from the heating. The net result is that the electrode "sees" a Po_2 close to arterial Po_2.

The problem of oxygen consumption by the electrode and slow diffusion through the skin has been tackled in two ways. In one electrode system a membrane with com-paratively low oxygen permeability is used. This results in a relatively long response time and a low current from the electrode. An alternative approach is to use a more permeable membrane material but to decrease the size of the cathode.

The main disadvantage of cutaneous measurements is that they are very sensitive to small changes in skin blood flow and thus become quite unreliable in shock. Changes in circulatory status seem to be of less importance in neonates than in adults, so that transcutaneous Po_2 monitoring will probably prove to be a useful adjunct to intermittent blood–gas analysis in neonates (Huch *et al.* 1977). Successful application of percutaneous monitoring has been re-ported in adults but its role in clinical prac-tice has yet to be determined (Severinghaus

et al. 1978). The membrane of most elec-trodes needs to be changed every 24 hours or so and it seems probable that the incid-ence of skin reactions can be decreased by changing the position of the electrode at regular intervals. Some of the commercially available electrodes are also sensitive to nitrous oxide and halothane so that their use as a monitor during anaesthesia may be limited (Gøthgen & Jacobsen 1978).

O₂ saturation

The standard method of determining oxygen saturation is to measure the oxygen content and capacity of the red cells. Then

$$\% \text{ saturation} = \frac{\text{oxygen content}}{\text{oxygen capacity}} \times 100.$$

The oxygen content of the red cells is obtained by analysing the sample on the Van Slyke apparatus and subtracting an appropriate value for dissolved oxygen. Oxygen capacity is obtained by a similar analysis of another sample of the patient's blood which has been fully saturated by equilibration with oxygen. Again, a correc-tion for dissolved oxygen must be applied. Since analyses on the Van Slyke apparatus are time-consuming and require great technical skill, most measurements of oxygen saturation are now made by oxi-metry, a method which measures the ab-sorption or reflectance of light by the pigment oxyhaemoglobin. Unfortunately, the Beer–Lambert laws (see Chapter 8) can only be applied to situations in which there is no scattering of light waves: it is therefore strictly applicable only to haemolysed blood. However technical developments have now circumvented this problem so that satisfactory measurements can be made not only on whole blood, but also on tissues containing blood.

The saturation of the red cell depends on the ratio of oxyhaemoglobin to reduced haemoglobin. These two pigments have

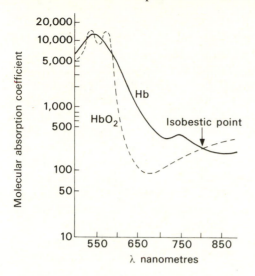

Fig. 18.15. Absorption spectra for oxygenated (HbO$_2$) and reduced (Hb) haemoglobin.

different absorption spectra (Fig. 18.15). By simultaneously measuring absorption or reflection at the wavelength at which their absorption coefficients are equal (the iso-bestic point) and at a point at which the coefficients differ, it is possible to estimate saturation without knowing the thickness of blood through which the light passes. The use of this principle enables saturation to be measured, not only in blood samples, but also *in vivo*.

REFLECTION OXIMETERS

The American Optical Company's oximeter is an example of this type of apparatus. A small quantity of blood is placed in a cuvette and stirred mechanically. A beam of light is shone on to the bottom of the cuvette and the reflected light is passed through two filters which transmit light with wavelengths close to 805 or 650 nm. The intensity of these two beams of light is measured simultaneously by two photocells. The operator balances the circuit until a null-deflection is observed on the meter and the percentage saturation is then read directly from a calibrated scale. The amount of light reflected at 805 nm (the isobestic point) is related to the haemoglobin concentration whilst the reflection at the 605-nm wavelength is related to the oxy-haemoglobin concentration. The instrument is reliable, simple to operate and obviates the need to haemolyse the blood sample. It is reasonably accurate but tends to read high when compared with the Van Slyke apparatus, particularly below 40% satura-tion (Cole & Hawkins 1967). Attempts have been made to use reflection oximetry to measure the saturation of blood in an arterialized area of skin but have not met with success. However the principle has been applied successfully to measure the saturation of blood in the right heart, the light being transmitted and received via fibre-optic bundles contained in a cardiac catheter (Enson *et al.* 1962).

TRANSMISSION OXIMETERS

These instruments are usually capable of greater accuracy than reflection oximeters but the blood must be haemolysed before measurements are made. Measurements of light transmission are first made with the infrared filter at approximately 805 nm and then at a wavelength of 620–650 nm. Three commercial instruments with special attri-butes must be mentioned. The Radiometer OSM2 can be operated with very small samples which can be taken from a heel prick into a capillary tube (Siggaard-Andersen 1977). The blood is haemolysed by freezing and thawing and is then drawn by capillary action under the cover slip of the cuvette which is similar to a haemo-cytometer slide. Readings are then taken at 505 and 598 nm and the percentage satura-tion read from a nomogram. Agreement with the Van Slyke is good (Cole & Hawkins 1967). Another instrument, the IL Co-Oximeter is completely automatic. A heparinized blood sample of about 0.5 ml is injected directly into the instrument. The sample is automatically diluted, haemolysed and propelled into the measuring cuvette where simultaneous readings are taken at 548, 568 and 578 nm. The optical trans-missions are automatically computed and presented as digital readouts of total haemo-globin, percentage O_2 saturation and per-centage carboxyhaemoglobin. The machine is accurate and fairly simple to use (Cole & Williams 1976).

A number of transmission oximeters have measuring units which can be attached to the arterialized ear lobe so that continuous *in vivo* monitoring can be carried out. Whilst these instruments provide a continuous monitor of saturation, calibration has always proved difficult and the absolute values have therefore been open to question. The new Hewlett–Packard instrument (47201A) appears to overcome many of the previous problems. The instrument measures light transmission in the ear at eight different wavelengths between 650 and 1050 nm by rotating filters in front of the light source, the light being transmitted to the ear in fibre-optic bundles. The use of a large number of different wavelengths enables the effects of pigmentation and different ear thickness to be discounted so that movement artefacts are reduced to a minimum. The machine is easily calibrated with an 'artificial ear' and the patient's ear is maintained at 41°C, which is a comfort-able temperature for the patient. The machine is expensive but its accuracy appears to be superior to most other ear-piece oximeters (Saunders, Powles & Rebuck 1976).

Oxygen dissociation curve analysers

Simultaneous measurements of saturation, Po_2 and pH are required in the determina-tion of the oxygen dissociation curve of whole blood and a number of instruments are now available which permit both the position and shape of the curve to be defined with reasonable accuracy. The original analyser was described by Duvelleroy *et al.* (1970) and modifications have been described by Hahn, Foëx & Raynor (1976). Simpler methods based on the determination of one fixed point have been described by Kirk, Raber & Duke (1975) and Aberman *et al.* (1975).

O_2 content

THE VAN SLYKE APPARATUS

Although both volumetric and manometric methods have been described, it is the manometric technique which has been most commonly used for measuring oxygen or carbon dioxide content, for its accuracy is greater than the volumetric method (Van Slyke & Neill 1924). The apparatus consists essentially of a burette of known volume and a mercury column for measuring the pressure in the burette. A mercury reservoir is used to aspirate the reagents into the

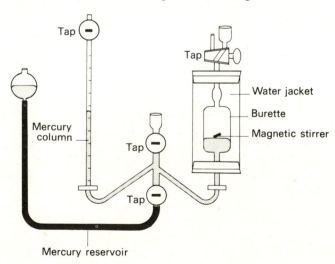

Fig. 18.16. The manometric Van Slyke apparatus.

measuring chamber; it can also be used to create a vacuum in the burette (Fig. 18.16). After checking the apparatus for leaks, the chemical reagents to be used are de-gassed by shaking under reduced pressure in the burette. The gases are driven off and the reagents stored anaerobically in separate burettes. One millilitre of blood is then introduced into the Van Slyke burette with an Ostwald pipette and an acid–saponin mixture is added to haemolyse the blood and drive off all the gases. The mixture is shaken under reduced pressure and the total volume of the extracted gases is measured by recording the pressure on the manometer after the gases have been reduced to a known volume in the burette by means of the mercury reservoir. An absorbent solution is then added to the contents of the burette and the drop in pressure recorded. By using different solutions for the absorption of CO_2 and O_2 and noting the resultant drops in pressure it is possible to calculate the volumes of CO_2 and O_2 in the original blood sample.

The method is technically difficult, slow and inaccurate in the presence of anaesthetic gases. The accuracy obtainable is about 0.1 vol % for oxygen and 0.2 vol % for CO_2 under the very best conditions, but it takes the average technician several months to attain this degree of competence.

GALVANIC CELL ANALYSER

The system used in a commercial analyser (the Lex–O_2–Con CL) is shown in Fig. 18.17. A 1% carbon monoxide and 2% hydrogen in nitrogen gas mixture is passed over a palladium catalyst to free it of oxygen and then bubbled continuously through a column of distilled water. Twenty microlitres of blood are aspirated into a Hamilton syringe and then injected through a rubber diaphragm into the water column. The red cells are immediately haemolysed and carboxyhaemoglobin formed. The released oxygen is carried by the gas stream over the galvanic cell which yields an electrical output which is proportional to the number of oxygen molecules present in the blood sample. The output from the cell is integrated electronically over the wash-out period of 5 min and the result displayed digitally. The apparatus is calibrated by injecting a known volume of air at known temperature and pressure into the column. Great care is required when handling the blood samples to ensure that the cells and plasma are continuously mixed and transferred anaerobically to the Hamilton syringe, but if care is taken an accuracy of ±0.3 vol % can be achieved (Selman, White & Tait 1975; Douglas et al. 1975; Cole & Williams 1976).

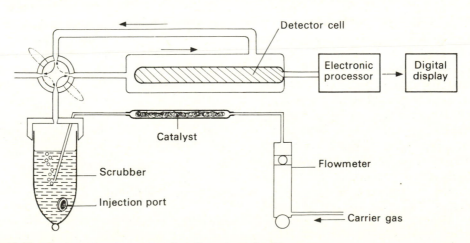

Fig. 18.17. The Lex–O_2–Con galvanic cell analyser for O_2 content.

METHODS BASED ON MEASUREMENT OF Po_2

The first successful methods were described by Linden, *et al.* (1965) and by Laver *et al.* (1965). A small sample of blood (varying from 50 μl to 0.5 ml) is mixed with a large volume of potassium ferricyanide solution which haemolyses the red cells and drives the oxygen into solution. The Po_2 of the solution is recorded before and after the addition of the blood and from the known solubility of O_2 in the solution the oxygen content of the blood sample can be calculated. Klingenmaier, Behar & Smith (1969) used a solution of saline saturated with carbon monoxide to displace the oxygen from the cells but like most of the earlier workers, they also found a small systematic difference from the O_2 content determined by the Van Slyke apparatus. Further modifications of the technique have been described by Horabin & Farhi (1978).

Automated blood–gas analysis systems

A number of automated and semi-automated systems have now been produced. A completely automated system (such as the Radiometer ABL 2) contains three functional subunits; a calibration system, a measuring system and a control system. The *calibration system* produces two fluids of known pH, Pco_2 and Po_2 for the calibration of the electrodes. These are prepared by equilibrating two calibrating solutions with two different gas mixtures, the gas mixtures in turn being generated by mixing CO_2 and air in different proportions. The *measuring system* contains the pH, Pco_2 and Po_2 electrodes, a photometer for haemoglobin estimation and a barometer. The *control system* consists of a microprocessor combined with a data-logger, display, printing and control hardware.

The computer has three modes of operation: calibrate, sample and rinse. The initial calibration sequence is initiated when the machine is switched on and includes a checking procedure to ensure that the electrodes are functioning correctly. If they are not, a warning system operates. Subsequent calibrations are initiated by the computer every 2 hr and the results displayed on the printed output. The calibration data are stored in a memory and used to correct subsequent blood–gas measurements. A new calibration may be initiated at any time by the operator.

In the sample mode, a blood sample is aspirated into the measuring cuvette and at the end of a preset period the outputs from the electrodes are 'read', the data are corrected from the calibration curves and displayed in digital form on illuminated panels, and the derived data (base excess, standard bicarbonate etc.) are calculated. The complete results are then printed out and a rinse sequence is initiated. The full analysis cycle takes about 4 min, the calibration cycle about 6 min and the rinse cycle about 1 min.

Although such systems are expensive they have many advantages. Being automatic they can be used by relatively unskilled staff who can be engaged in other work whilst the analysis is proceeding. The regular rinse and calibrate sequences ensure that the machine does not become clogged with blood and that it is always ready for use. The accuracy compares well with the standard electrode systems operated by skilled technicians and the likelihood of errors due to inaccurate readings is reduced by the printed output (Selman & Tait 1976). Nevertheless undetected errors do occur and some degree of user training and technical control is essential (Rubin, Bradbury & Prowse 1979).

Temperature corrections

In clinical practice it is convenient to run the electrode system at 37°C and to apply correction factors to the measured Po_2,

P_{CO_2} and pH if the patient's blood was sampled at a different temperature.

For P_{O_2} and P_{CO_2} the factors of Kelman & Nunn (1966) are usually used. For pH the correction factor suggested by Rosenthal (1948) is customarily applied. This factor is $+0.0147$ pH units for each $1°C$ fall in temperature. Burton (1965) showed that this factor depends on the original pH.

Since the significance of pH measurements at low temperatures is not clear, most clinicians correct P_{O_2} and P_{CO_2} to body temperature but measure the non-respiratory component of acid–base balance at $37°C$.

Blood sampling and storage

The samples used in blood–gas analysis may be venous, capillary or arterial. Venous samples taken with a tourniquet should never be used, since stasis markedly influences pH. Venous blood taken without stasis may be used to determine the non-respiratory component, but a correction for the arterial desaturation should be applied. 'Arterialized' venous blood obtained from the back of the hand after thorough warming of the limb may provide a useful estimate for P_{CO_2} and pH, but not P_{O_2}. Capillary blood obtained from the vaso-dilated earlobe in adults or from a heel prick in babies may also yield satisfactory results for P_{CO_2} and pH if the skin flow is brisk and there are no other influences, such as pain or blood-loss, which are producing vasoconstriction.

Since all these samples are subject to error and none are really satisfactory for P_{O_2} measurement, arterial samples are used whenever possible. Arterial blood may be sampled by intermittent puncture using a standard No. 1 (S.W.G. size 21) needle or by indwelling catheter. Catheters may be of the disposable type inserted over a needle or may be inserted by the Seldinger (1953) technique. To minimize complications catheters should be made of Teflon and should have parallel sides, the diameter being no greater than 20 gauge (Bedford & Wollman 1973; Bedford 1975). Catheters may be left in the radial or brachial arteries for 24–48 hr provided they are inserted carefully and are flushed with small quantities ($\frac{1}{2}$–1 ml) of heparinized saline (10 I.U./ml) at intervals of $\frac{1}{2}$–1 hr or are connected to a continuous flush apparatus.* When the needle or catheter is removed firm pressure must be applied to the site of puncture for at least 3–4 min. Non-occlusive pressure is then applied for a further 2–3 min and, if there is then no sign of haematoma formation, a firm pressure-dressing is applied.

Blood may be taken into glass or plastic syringes. A small quantity of heparin is drawn into the syringe which is held with the nozzle uppermost whilst the plunger is moved up and down to wet the sides of the cylinder. All air bubbles are now carefully expelled, only the dead space being left filled with heparin. The blood sample should be withdrawn slowly (preferably over a period of 1–2 min), the syringe is then capped and rotated rapidly between the palms of the hands. The sample is stored in a thermos flask containing ice and water if analysis is likely to be delayed for more than 30 min. Plastic syringes should not be used for prolonged storage since gases diffuse through their walls (Scott, Horton & Mapleson 1971a, b).

* e.g. 'Intraflo' Sørensens, P.O. Box 15588, Saltlake City, Utah, USA.

References

ABERMAN A., CAVANILLES J.M., WEIL M.H. & SHUBIN H. (1975) Blood P_{50} calculated from a single measurement of pH, P_{O_2} and S_{O_2}. *Journal of Applied Physiology*, **38**, 171.

ADAMS A.P. & MORGAN-HUGHES J.O. (1967) Determination of the blood–gas factor of the oxygen electrode using a new tonometer. *British Journal of Anaesthesia*, **39**, 107.

ADAMS A.P., MORGAN-HUGHES J.O. & SYKES M.K. (1967) pH and blood–gas analysis. Methods of measurement and sources of error using electrode systems. Part 1, *Anaesthesia*, **22**, 575.

ADAMS A., MORGAN-HUGHES J.O. & SYKES M.K. (1968) pH and blood–gas analysis. Methods of measurement and sources of error using electrode systems. Part 2, *Anaesthesia*, **23**, 47.

ALBERY W.J., BROOKS W.N., GIBSON S.P. & HAHN C.E.W. (1978) An electrode for P_{N_2O} and P_{O_2} analysis in blood and gas. *Journal of Applied Physiology: Respiratory, Environmental and Exercise Physiology*, **45**, 637.

BEDFORD R.F. & WOLLMAN H. (1973) Complications of percutaneous radial artery cannulation. *Anesthesiology*, **38**, 228.

BEDFORD R.F. (1975) Percutaneous radial-artery cannulation-increased safety using Teflon catheters. *Anesthesiology*, **42**, 219.

BIRD B.D. & HENDERSON F.A. (1971) The use of serum as a control in acid-base determination. *British Journal of Anaesthesia*, **43**, 592.

BIRD B.D., WILLIAMS J. & WHITWAM J.G. (1974) The blood–gas factor: a comparison of three different oxygen electrodes. *British Journal of Anaesthesia*, **46**, 249.

BLACKBURN J.P. (1978) What is new in blood–gas analysis? *British Journal of Anaesthesia*, **50**, 51.

BURTON G.W. (1965) Effects of the acid-base state upon the temperature coefficient of pH of blood. *British Journal of Anaesthesia*, **37**, 89.

CAMPBELL E.J.M. & HOWELL J.L.B. (1962) Rebreathing method for measurement of mixed venous P_{CO_2}. *British Medical Journal*, **2**, 630.

CHALMERS C., BIRD B.D. & WHITWAM J.G. (1974) Evaluation of a new thin film tonometer. *British Journal of Anaesthesia*, **46**, 253.

CLARK L.C. (1956) Monitor and control of blood and tissue oxygen tension. *Transactions of the Society for Artificial Internal organs*, **2**, 41.

COLE P.V. & HAWKINS L.H. (1967) The measurement of the oxygen content of whole blood. *Biomedical Engineering*, **2**, 56.

COLE P. & WILLIAMS J. (1976) Apparatus for blood–gas analysis. *British Journal of Clinical Practice*, **1**, 267.

DENT J.G. & NETTER K.J. (1976) Errors in oxygen tension measurements caused by halothane. *British Journal of Anaesthesia*, **48**, 195.

DOUGLAS I.H.S., MacDONALD J.A.E., MILLIGAN G.F., MELLON A. & LEDINGHAM I.McA. (1975) A comparison of methods for the measurement of cardiac output and blood oxygen content. *British Journal of Anaesthesia*, **47**, 443.

DOUGLAS I.H.S., McKENZIE P.J., LEDINGHAM I.McA. & SMITH G. (1978) Effect of halothane on P_{O_2} electrode. *Lancet*, **ii**, 1370.

DUVELLEROY M.A., BUCKLES R.G., ROSENKAIMER S., TUNG C. & LAVER M.B. (1970) An oxyhaemoglobin dissociation analyzer. *Journal of Applied Physiology*, **28**, 227.

ENSON Y., BRISCOE W.A., POLYANI M.L. &

COURNAND A. (1962) *In vivo* studies with an intravascular and intracardiac reflection oximeter. *Journal of Applied Physiology*, **17**, 552.

EVANS M.C. & CAMERON I.R. (1978) Oxygen electrodes sensitive to nitrous oxide. *Lancet*, **ii**, 1371.

GØTHGEN I. & JACOBSEN E. (1978) Transcutaneous oxygen tension measurement. 2 The influence of halothane and hypotension. *Acta Anaesthesiologica Scandinavica Supplement*, **67**, 71.

HAHN C.E.W., DAVIS A.H. & ALBERY W.J. (1975) Electrochemical improvement of the performance of P_{O_2} electrodes. *Respiration Physiology*, **25**, 109.

HAHN C.E.W., FOËX P. & RAYNOR C.M. (1976) A development of the oxyhaemoglobin dissociation curve analyzer. *Journal of Applied Physiology*, **41**, 259.

HAHN C.E.W. & SMITH A.C. (1975) Studies with the "Severinghaus" P_{CO_2} electrode II: Carbon dioxide measurements using a single control analyser. *British Journal of Anaesthesia*, **47**, 559.

HEESE H.deV. & FREESEMAN C. (1964) Determination of mixed venous P_{CO_2} in infants and children. *British Medical Journal*, **1**, 1290.

HORABIN A.L. & FARHI L. (1978) Measurement of blood O_2 and CO_2 concentrations using P_{O_2} and P_{CO_2} electrodes. *Journal of Applied Physiology: Respiratory, Environmental and Exercise Physiology*, **44**, 818.

HUCH A., HUCH R., SCHNEIDER H. & ROOTH G. (1977) Continuous transcutaneous monitoring of fetal oxygen tension during labour. *British Journal of Obstetrics & Gynaecology*, **84**, Suppl. 1, 1.

KELMAN G.R., COLEMAN A.J. & NUNN J.F. (1966) Evaluation of a microtonometer used with a capillary glass pH electrode. *Journal of Applied Physiology*, **21**, 1103.

KELMAN G.R. & NUNN J.F. (1966) Nomograms for correction of blood P_{O_2}, P_{CO_2}, pH and base excess for time and temperature. *Journal of Applied Physiology*, **21**, 1484.

KIRK B.W., RABER M.B. & DUKE K.R. (1975) A simplified method for determining the P_{50} of blood. *Journal of Applied Physiology*, **38**, 1140.

KLINGENMAIER C.H., BEHAR M.G. & SMITH T.C. (1969) Blood oxygen content measured by oxygen tension after release by carbon monoxide. *Journal of Applied Physiology*, **26**, 653.

LAMBIE A.T. (1980) Measurement of sodium and potassium in body fluids. *British Journal of Clinical Equipment*, **5**, 70.

LAVER M.B., MURPHY A.J., SIEFEN A. & RADFORD E.P. (1965) Blood oxygen content measurements using the oxygen electrode. *Journal of Applied Physiology*, **20**, 1063.

LINDEN R.J., LEDSOME J.R. & NORMAN J. (1965) Simple methods for the determination of the concentration of carbon dioxide and oxygen in blood. *British Journal of Anaesthesia*, **34**, 77.

MCEVOY J.D.S., JONES N.L. & CAMPBELL E.J.M. (1974) Mixed venous and arterial P_{CO_2}. *British Medical Journal*, **4**, 687.

NATELSON S. (1951) Routine use of ultra-micromethods in the clinical laboratory. *American Journal of Clinical Pathology*, **21**, 1153.

PARKER D., DELPHY D. & LEWIS M. (1978) Catheter tip electrode for continuous measurement of P_{O_2} and P_{CO_2}. *Medical & Biological Engineering and Computing*, **16**, 601.

PLESCH J. (1909) Hamodynamisch studien. *Zeitschrift für Experimentelle Pathologie und Therapie*, **6**, 380.

ROLFE P. (1976a) Monitoring equipment for the neonate. *British Journal of Clinical Equipment*, **1**, 189.

ROLFE P. (1976b) Arterial oxygen measurement in the newborn with intravascular transducers; in *IEE Medical Electronics Monographs* 18–22 (eds D.W. Hill & B.W. Watson) p. 126. Stevenage: Peter Perigrinus.

ROSENTHAL T.B. (1948) The effect of temperature on the pH of blood and plasma *in vitro*. *Journal of Biological Chemistry*, **173**, 25.

RUBIN P., BRADBURY S. & BROWSE K. (1979) Comparative study of automatic blood–gas analysers and their use in analysing arterial and capillary samples. *British Medical Journal* **1**, 156.

SAUNDERS N.A., POWLES A.C.P. & REBUCK A.S. (1976) Ear oximetry; accuracy and practicability in the assessment of arterial oxygenation. *American Review of Respiratory Disease*, **113**, 745.

SCOTT P.V., HORTON J.N. & MAPLESON W.W. (1971a) Mechanism and magnitude of leakage of oxygen from blood and water samples stored in plastic syringes. *British Journal of Anaesthesia*, **43**, 717.

SCOTT P.V., HORTON J.N. & MAPLESON W.W. (1971b) Leakage of oxygen from blood and water samples stored in plastic and glass syringes. *British Medical Journal*, **3**, 513.

SELDINGER S.I. (1953) Catheter replacement of the needle in percutaneous arteriography. *Acta radiologica (Stockholm)*, **39**, 368.

SELMAN B.J. & TAIT A.R. (1976) Towards blood–gas autoanalysis; an evaluation of the Radiometer ABL1. *British Journal of Anaesthesia*, **48**, 487.

SELMAN B.J., WHITE Y.S. & TAIT A.R. (1975) An evaluation of the Lex–O_2–Con oxygen content analyser. *Anaesthesia*, **30**, 206.

SEVERINGHAUS J.W. (1962) Electrodes for blood and gas P_{CO_2} and blood pH. *Acta anaesthesiologica Scandinavica Supplement*, **11**, 207.

SEVERINGHAUS J.W., PEABODY J., THUNSTROM A., EBERHARD P. & ZAPPIA E. (eds) (1978) Workshop on methodologic aspects of transcutaneous blood gas analysis. *Acta Anaesthesiologica Scandinavica Supplement 68*.

SEVERINGHAUS J.W., WEISKOPF R.B., NISHIMURA M. & BRADLEY A.F. (1971) Oxygen electrode errors due to polarographic reduction of halothane. *Journal of Applied Physiology*, **31**, 640.

SKEATES S.J. (1978) The non-invasive measurement of arterial oxygen. *British Journal of Clinical Equipment*, **3**, 63.

SIGGAARD-ANDERSEN O. (1962) The pH-log P_{CO_2} blood acid-base nomogram revised. *Scandinavian Journal of Clinical and Laboratory Investigation*, **14**, 598.

SIGGAARD-ANDERSEN O. (1971) An acid-base chart for normal and pathophysiological reference areas. *Scandinavian Journal of Clinical and Laboratory Investigation*, **27**, 239.

SIGGAARD-ANDERSEN O. (1977) Experiences with a new direct-reading oxygen saturation meter using ultrasound for haemolyzing the blood. *Scandinavian Journal of Clinical and Laboratory Investigation*, **37**, *Supplement 146*.

SMITH A.C. & HAHN C.E.W. (1975) Studies with the Severinghaus P_{CO_2} electrode, I: Electrode stability memory and S plots. *British Journal of Anaesthesia*, **47**, 553.

SYKES M.K. (1960) Observations on a rebreathing technique for the determination of arterial P_{CO_2} in the apnoeic patient. *British Journal of Anaesthesia*, **32**, 256.

VAN SLYKE D.D. & NEILL J.M. (1924) The determination of gases in blood and other solutions by vacuum extraction and monometric measurement. *Journal of Biological Chemistry*, **61**, 523.

ZICK G.L. (1976) Determination of oxygen tension by measurement of net charge transport. *IEE Transactions on Biomedical Engineering*, **23**, 472.

Further reading

FLENLEY D.C. (1978) Clinical physiology: interpretation of blood–gas and acid-base data. *British Journal of Hospital Medicine*, **19**, 384.

SYKES M.K., MCNICOL M.W. & CAMPBELL E.J.M. (1976) *Respiratory Failure*. Oxford: Blackwell Scientific Publications.

Chapter 19
Thermometry, Thermography and Humidity Measurement

Thermometry

Spontaneous and controlled changes in body temperature are now so commonly encountered in clinical practice that temperature monitoring has become routine in the operating theatre and intensive care situations. Thermometry is also used to monitor the function of therapeutic devices such as humidifiers and extracorporeal circulation equipment, and ancillary equipment such as autoclaves, refrigerators and laboratory apparatus.

TEMPERATURE SCALES AND CALIBRATION

In 1714 the German physicist Fahrenheit developed the first thermometer using mercury in a closed tube. There is some doubt about the fixed points on his scale of temperature but it is believed that he set the zero point with a mixture of sodium chloride and ice and assumed that body temperature was 100°F. The temperature of melting ice then read 32°F and that of boiling water 212°F. In 1742 the Swedish astronomer Anders Celsius adopted a different scale which, in its final form, utilized the temperature of melting ice and boiling water as the two fixed points on the scale. This scale was divided into a hundred

steps and so became known by the Latin equivalent 'centigrade'. However in 1948 the scale was renamed the Celsius scale (°C) in honour of its inventor. The conversions between the two scales are given by:

$$°F = \left(°C \times \frac{9}{5}\right) + 32$$

and

$$°C = (°F - 32) \times \frac{5}{9}.$$

Normal body temperature is thus 37°C or 98.4°F.

When dealing with gas law equations it is necessary to employ yet another scale of temperature, the Absolute or Kelvin temperature scale. On this scale the zero is the Absolute zero, which is the lowest temperature it is theoretically possible to attain. This is -273.16°C. The unit of the Kelvin scale used to be called the degree Kelvin but in the SI system is now simply called the kelvin (K). It is defined as 1/273.16 of the thermodynamic temperature of the triple point of water (the point where the solid, liquid and vapour forms of water co-exist). Thus 0°C is equivalent to 273 K and 100°C to 373 K. Since each degree Celsius is equal to a kelvin, K = °C + 273 (Fig. 19.1).

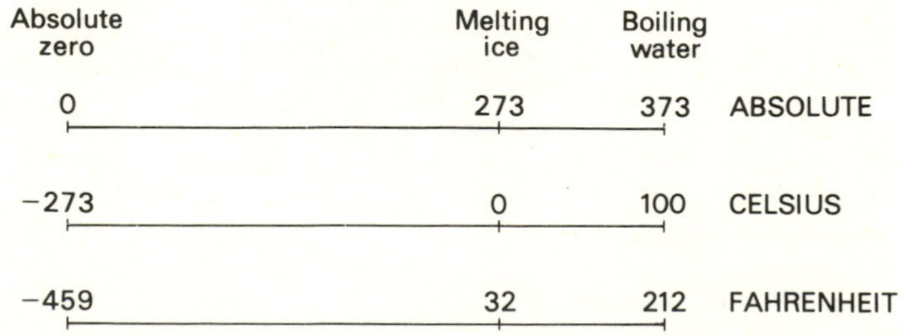

	Absolute zero		Melting ice	Boiling water	
	0		273	373	ABSOLUTE
	−273		0	100	CELSIUS
	−459		32	212	FAHRENHEIT

Fig. 19.1. Absolute, Celsius and Fahrenheit temperature scales.

264

The fixed points on most thermometers can be set with melting ice and boiling water. However the accuracy of intermediate points can only be ensured by checking that the scale is linear. Furthermore some thermometers have a limited scale length so that the 0°C and 100°C points cannot be established. Thermometers are therefore calibrated by reference to a thermometer whose accuracy has been certified by the National Physical Laboratory at Teddington.

Types of thermometers

DIRECT READING INSTRUMENTS

Liquid expansion thermometers

These are the simplest and most reliable devices for measuring temperature. The instrument consists of a glass bulb, connected to an evacuated, closed capillary tube. The bulb is filled with a liquid (generally alcohol or mercury) and the temperature is indicated by the position of the meniscus in the capillary tube. If the cross-sectional area of the capillary is uniform throughout its length a linear calibration can be achieved.

The coefficient of expansion of mercury is relatively small (about 1.8 % of its volume between 0 and 100°C) so that the clinical thermometer requires a large bulb and a very narrow capillary to increase sensitivity. The narrow capillary is rendered more easily visible by shaping the thermometer so that the glass forms a lens and by incorporating

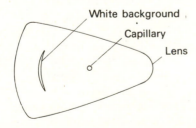

White background
Capillary
Lens

Fig. 19.2. Cross-section through a clinical thermometer.

a strip of white glass behind the capillary (Fig. 19.2). A constriction in the capillary tube permits the mercury to expand but hinders its return to the bulb so that the reading is preserved until the mercury is shaken down into the bulb. This type of thermometer has several disadvantages. It is fragile, has a large thermal capacity and so is slow to respond, is difficult to read and to reset, is unsuitable for insertion into body cavities and cannot be used for remote reading or recording. Most clinical thermometers also have a limited scale length so that special low-recording thermometers must be used when hypothermia is suspected.

Dial thermometers

It is possible to separate the display from the site of temperature measurement by using liquid or gas expansion thermometers in which the expansion is detected by a pressure-measuring device such as a Bourdon gauge (p. 151). The temperature sensing bulb is connected to the pressure gauge by a narrow metal tube and the cavity is filled either with a liquid or with a volatile liquid and its saturated vapour. The change in pressure produced by the alteration in temperature is sensed by the gauge and displayed on the dial. The volume of the bulb must be large compared with the volume of the connecting tube and gauge (to minimize the effects of changes in ambient temperature on the reading) and the connecting tube must not be bent or narrowed after calibration has been performed. This type of thermometer is relatively cheap and robust but not very accurate. It is therefore generally employed to measure fairly large temperature changes e.g. in humidifiers, water baths or autoclaves.

Bimetallic thermometers

If strips of two metals with different coefficients of expansion are fastened together throughout their length, the combined strip will bend when heated. In thermometers based on this principle the bimetallic strip is usually twisted into a spiral or coil and one end is fixed whilst the other end is attached to a pointer lying in front of a dial. A change in temperature causes the coil to wind or unwind so moving the pointer across the dial. This principle is used in cheap, but not very accurate thermometers for measuring air temperature. A bimetallic strip is also used in a number of anaesthetic vaporizers to compensate for changes in the temperature of the liquid being vaporized. The strip opens and closes an orifice which varies the proportion of gases passing through the bypass tube and vaporizing chamber. It thus maintains a constant output concentration of vapour despite changes in vapour pressure due to changes in temperature of the volatile agent.

Chemical thermometers

One clinical instrument consists of an aluminium strip with a transparent cover. The strip contains several rows of small cells along its length. Each cell is filled with a unique mixture of chemicals which melts at a particular temperature, the number of cells being chosen to suit the desired accuracy and temperature range. The chemicals melt within about 30 s and, in doing so, release a dye. The temperature is indicated by the number of cells which have changed colour. By incorporating 50 such cells in one strip it is possible to cover the range 35.5–40.4°C with an accuracy of ±0.1°C. The method is somewhat expensive because a fresh thermometer is required for each temperature reading; however the use of disposable thermometers eliminates the danger of cross-infection.

Reversible chemical thermometers are also available. These contain a number of cells filled with liquid crystals, (long-chain polymers), each cell having a slightly different composition from the next. At a critical temperature the optical properties change due to a re-alignment of the molecules, causing reflection instead of absorption of incident light. By selecting suitable

materials, temperature intervals of about 0.5°C can be differentiated (Lees *et al.* 1968).

REMOTE READING INSTRUMENTS

Resistance-wire thermometers

These are based on the principle that the resistance of certain metal wires increases as their temperature increases. The metal most commonly used for this purpose is platinum, since it resists corrosion and has a large temperature coefficient of resistance. Over the range 0–100°C the change in resistance is linearly related to the change in temperature and is about 0.4 ohm per °C for a 100 ohm resistance element. Copper and nickel are also used. The change in resistance of the wire due to the change in temperature is usually measured by a Wheatstone bridge circuit (Chapter 3). This may be used on the null deflection principle or as a direct readout.

Platinum resistance thermometers can be made to sense very small differences in temperature (±0.0001°C), but the instrument then becomes somewhat fragile and slow to respond. Resistance wire thermometers are not commonly used in clinical practice.

Thermistor thermometers

Thermistors are semiconductors made from the fused oxides of heavy metals such as cobalt, manganese and nickel, and can be made to have positive (PTC) or negative (NTC) temperature coefficients. Their resistance varies markedly with temperature (about 5% per °C) but the change is nonlinear. However this can be corrected over a limited temperature range by suitable electronic circuitry. Thermistors have several other disadvantages. First, the resistance of individual thermistors in a batch tends to vary. Second, thermistors tend to 'age' or show a change in resistance with time. Third, they tend to exhibit a 'memory' of the previous temperature so that the value of a given temperature recorded during a heating cycle is less than the value recorded at the same temperature during a cooling cycle. This is termed hysteresis. These disadvantages can be minimized by purchasing matched, pre-aged thermistors which display a much smaller hysteresis effect.

The temperature coefficient of a thermistor is much greater than that of a resistance wire element so that thermistors can be used to detect very small temperature changes. Furthermore the beads are extremely small (about the size of a pinhead) so that they respond very quickly. They are therefore ideally suited for detecting the change in temperature of pulmonary arterial blood in the thermal dilution method of cardiac output measurement. They have also been used to detect changes in temperature between inspired and expired gas in respiration monitoring and have been incorporated into endoradiosondes or 'radio pills' which are swallowed and then transmit the deep body temperature of mobile patients or free-ranging animals.

Thermocouple thermometers

If two dissimilar metals are joined to create an electrical circuit and the junctions are at different temperatures, a current will flow from one metal to the other, the e.m.f. generated being a function of the temperature difference between the two junctions (Fig. 19.3). This phenomenon was first described by Seebeck in 1823 and is known as the Seebeck effect. Common combinations of metals used to make thermocouples are copper and constantan, or iron and constantan (constantan is 60% copper and 40% nickel). The e.m.f. generated by these junctions is relatively small so that a sensitive measuring instrument is necessary. Furthermore, it is essential to maintain the cold junction at a constant temperature (e.g. ice water) or to include some electronic or mechanical compensating device which will correct for changes in ambient temperature (Krog 1962).

The output from a copper-constantan junction is relatively small (about $40 \mu V$ per °C temperature difference between the junctions) but can be sensed with sufficient accuracy by a galvanometer or digital voltmeter. The supreme advantage of the thermocouple is that all junctions made from the same materials behave identically, and are very inexpensive, so that multichannel thermometers can be economically constructed.

DIRECT HEAT/ELECTRICITY GENERATORS

The Seebeck effect is also observed with some semiconductors and has now been utilized in applications other than thermometry. For example small electrical generators can be built to convert heat directly into electric current. The reverse phenomenon is the Peltier effect. If a current is passed through the junctions between two dissimilar metals a temperature difference will develop between them. If the 'hot' junction is kept cold, the 'cold' one will be even colder. This effect is used in cryoprobes utilized for cryosurgery. (Many such junctions, connected in series, are necessary to produce useful cooling.)

Site of body temperature measurement

Small gradients of temperature between different parts of the body exist in normal

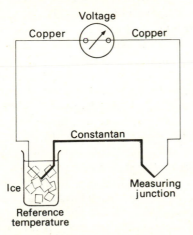

Fig. 19.3. Principle of a thermocouple thermometer.

subjects but these gradients are often accentuated in disease and when the body is rapidly cooled or heated by external means (Cooper & Kenyon 1957).

The highest temperature is normally recorded in the rectum. This is usually assumed to represent 'core' temperature but may prove unreliable if faeces are present. The oesophageal temperature is mainly dominated by the temperature of the blood in the heart and is usually 0.5°C lower than rectal temperature. However if the probe is situated in the upper oesophagus and the patient is vigorously hyperventilated through a tracheostomy or an endotracheal tube oesophageal temperature may be several degrees below rectal (Whitby & Dunkin 1968; 1969; 1970). Oesophageal probes should therefore lie about 25 cm below the laryngeal orifice. Tympanic membrane temperature reflects brain temperature and is usually close to oesophageal (Dickey, Ahlgren & Stephen 1970; Holdcroft & Hall 1978). However there is a risk of bleeding and damage to the tympanic membrane (Webb 1973). To prevent such damage Keatinge & Sloan (1975) recommend that the probe should be placed on the anterior wall of the aural canal with a servocontrolled heating device on the outer ear to prevent local cooling. Nasopharyngeal temperature can be used to monitor brain temperature providing that the probe is maintained in apposition to the mucosa. However it frequently becomes displaced and the method is unreliable in practice (Whitby & Dunkin 1971).

Skin temperature varies widely and is markedly affected by skin blood flow. It thus provides a useful measure of tissue blood flow, the toe-core temperature difference often being used as a monitor of the adequacy of the circulation in shock or other low output states (Matthews, Meade & Evans 1974a, b). In the neonate the abdominal skin temperature decreases rapidly as the infant cools, thus providing a more sensitive index of body cooling than rectal temperature. This fact has been utilized in a number of servocontrolled heaters for neonates which control their heat output on the basis of the abdominal skin temperature.

Rapid changes in blood temperature, produced, for example, by extracorporeal circulation, are reflected immediately by changes in oesophageal temperature. Temperature changes in the organs receiving a high proportion of the cardiac output (brain, heart, kidney) lag slightly behind the changes in blood temperature whilst changes in muscle and rectal temperature may be considerably delayed. When rewarming by the bloodstream route it is therefore important to continue warming until full equilibrium between oesophageal and tissue temperature has been achieved, otherwise oesophageal temperature may fall when the extracorporeal circulation is discontinued. When skin cooling is used the gradient is reversed; with this technique cooling must be terminated at an oesophageal temperature 2–3°C higher than the final desired oesophageal temperature to allow for the redistribution of the colder blood from the superficial tissues.

Thermography

The human skin behaves almost exactly as a black-body radiator. This means that it emits infrared radiation with a predictable spectrum. The shortest wavelength emitted is about 3 μm, but the range extends up to several hundred micrometers. The emitted energy at all wavelengths increases as the temperature rises, and if a narrow range of frequencies can be detected, the amount of radiant emission is proportional to the fourth power of the temperature.

Detectors are of two basic kinds: temperature-sensitive devices such as thermistors and thermocouples, or photon-sensitive devices. The former have a high sensitivity but the response time is slow. They are thus suitable for measuring the temperature of a small but uniform area whose temperature is not changing quickly, but are unsuitable for use in scanning cameras.

For heat scans the most versatile photosensitive material is indium antimonide, which is a photo-conductive material which produces a small current when infrared radiation between 1 μm and 6 μm impinges on it. The detector has to be kept very cold in liquid nitrogen to eliminate thermal noise arising in the detector itself. Filters are used to minimize the effects of other wavelengths, such as reflected sunlight, and the elements are shielded from ambient temperatures.

The field is scanned, rather like a television picture, successively, both vertically and horizontally (Fig. 19.4). The speed of response is such that as many as a hundred individual points in a frame can be scanned four times a second. The information can be displayed on a cathode-ray oscilloscope, intensity modulated, so that hotter areas appear brighter.

The main fields of application of thermographic scanning have been in the diagnosis of breast tumours, the location of deep perforating varicose veins of the leg, the site of vascular occlusions, and the location of the placenta. No direct applications to anaesthesia have yet been reported, but the measurement of changes in blood flow in the intensive care unit is an obvious possible future application.

Measurement of humidity

There are several situations in clinical practice in which the control of humidity is of the utmost importance. One is in the operating theatre where a high relative humidity is maintained to decrease the risk of static sparks. Another is when a patient breathes through an endotracheal or tracheostomy tube and extra humidity must be provided to prevent crusting of secretions and to maintain ciliary activity. Relative humidity is an important determinant of body heat loss so that careful control is also required when the patient is isolated in special environments, e.g. in plastic isolators, or in the treatment of widespread burns.

Two measures of humidity are in common use. *Absolute humidity* is the actual amount of water vapour contained in a given volume of gas at a given temperature and pressure. It is expressed in grams of water vapour per cubic metre of gas. *Relative humidity* is the actual amount of water vapour present in the gas expressed as a percentage of the amount that the same volume of gas would

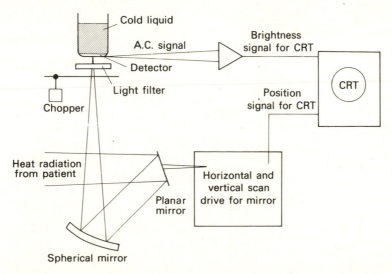

Fig. 19.4. Principle of a thermographic unit.

contain at the same temperature and pressure if it were fully saturated. The amount of water vapour required to saturate a given volume of air increases with temperature (Fig. 19.5). Consequently, air which is fully saturated at 20°C will be only about 30% saturated when warmed to 37°C. Normally, the additional moisture required to saturate the inspired air is added during its passage through the nose, mouth and trachea.

Measurements of humidity are made by instruments termed hygrometers.

REGNAULT'S HYGROMETER
(DEWPOINT HYGROMETER)

A silver tube is cooled gradually by the evaporation of liquid ether. When the tube cools to the dewpoint of the surrounding air (i.e. the point at which the air becomes fully saturated), small droplets of water will condense on the outside of the silver tube. If the temperature of the ether is now

measured the absolute humidity can be read from the graph (Fig. 19.5) or from tables.

Hair hygrometer

A human hair increases in length as the humidity of the surrounding air increases. If one end of the hair is fixed and the other is attached to a light lever system which magnifies the change in length, the scale can be suitably calibrated and a direct reading of relative humidity obtained. The range is limited to 15–85% relative humidity and the accuracy is not high.

Wet and dry bulb thermometer

Two mercury-in-glass thermometers are mounted side by side. The bulb of one is exposed to the air whilst the bulb of the other is surrounded by a small wick which dips into a water reservoir. The temperature of the wet bulb depends on the rate of evaporation, and hence on the humidity of

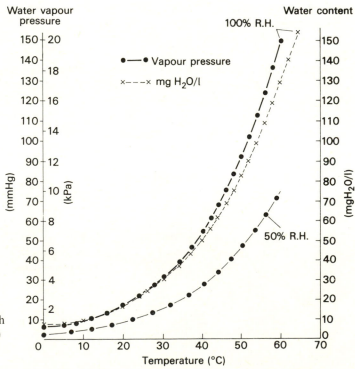

Fig. 19.5. Water vapour pressure and absolute humidity (mg H_2O/l) curves for gas which is fully saturated (R.H. = 100%) and gas which is half saturated (R.H. = 50%).

the surrounding air, and is therefore lower than the temperature of the dry bulb. There must, of course, be a minimum airflow over the wet bulb. As humidity is increased the rate of evaporation becomes less and the temperature difference between the two bulbs decreases. The relative humidity is determined from tables which relate the dry and wet bulb temperatures to the humidity.

The *whirling hygrometer* works on an identical principle, but is actively 'whirled' in the air in which humidity is to be measured before a reading is made. The tables for this forced-draught device are different from the still-air hygrometer, as evaporation from the wet bulb is greater. The device is insensitive to room-air movements, and therefore marginally superior.

Humidity transducers

These utilize the change in electrical characteristics which occurs in a substance when it absorbs water. The substance is usually incorporated into an electronic circuit as a resistor or as the dielectric portion of a capacitor, and the change in resistance or capacitance is detected. Such an instrument can be made extremely sensitive and can be used as part of a servo-system to control humidity in air-conditioning systems. However such transducers do tend to display hysteresis and this feature makes them unsuitable for critical applications.

Weighing

When water droplets are present in the air the absolute humidity may exceed the value for saturated air at that temperature. The measurement of humidity can then only be accomplished by either warming the air so that all the droplets are evaporated or by condensing the water vapour and weighing the quantity of water in a known volume of air. Allowance must then be made for the water vapour still present in the saturated vapour over the condensed water. An alternative technique is to absorb the water vapour in concentrated sulphuric acid, silica gel or anhydrous calcium chloride and again to determine the quantity present by weighing. If these methods are used the air must be passed through a number of chambers arranged in series, so that the completeness of absorption can be checked. (There should be no weight gain in the terminal chamber.)

Mass spectrometer

This instrument (see page 234) can be used to measure the water vapour pressure (Hayes & Robinson 1969) and is the only instrument which is sufficiently rapid to follow breath-by-breath changes. However, the expense of such an instrument precludes its general use.

References

COOPER K.E. & KENYON J.R. (1957) A comparison of temperatures measured in the rectum, oesophagus and on the surface of the aorta during hypothermia in man. *British Journal of Surgery*, **44**, 616.

DICKEY W.T., AHLGREN E.W. & STEPHEN C.R. (1970) Body temperature monitoring via the tympanic membrane. *Surgery*, **67**, 981.

HAYES B. & ROBINSON J.S. (1970) An assessment of methods of humidification of inspired gas. *British Journal of Anaesthesia*, **42**, 94.

HOLDCROFT A. & HALL G.M. (1978) Heat loss during anaesthesia. *British Journal of Anaesthesia*, **50**, 157.

KEATINGE W.R. & SLOAN R.E.G. (1975) Deep body temperature from aural canal with servo-controlled heating to outer ear. *Journal of Applied Physiology*, **38**, 919.

KROG I. (1962) Electrical measurements of body temperature. In: Electrical Measurements in Anesthesiology (ed. H. Poulsen). *Acta Anaesthesiologica Scandinavica*, Supplement XI.

LEES D.E., SCHUETTE W., BULL J.M., WHANG-PENG, J., ATKINSON E.R. & MACNAMARA T.E. (1968) An evaluation of liquid–crystal thermometry as a screening device for intra-operative hyperthermia. *Anesthesia and Analgesia*, **57**, 669.

MATTHEWS H.R., MEADE J.B. & EVANS C.C. (1974a) Peripheral vasoconstriction after open-heart surgery. *Thorax*, **29**, 338.

MATTHEWS H.R., MEADE J.B. & EVANS C.C. (1974b) Significance of prolonged peripheral vasoconstriction after open-heart surgery. *Thorax*, **29**, 343.

WEBB G.E. (1973) Comparison of esophageal and tympanic temperature monitoring during cardiopulmonary bypass. *Anesthesia and Analgesia, Cleveland*, **52**, 729.

WHITBY J.D. & DUNKIN L.J. (1968) Temperature differences in the oesophagus: preliminary study. *British Journal of Anaesthesia*, **40**, 991.

WHITBY J.D. & DUNKIN L.J. (1969) Temperature differences in the oesophagus. The effects of intubation and ventilation. *British Journal of Anaesthesia*, **41**, 615.

WHITBY J.D. & DUNKIN L.J. (1970) Oesophageal temperature differences in children. *British Journal of Anaesthesia*, **42**, 1013.

WHITBY J.D. & DUNKIN L.J. (1971) Cerebral, oesophageal and nasopharyngeal temperatures. *British Journal of Anaesthesia*, **43**, 673.

Further reading

BENZINGER T.H. (1969) Heat regulation: homeostasis of central temperature in man. *Physiological Reviews*, **49**, 671.

HALL G.M. (1978) Body temperature and anaesthesia. *British Journal of Anaesthesia*, **50**, 39.

Part 3
Statistics

Chapter 20
Descriptive and
Deductive Statistics

It would be presumptuous to suppose that it is possible to more than skim the subject of statistics in two chapters. Nevertheless, the acquisition of numerical data should create an interest in the degree of significance which can be attached to the measurements, and should encourage an appreciation of the techniques of summarizing them and drawing inferences from them.

The purpose of this section is to give an outline of the statistical methods which are most used in anaesthesia and in the anaesthetic literature. No initial knowledge of mathematics beyond simple arithmetic and algebra is assumed, and the approach will be to try to explain the scope and purpose of the subject in an intuitive fashion, rather than merely to supply formulae.

The present chapter is concerned with descriptive statistics and with the concepts involved when making deductions about a population from which samples of data have been drawn. The evolution of inferential statistics, such as tests of significance, is discussed in Chapter 21. Throughout both chapters words or phrases which have a special meaning in statistics are written in italics when first used, but they are only defined if the meaning is not clear from the context in which they appear.

BASIC TERMINOLOGY

Any observation is termed a *variable*, and in formulae is usually denoted by x. Any calculation applied to a *sample* of x values, is a *statistic*. Samples are always drawn from a *population*, and any measurement which relates to a population is a *parameter*.

In statistical terms, a population is a theoretical concept, and is the total number of all the similar observations which might have been sampled.

In order to derive the characteristics of the population it is necessary to *estimate* the population parameters from the sample statistics. The conventional notation uses lower-case Greek letters to denote actual population parameters whereas the estimates of population parameters, which are based on samples, are given lower-case English letters. Sample statistics, rather confusingly, are often likewise denoted, but in this text, they will be given in full, or in English abbreviations. For convenience a glossary of the abbreviations is given in Appendix 1.

Descriptive statistics

It is difficult to comprehend a large body of raw data or to comprehend its significance. If one casts an eye over a hundred values of Po_2 it is possible to get only a rough idea of the average value and scatter of results. Descriptive statistics are designed to express the important features of such data in a way that will enable useful deductions to be made subsequently. They also reduce the bulk of the data, which is of particular practical importance in scientific journals. Descriptive statistics are either *measures of central tendency* or *measures of dispersion.*

MEASURES OF CENTRAL TENDENCY

The commonest measure of central tendency is the arithmetic *mean,* or average. The mean is an everyday concept which needs no special explanation. The mean of a group of x values is denoted $\bar{x}$ (called x-bar) and is calculated from the equation:

$$\bar{x} = \frac{x_1 + x_2 \ldots x_N}{N}$$

or more simply

$$\bar{x} = \frac{\Sigma(x)}{N}$$

The symbol Σ is the Greek capital 'sigma' and stands for 'the sum of', and 'N' is the number of x values which are added together in order to derive the mean.*

The mean tells us around what central value the individual values lie. Looked at another way, it *locates* the point on a progressive scale around which the values lie. Measures of central tendency are, therefore, sometimes called measures of *location.* If the mean weight of one group is found to be 70 kg and the mean of another is found to be 60 kg, one is now able to locate where on the scale of weight the two groups lie. The mean values act as representatives of their groups.

The mean of a group of values is, perhaps, the easiest statistic to calculate, but this

* It is an exceedingly valuable discipline to verbalize any equation on first acquaintance, and see if it appears to 'make sense': this is particularly necessary when the equation contains specialized symbols or foreign letters. In this instance the equation says, 'to find the arithmetic average of a group of values, add up all the individual values and divide by the number of values'.

does not justify its universal employment. If groups of patients each include infants and octogenarians, the mean ages of the groups, even if different, may have little relevance. Similarly, a mean of 1.8 doses of relaxant per anaesthetic cannot possibly represent any of the actual values which must have all been either one, two, three or more doses. Since the object is description, it is more helpful to say how many individuals had each number of doses. Where the distribution of the values is not broadly symmetrical, the arithmetic mean is also frankly misleading. In such circumstances other measures of location (Fig. 20.1), such as the *mode* (the most commonly occurring value), the *mid-range* (the middle of the range) and the *median* (the value of the middle observation, when they are arranged in order of size) may convey the necessary information more accurately. There is a rough relationship between these measures: Mode = mean − 3 × (mean − median). Still other types of mean may have to be calculated for other applications.

Information about distributions may often be conveyed better by using *histograms*. The frequency histogram not only conveys information about location, it also indicates the extent of dispersion. Figure 20.2 is an example. Providing all the columns are of the same width, both the height and area of each column represent the frequency of each occurrence. Such a method of display not only shows clearly which is the commonest value, but also gives a visual

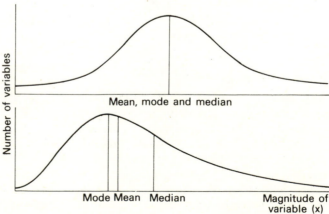

Fig. 20.1. Measures of location. The upper curve is symmetrical: the lower curve is positively skewed.

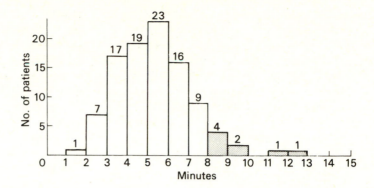

Fig. 20.2. Histogram of sleep time of one hundred patients after thiopentone (grouped in minute intervals).

impression of the variability of the values. If Fig. 20.2 is compared with Fig. 20.3, for instance, it is clear that not only is the mean sleeping time after propanidid much shorter than with thiopentone, but there is much less variation between patients.

MEASURES OF DISPERSION

It would obviously be desirable to have a numerical way of expressing the degree of variability of a given set of figures. There are several ways in which variability can be represented, and they all have their uses in different circumstances.

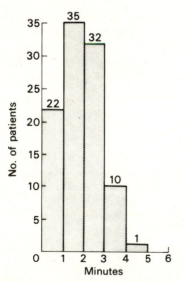

Fig. 20.3. Histogram of sleep time of one hundred patients after propanidid (grouped in minute intervals).

For example, it may be appropriate to quote the *range*, that is, the difference between the largest and the smallest value. The weakness of this method is that this measurement depends on only two of the values. If one of the subjects in Fig. 20.3 had slept for 13 min, the range would have been the same in both the thiopentone and propanidid groups but the overall variability of the subjects would have been little different. For this reason one needs some parameter which utilizes all the values.

One obvious solution is to subtract each value from the mean value, ignoring the sign, and then to average all these deviations from the mean. This value, which is the *mean absolute deviation*,* whilst a perfectly valid statistic which uses all the data, has limitations from both practical and theoretical points of view.

From a practical point of view, it may sometimes be convenient to combine two sets of data. Deriving a new mean absolute deviation for the amalgamated data requires the calculation of a new grand mean, and subtraction of all the values from it before one can start to calculate a new value. This is much more laborious than the alternative discussed below. From a theoretical point of view, the statistic gives too little weight to

* This is written

$$\frac{\Sigma |x - \bar{x}|}{N}$$

the vertical lines indicating that the deviation is always taken as positive.

the extremely deviant values if one wishes to make valid deductions about the population from which the sample has been taken.

Both these objections are overcome if one *squares* all the deviations from the mean before dividing by the number in the sample (*N*). The statistic then obtained is the *mean squared deviation,* which is customarily known as the *sample variance:*

$$\mathrm{var}(x) = \frac{\Sigma(x - \bar{x})^2}{N}. \quad *$$

Several practical and theoretical advantages accrue from the use of this concept. Firstly, although the terms are derived by squaring the difference between each value and the mean value, the sum of these terms (called the *sum of squares,* or *SS*) can be obtained by a simple method of calculation which does not require a knowledge of the mean value. (The formula for doing this is derived in Appendix 2.) This makes it relatively easy to apply tests of significance to data as it accumulates. This is particularly valuable when one is trying to limit the total number of experiments by testing for a significant result after each one. It is merely necessary to add the extra observed value, and the square of the value to existing totals in the computation and then to divide by the new value of *N*.

Secondly, the square root of the variance (called the standard deviation—*see below*) is a term in the equation which describes the shape of one of the commonest distributions found in biological measurement (the normal distribution) and is most useful in drawing deductions about the parameters of such data.

Variances are additive: in any group of measurements, not only is there the inherent variability of the values in the population but variability in the accuracy of the instruments, the reproducibility of the instruments, reading errors, observer errors etc. which all contribute to the total variability. The proportion of the variance which is contributed by each factor can be calculated by an *analysis of variance.*

Whilst the variance is a fundamental,

independent measure of variability which can be handled by a simple arithmetical method it does have the disadvantage that its dimensions are not the same as the original measurements. If the measurements were say, in minutes, the variance would be in square minutes, a term with no common sense meaning. To obviate this the square-root of the variance is usually taken to give the *standard deviation* (s.d.). The s.d. of a sample, then is defined as:

$$\mathrm{s.d.} = \sqrt{\frac{\Sigma(x - \bar{x})^2}{N}} \quad *$$

It can be seen from the formula that, if the majority of the values are near the mean (i.e., $x - \bar{x}$ is small), then the variance and standard deviation are small.

It should be noted that the values for the s.d.'s of different samples do not measure their relative variability. For example, the mean weight of a group of men might be 68 kg with an s.d. of 3.1 kg, and that of a group of women might be 59 kg with a s.d. of 2.9 kg. On the face of it, the men appear to be more variable. However, since the means are different, the s.d.'s can only be compared by expressing them as a percentage of the mean. This quantity is called the *coefficient of variation.* In the case mentioned above the coefficient of variation of men is

$$\frac{3.1 \times 100}{68} = 4.6\%$$

and that of women is

$$\frac{2.9 \times 100}{59} = 4.9\%$$

so that in fact the height of women, on these figures, is more variable than that of men.

Deductive statistics

If one wishes to discover a general truth, one can obviously make such a large

*As will be discussed on page 281, for most purposes *N*–1 is used as the denominator rather than *N*.

number of observations that the results can be assumed to be true of the population in general. When the 'population' of interest is restricted, say, to those who have received a particular treatment, this is rarely possible. Only a *sample* of all the theoretically possible number of observations can be obtained. In presenting the results on such a sample, mere description is not the most important objective of using statistical methods; the experimenter mainly wishes to deduce from the results of the sample, what is likely to be generally true about the population from which the sample was taken. We want to know what is the 'normal' range of fasting blood sugar or the arterial carbon dioxide tension of patients who have had an injection of a new analgesic. These generalizations can be made with more or less *confidence*, on the basis of the results obtained from the sample. It is for this reason that the design of clinical trials and the selection of subjects is so important. Unless the sample is randomly obtained from the population so that it is without bias, it is erroneous and misleading to use sample data to estimate the parameters of the population.

DISTRIBUTIONS

Data which is subjected to statistical analysis is of two kinds. In one case, the magnitude of each variable could theoretically take any one of an infinite number of values, the number of values being limited only by the accuracy of the measuring instrument. Such variables form a *continuous distribution*. For example, values of P_{O_2} of 10 kPa and 11 kPa could have been 10.1 kPa and 11.2 kPa or 10.092 kPa and 11.236 kPa. Only the limitations of apparatus, time and commonsense dictate that one chooses to limit the number of values to, say, the nearest 0.1 of a kilopascal. On the other hand, the number of radioactive counts recorded on one occasion may be 1007, or 1008, but can never be anything in between. Likewise, either six or seven out of nine patients may complain of pain during an intravenous injection, although such a *discontinuous distribution* may be disguised by reporting it as 66.67% or 77.78% of patients, respectively. In practice, most instrumental measurements yield values which are on a theoretically continuous scale. Even when the distribution of measurements is discontinuous, provided there are a large number of increments and at least 30 or so observations, the statistical methods are essentially similar; consequently, a thorough understanding of the most common continuous distribution, the 'normal' distribution, is of general value.

THE NORMAL DISTRIBUTION

It will be recalled that the area under a frequency histogram indicates the frequency of occurrence of events. For instance, in Fig. 20.2 the total area represents the

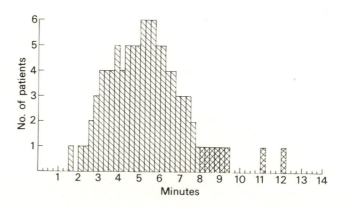

Fig. 20.4. Histogram of sleep time of same one hundred patients as in Fig. 20.2, but grouped in 15 s intervals.

sleeping time of the 100 patients. It can be seen that eight patients slept longer than 8 min: since the columns are of similar width, the shaded area to the right of the 8-min mark is 8% of the total area. One could also say that if one picked one of the patients' records at random, there are eight chances in a hundred that it would be from a patient who slept more than 8 min.

If the measurement interval had been not 1 min but 15 s, there would have been four times as many columns, with less patients per column. It might have looked like Fig. 20.4. Extending this idea, if the number of possible values is infinite and the number of observations is large, a smooth curve will be obtained. This is a *frequency distribution curve*: just like the histogram, the area under the curve is proportional to the number of observations.

If one repeatedly makes some measurement which is subject to random errors, or measures a quantity which is subject to biological variation, and then plots the frequency with which each value occurs, the frequency–distribution curve which is obtained has a characteristic 'bell' shape, and is often referred to as either the normal curve, the error curve or the Gaussian curve.

Figure 20.5 for example is a hypothetical example showing the frequency with which various values of vital capacity are found in 1000 men (a sample large enough to enable us to assume that it is synonymous with the theoretical population). The mean value is 5 litres, the majority of patients falling between 4 and 6 litres. If one wants to know what is the chance of any person taken at random from this population having a vital capacity greater than, say 6.2 litres it can be seen that it corresponds to the proportion of the shaded area under the graph to the whole area.

It would be very laborious to measure or calculate the appropriate area afresh for every such problem. Fortunately, it is not necessary. The equation which describes this curve contains only two variables, the *mean* which locates the curve on the *x*-(or horizontal) axis, and the *standard deviation* (σ-sigma) which describes its breadth. One standard deviation along the *x*-axis coincides with the inflection on the curve (marked *I* in Fig. 20.5) which in this case corresponds to 1 litre either above or below the mean.

Since areas under curves can be computed if the equation is known, this has been done for a standardized curve and the results are available in tables. To obtain the area for any particular set of results from the tables of the standard normal curve, the tables

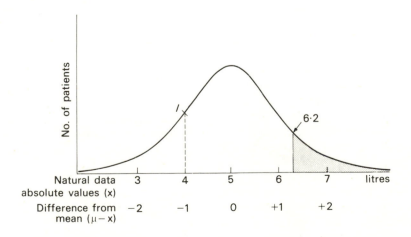

Fig. 20.5. The normal (Gaussian) distribution curve.

must be entered in terms of the number of standard deviations rather than in the original units. It turns out that just over 68% of the observations in a normal population lie within one standard deviation of the mean, i.e. between 4 and 6 litres in this example. Approximately 96% of the observations lie within twice these limits and well over 99% fall within 3 s.d.'s above or below the mean.

More commonly, we need the information the other way round and wish to know what are the limits, in standard deviations, that will include 95% or 99% of the values (which is the same as the limits that *exclude* 5% or 1%, respectively).

Table 1 in the Appendix is laid out in this way. This shows that 1.96 s.d.'s exclude 5% (or include 95%) and 2.58 s.d.'s exclude 1%. The co-ordinates are laid out as probabilities, since there is a 5% probability that a value will lie outside the range: mean $\pm$ 1.96 s.d. and a 1% probability that it will lie outside the range: mean $\pm$ 2.58 s.d. Thus by quoting the mean and standard deviation of a population, we are in a position to predict what proportion of individual values will fall within specified limits, or what is the *probability* of obtaining a value falling outside or inside certain limits.

SAMPLING FROM A NORMAL POPULATION

In the first part of this chapter, it was shown that the mean and standard deviation could be used to describe a sample or a population. In the case of a population, it is rarely practicable to measure the parameters and we are driven to estimate them from the statistics of a sample drawn from the population. If the sample is large (more than about 30 observations), then no practical error will arise if one assumes that the sample statistics are the same as the population parameters, and therefore the sample mean and variance of such samples can be used as population mean and variance.

However, when the samples are small, this is not acceptable. The sample mean ($\bar{x}$) is

the only estimate that can be obtained of the population mean (μ),* but the sample variance more often *underestimates* the population variance than overestimates it. The reason for this is that the small sample is unlikely to contain an extreme value and so will underestimate the population variance, although on rare occasions, the inclusion of an extreme value in the sample will cause the sample variance to overestimate the population variance. There is, of course, no way of knowing, but because the former error is much more common, it is customary to 'correct' the sample variance by making it larger and using that figure as the *best estimate* of the population variance. How much larger? Since it is a correction whose magnitude needs to be associated with sample size, one divides the sum of squared deviations by $N - 1$, instead of N. A larger calculated value for the variance is obtained, and it can be shown that this value is more likely to approximate to the true population variance than the original sample variance.

Note that when N is large, say over 30, this correction makes virtually no difference, which is another way of saying that sample statistics for big samples can be used as population parameters.

One can accordingly estimate the population variance from any sample size as

$$s^2 = \frac{\Sigma(x - \bar{x})^2}{N - 1}.$$

(Note that s^2 is used instead of σ^2 because this is an estimate of the population variance based on a sample.)

STANDARD ERROR OF THE MEAN

Whilst presenting the mean and standard deviation usefully describes one's results, the question that should be uppermost in the reader's mind is what degree of confidence can he have in these statistics? You have, for example, discovered the mean Pa_{CO_2} of 20 patients who have been

* The Greek 'm', μ (pronounced 'mew'), is used because we are talking about a population.

prescribed a new analgesic to be 4.2 kPa (31.5 mmHg). Is this generally true? If you examined a much larger sample of patients, would the mean then turn out to be 4.8 kPa (36 mmHg)? Put another way, if you repeated the experiment, within what range of values would you expect the mean to fall, and how confident could you be of this opinion? These are clearly important questions if one is to make any generalized assertions about the 'truth' on the basis of a limited sample. Common sense tells us that the bigger the sample, the closer to the population mean the sample mean is likely to be. The greater, in fact, is the likelihood that random high and low extreme values will have cancelled each other out. A large sample, therefore, gives us increasing confidence in the accuracy of the mean. Furthermore, the smaller the variance, the less likely is it that a further value or two (if we had obtained them) would have seriously disturbed the mean.

If, on the other hand, the values are all over the place (the variance and standard deviation being large), one fears that another one or two measurements could easily alter the mean. The statistic we are looking for then is one which takes account of both sample size and population variance. Such a statistic is the standard deviation of the mean, more commonly called the *standard error of the mean*, sometimes abbreviated to standard error (s.e.). In fact, the standard error is the resultant of dividing the s.d. by $\sqrt{N}$.* It is therefore large when the s.d. is

large and when N is small and conversely, it is small when the s.d. is small and N is large. The importance of the magnitude of the s.e. is that it serves the same function for the distribution of *means* as the s.d. does for the distribution of *values*. Thus, we can expect 68% of sample means to lie within 1 s.e. of the true population mean, 96% within 2 s.e.'s and 99.7% within 3 s.e.'s. Or, looking at it the other way around, a sample mean will only fall by chance outside ± 1.96 s.e.'s once in twenty times (5% of the time) or outside 2.58 s.e.'s once in a hundred times. We are thus in a position to say that we are 95% confident that the population mean lies between the limits, the mean $(\mu) \pm (1.96 \times \text{s.e.})$.

Strictly speaking, in calculating the s.e., one should use the estimate of population variance (s^2) as derived above and take the square root to obtain the estimated population standard deviation before dividing by sample size. Thus, the formula is:

$$\text{s.e.} = \sqrt{\frac{\Sigma(x - \bar{x})^2}{(N-1)/N}}.$$

The s.e. calculated above, then, is a statistic which indicates the degree of reliability with which we can regard the sample mean as representing the true mean. Just as 96% of all values in the sample lie within ± 2 s.d. of the mean, so there is a 96% chance that the population mean will lie within ± 2 s.e. of the sample mean. This statistic is used

---

* For those who do not wish to accept this on trust, the reasoning is as follows: from any group of values, the variance can be calculated. Suppose that the values are now added together randomly in pairs and averaged to give means of samples of two. This will give a new set of values, half as many, but with a smaller variance. Some of the variability will have disappeared in the averaging, since some high values will have been combined with less high, or even low, values to produce a value which is closer to the mean. The further away from the mean any value was, the more likely is it that combining it with any other value will have produced a new value

closer to the mean. Because the values have moved closer to the mean, recalculation of the variance must give a lower value. In fact, the variance will be exactly halved. If the values had been combined in tens, the variance of the means so created would have been ten times smaller than the original variance, i.e.

$$\text{Var}_{(\bar{x})} = \frac{\sigma^2}{N}$$

Therefore,

$$\text{s.d.}_{(\bar{x})} \text{ (i.e. s.e.)} = \frac{\sigma}{\sqrt{N}}.$$

in the calculation of confidence intervals, and in tests of significance, as outlined in the next chapter.

Although we have started from the assumption of a normally-distributed population of values, it can be shown that even if the population is *not* normal, the means of samples of a reasonable size (over 30) *are* normally distributed, thus allowing this kind of deduction without postulating a normally-distributed population of values.

METHODS OF REPORTING QUANTITATIVE DATA

It is relevant at this point to consider what statistics should be quoted in scientific papers when the data are too numerous to be given in full. The basic principle is that enough data should be provided to enable the reader to calculate further statistics for himself. This is satisfied by quoting at least the mean, the number of observations and either the standard deviation or the variance. The provision of further information is largely dependent on the conclusions one is trying to draw, and where the major interest resides. If the variability of the data is of interest it is helpful to quote the coefficient of variation; if the interest in the mean is in its use as an indication of the likely true value of the mean of the population, then the standard error of the mean, depending as it does on the number of observations, will give the reader a better impression of the possible range of the true value.

Chapter 21
Inferential Statistics

It was shown in the previous chapter that the calculation of the mean, variance and standard error of the mean on a sample enables us to infer something concerning the population, and to give a numerical value to the range in which the mean of any sample of similar data will lie at any desired level of probability. The concept of probability is quite an everyday one; in statistical nomenclature it is always denoted by P, and expressed on a scale from 0 to 1. $P = 0$ means that an *event* never occurs, and $P = 1$ implies that it always occurs. $P = 0.5$ describes a situation in which an event is as likely as not to occur. The probability of tossing heads when spinning a coin is 0.5. The sum of all possible outcomes of mutually exclusive events comes to $P = 1$. In some situations such as coin tossing, or card selection, the probability of certain events can be worked out in advance. In medical work this is rarely the case, and by probability one can only mean the frequency of an event to which all *trials* tend to converge in the long term. Examples of this are the five-year survival of a certain disease, or the operative mortality of a particular procedure. In the previous chapter, the probabilities were neither inherently predictable, nor dependent on long-term experience, but were mathematical predictions based on a particular sample. In asserting that 95% of all means of samples of a given size will be within 1.96 times the standard error of the mean, one is inevitably implying that the real situation is adequately represented by the mathematical notion of the normal distribution; if a particular sample has a mean outside that range, one can claim that the probability of drawing such a sample at random from a normal

population is less than once in twenty times. P is less than 0.05 ($P < 0.05$) and this is therefore asserted to be a *statistically significant* difference which may then be ascribed to special factors, such as treatment, or age. Note, however, that once in every twenty identical experiments such a result should occur in the absence of any difference between the sample and the population. A significant result is not certainly true. Once in every twenty times we shall assert a significant effect when in fact none exists, merely on the results of sampling error. This false positive is called a type-α (alpha) error, and this is the value usually chosen when selecting a level of significance.

A more stringent level of significance would be a lower P value, i.e. $P < 0.01$, which would assert that there is only one chance in a hundred of making a type-α error, i.e. of falsely concluding that the result was significant when in fact it was due to random sampling effects.

It might be thought that it would be desirable to select a very low value of P, to minimise the possibility of this error. This is not necessarily so, for there is another kind of error over which the experimenter has less control, this is called a type-β (beta) error. This error occurs when it is concluded that there is no difference between the treatment group and the control group, when in fact a difference does exist, i.e. a false negative. The probability of making this error depends on the interaction of two effects. The first is the magnitude of α error that has been selected. The smaller this is, the further out into the 'tail' of the distribution curve a result has to fall before it is considered 'significant'. This leaves a bigger range of potentially real differences which would normally be regarded as being due to the effects of random sampling. If the difference between the populations of treated and nontreated patients is not great, the two distributions overlap to a considerable extent. This difference can then only be resolved by taking larger samples since this causes curves of the sample means to become taller and narrower, so that the overlap of the two distributions is reduced.

Thus we have a two-way conflict. We can increase the likelihood that we do not make an unjustifiable conclusion that treatment is effective by taking a very low level of α, but only at the cost of not detecting real but small effects. We can only avoid this conflict by taking bigger samples, which means more experiments, more expenditure of time, money and patient material. It is customary in biological work to make α, and therefore P to be 0.05, and let β be what it will on the assumption that it is not worthwhile to expend a great effort to unearth minor changes. Conversely, when the experiments are costly or difficult to perform, a higher level of P, say $P = 0.1$, might be quite acceptable, particularly when the consequences of falsely assuming that the treatment is beneficial are not likely to be harmful.

Remember, $P = 0.15$ is conventionally nonsignificant, and the reader is inclined to dismiss it entirely. However, although there are fifteen chances in a hundred that the result could have occurred by chance, there are eighty-five chances that it did not, and such a value may, on occasion, be enough to justify the acquisition of more data.

CONFIDENCE INTERVALS

In the previous chapter it was stated that the means of large samples taken from the normal population are themselves normally distributed. It was shown that such means had a standard deviation which was equal to the population standard deviation divided by $\sqrt{N}$ and that this statistic is called the standard error of the mean. By using this statistic, we could infer that, for example, 68% of sample means lie within one s.e. either side of the mean. Other ways of looking at this statement would be to say that there is a 68% chance of any similar sample mean lying within one s.e. of the sample mean or that we are 68% sure that the true mean lies within one s.e. of the sample mean.

In line with our customary and arbitrary selection of $P < 0.05$ and $P < 0.01$ as statistically significant and statistically highly significant respectively, we normally calculate 95% and 99% confidence limits. By analogy with the treatment of sample data (see pages 280–281) to define the area under the frequency curve which will include 95% of all sample means, we need to set the limits at plus or minus 1.96 standard errors. To include 99%, the limits must be wider, ± 2.58 standard errors. Thus, if one wishes to be 99% confident about the limits within which the mean lies, one has to accept quite a wide range.

The foregoing is correct if the sample size is large and if the population variance can be taken to be the same as the sample variance. However, with small samples, *the means are not distributed normally*, and for each succeeding smaller sample size the curve becomes slightly flatter and broader.* Consequently, one needs to take wider limits along the x axis in order to encompass the same area as under the normal curve. These curves have an area distribution which has been tabulated for all sample sizes. This is the '*t*' distribution. The value of t chosen for any required area is obtained from a table such as Table 3 in the Statistical Tables, which gives the most commonly-used values for each level of significance and for each sample size. Sample size is listed as *degrees of freedom*, a term which will occur again. It refers to the number of items in the data which can

---

* This is due to the impossibility of obtaining a truly representative sample of the data in any *small* sample.

vary. Once the mean is specified, $N - 1$ items could vary without changing the mean value, but the last value would be predetermined by the others and the mean. In a collection of numerical data, therefore, the degrees of freedom (df) are one less than the sample size.

The procedure, then, is to find the t-value for the correct degrees of freedom, for the desired area (i.e. probability); this will give the desired *confidence interval for the mean*. For example, with a sample of four values (3df) the t value which includes 95% of the area is 3.18. This should be compared with the figure which applies to the normal distribution curve which for 95% area is 1.96. The t value is much greater because the distribution curve of the means of samples of only four is much flatter and broader than the normal curve, and therefore a greater distance along the x axis is necessary to encompass the same area. As with the normal curve, the confidence interval is derived by multiplying the t value by the standard error, which has in turn been derived by estimating the population variance from the sample data:

$$s_{\bar{x}} = \sqrt{\frac{\Sigma (x - \bar{x})^2}{(N - 1)/N}}.$$

Note that when df is 60, the 95% area for $t = 2.00$, and the t distribution becomes almost synonymous with a normal distribution, as one would expect.

TESTS OF SIGNIFICANCE –
STUDENT'S 't'

One of the commonest situations which presents itself is the possession of data related to two or more fairly small samples, and the question that arises is whether or not they differ significantly from each other. Commonsense tells us that the greater the difference between the mean values of the two groups, the less likely they are to be from the same parent population. Similarly, the more values the individual means are derived from, the more reliance we can place on the difference between them. If we divide the actual difference between the means by 'the standard error of this difference' (remember that a 'standard error' is a quantity which decreases as the sample size increases) we can compute a figure which will be larger both when the actual difference is larger and when the sample size is larger. This statistic is Student's 't' and is computed using the formula

$$t = \frac{|\bar{x} - \bar{x}'|}{s_{(\bar{x} - \bar{x}')}}$$

where $|\bar{x} - \bar{x}'|$ is the absolute difference between the sample means, and $s_{(\bar{x} - \bar{x}')}$ is an estimate of the standard error of the difference between the means. The numerator of this fraction is self evident; it is the denominator that requires a moment's analysis.

What hypothesis is being tested? As is so often the case, one puts up the *null hypothesis* that there is really no difference between the populations. If this were so, the mean and the variance of both samples would be similar, although of course one would be surprised if they were identical in small samples.

The hypothesis, then, is that the difference between the means is really zero. One is also implicitly making the hypothesis that any difference between the two variances is due to random sampling effects. Before one can test the significance of the difference in means, it is necessary to examine the variances from this point of view.

If the variance of the two samples were identical, the ratio of one to the other would be unity. As the variances increasingly differ, dividing the larger variance by the smaller will give an increasingly large number. There comes a time when the number so obtained is so big that one is forced to conclude that the samples are from different populations, and a straight comparison of their means is not valid. This is the basis of the variance ratio, or F-test. Again sample size must be relevant, since the inherently greater variability of small samples must be allowed for, so the table for the appropriate level of significance is entered with the degrees of freedom appropriate to each sample, and if the variance ratio is less than the value tabulated (Table 2 in the Statistical Tables) then the variances are sufficiently similar to allow one to assume that they are from the same population, and one is at liberty to proceed with the analysis.

The next logical step is to argue that since the two samples have similar variances, combining the data would give a better estimate of the population variance than could be obtained from each individual sample alone. It will be recalled that the best estimate of <u>population variance is</u> <u>obtained by dividing the sum of the squared</u> <u>deviations by $N - 1$.</u> In this case we can add the sum of squared deviations (SS) for each sample, and divide by $N - 1$ for each sample.

$$s^2 = \frac{SS + SS'}{(N - 1) + (N' - 1)}.$$

Having calculated the best estimate of the population variance we can use it to obtain a more accurate value for the variance ($s_{\bar{x}}^2$) and standard error ($s_{\bar{x}}$) of each sample mean by dividing it by the number in that sample:

$$s_{\bar{x}}^2 = \frac{s^2}{N} \quad \text{s.e.} (s_{\bar{x}}) = \frac{s}{\sqrt{N}}$$

and

$$\text{and} \quad s_{\bar{x}'}^2 = \frac{s^2}{N'} \quad \text{s.e.} (s_{\bar{x}'}) = \frac{s}{\sqrt{N'}}.$$

We now have the standard errors of the means of each sample; what is the standard error of the difference between the means? Again, it is best to look at the problem intuitively.

If both the standard errors are very small, the true mean of each sample lies between small limits. The difference between the two mean values is therefore known fairly accurately, and the standard error of the difference (which delineates the range within which the true difference lies) will also be small. For example, if there is a 95% probability that the mean weight of one group of men lies between 69.8 kg and 70.2 kg, and the mean weight of another group lies between 71.4 and 71.8 kg, then we feel reasonably certain that the true difference lies between the smallest and largest probable differences, i.e. 1.2 and 2.0 kg (see Fig. 21.1). If however, the standard error of one group is large, the possible range for the difference increases. When both groups have large standard errors, the possible range for the true mean of the difference between the two means becomes doubly large.

Unfortunately, we cannot just add the two standard errors, but as was emphasized earlier, variances *can* be combined arith-

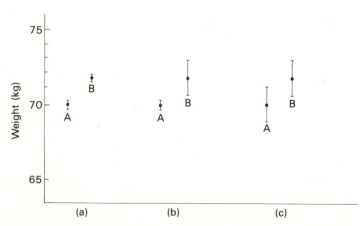

Fig. 21.1. Effect of standard error on confidence concerning the true difference between means. In each example the samples have the same means, A = 70.0 kg and B = 71.6 kg. In (a) the s.e. of both means is small and it seems intuitively probable that there is a difference, and the difference is between 1.2 kg and 2.0 kg. In (b) one s.e. is large and for a similar degree of confidence one would need to enlarge this estimate. In (c) both s.e.'s are large and one cannot even be sure there really is a difference.

metically, and if we add the two variances we get what could be called the variance of the difference, e.g.

$$s^2_{(\bar{x} - \bar{x}')} = \frac{s^2}{N} + \frac{s^2}{N'}.$$

If the samples are the same size, this simplifies to:

$$s^2_{(\bar{x} - \bar{x}')} = \frac{2s^2}{N}.$$

The standard error of the difference is therefore the square root of this quantity. This is the denominator of our fraction:

$$t = \frac{|\bar{x} - \bar{x}'|}{s_{(\bar{x} - \bar{x}')}},$$

i.e.

$$t = \frac{|\bar{x} - \bar{x}'|}{\sqrt{\dfrac{s^2}{N} + \dfrac{s^2}{N'}}}.$$

It has already been suggested that both a large difference in means and a *small* standard error of the difference increase the likelihood that the difference is significant, and this formula shows that both of these conditions will lead to larger values of t. If, therefore, the table of t-values (Table 3 in the Statistical Tables) is entered for the desired area (or P value) using the degrees of freedom contributed by samples $(N - 1) + (N' - 1)$ and if the value in the tables is *exceeded* by the calculated value, then the difference *is* significant at that P value, and the null hypothesis is rejected.

A worked example may be found in Appendix 3.

t-TEST FOR PAIRED OBSERVATIONS

The foregoing is often called an unpaired t-test because we are working on data derived from different samples. In some experimental situations it is possible to have data on two successive occasions in the same individual. For example, one may wish to compare some physiological variable before and after a particular drug. In this situation the 'between patient' variability is eliminated and one would expect to be able to detect much smaller differences. Instead of working with differences between the mean values of the two groups, one can work with the actual differences themselves. The null hypothesis is that there is a population of differences, with a mean difference of zero, and that the sample of differences which we have found could have occurred at random. The principle of the calculation follows the same logic as before. There is, in fact, a mean of the differences between the two sets of values ($\bar{d}$) whose value is not zero; if we divide this mean difference by the standard error of the difference ($s_{\bar{d}}$), we shall again get a t-value. The more the difference departs from zero the more likely is it to be significant, and the higher the t-value. Similarly, the more consistent the differences, and the more numerous the observations, the smaller will be the standard error of the difference and the higher the t-value. For paired samples, therefore,

$$t = \frac{\bar{d}}{s_{\bar{d}}}.$$

Again the numerator, the mean difference, presents no problem; the denominator is simply the square root of the best estimate of the variance of the population of differences, divided by the number of observations (see page 286).

$$s_{\bar{d}} = \sqrt{\frac{\Sigma(d - \bar{d})^2}{(N - 1)/N}}.$$

The table of t values is entered with the appropriate df which in this case is one less than the total number of *differences* (not two less than the total number of observations) and at the appropriate value of P. A worked example may be found in Appendix 3.

ONE- AND TWO-TAILED TESTS

In the preceding sections the problem was to determine whether or not the means of the two samples were significantly different, and this was done by comparing the magnitude of the difference with an estimate of the variability of the difference. No consideration was given to the problem of which of the two means was the larger for one was only interested in establishing that, at a chosen level of probability, the difference was outside the limits that could have occurred by chance in samples of that size and variability. The appropriate area under the *t*-distribution curve was therefore equally divided between both 'tails' of the distribution, and in the case of $P = 0.05$, there would have been a probability of $P = 0.025$, that A was larger than B, and $P = 0.025$ that B was larger than A. This is therefore called a 'two-tailed' test of significance.

Quite commonly, however, one has good reasons for expecting one mean to be greater than another. Indeed, it may only make clinical or physiological sense for one mean to be greater than the other. In this situation one should apply a one-tailed test and show that the value is in the appropriate area at one end of the curve. The *t*-value that is associated with 5% of the area at one end is, of course, the value that is tabulated for twice that area when distributed over both ends of the curve, or $P = 0.10$. This is always a *smaller* value of t, i.e. one easier to exceed.

Non-parametric tests

In many situations, it is necessary to test the significance of observations or judgements which can only be ranked and not measured. For example, several pathologists might be asked to give an opinion on the microscopic appearance of tumours and rank them in order of increasing malignancy. If these opinions were then going to be the basis of selection for therapy, which would be subsequently assessed for efficacy, it would be necessary to examine the consistency of the pathologists' judgements, both with one another, and on repeated attempts.

The ever increasing emphasis on quantitative measurement in physiological and pharmacological research makes the use of nonparametric tests for such purposes comparatively rare and they will not be considered further in that context. They are, however, of considerable value for rapid evaluation of experimental results for which parametric methods could also be used. They do not utilize the full value of the information contained in the data, but they are surprisingly accurate and give a useful guide to the likely value of a full-scale analysis by a Student's *t*, or other parametric test. Furthermore, they do not depend on assuming that the data follow a normal distribution. The most versatile of these are Willcoxon's Rank Sum test and Willcoxon's Signed Rank test for paired differences.

WILLCOXON'S RANK SUM TEST
(Mann-Whitney U test)

A common problem in measurement is the possession of two sets of numerical data which differ and we wish to know whether the difference is sufficient to warrant the conclusion that it is likely to be due to the effect of treatment.

As an example, let us consider the following simple experiment. It is suggested that patients coming to surgery in the afternoon are more anxious than those operated upon in the morning. Having eliminated sources of bias, preferably by allocating patients to morning or afternoon sessions on a random basis, we collect the pre-induction pulse rates. These are given in Table 21.1. The first step is to put all the results in descending order (irrespective of which group they are in) and give them a rank number. Ninety-five is the highest pulse rate and is therefore ranked 1, 92 is ranked 2, and so on. Ties are given a rank based on their average position: there are two 88's occupying the fourth and fifth positions, so they are both ranked

$$\frac{4 + 5}{2} = 4.5.$$

Table 21.1.

Morning patients		Afternoon patients	
Pulse rate/min	Rank order	Pulse rate/min	Rank order
61	22	68	19
66	20	64	21
91	3	95	1
84	6	92	2
75	11	76	10
72	13.5	80	7
79	8.5	88	4.5
69	17.5	69	17.5
74	12	70	16
71	15	79	8.5
72	13.5	88	4.5
$\bar{x}_1 = 74$	$n_1 = 142.0$	$\bar{x}_2 = 79$	$n_2 = 111.0$

Triple or larger ties, if there had been any, would be treated in the same way. These rank placings provide columns 2 and 4 in Table 21.1.

The rank numbers are now added for each group and come to 142 and 111 respectively. (As a check on the arithmetic so far, the sum of both totals – 253 – must be the same as the sum of the numbers 1–22, since there are 22 values and therefore 22 rank placings*.)

Now, if there were no difference between the groups, we would not expect any preponderance of high or low values in either group: the sum of each of the sets of ranks would therefore be much the same. In fact, they will differ: what is the probability of getting a difference as great as 111/142, which we have found in this instance?

Tables may be consulted (e.g. Documenta Geigy) which tabulate the range outside which the rank sums must fall before the null hypothesis can be rejected. These tables

* The sum of the first n natural numbers can be calculated from the formula

$$\frac{n(n + 1)}{2}$$

in this case, $n = 22$, so we have

$$\frac{22 \times 23}{2} = 253.$$

allow for different sizes of samples (up to 50 in one sample, and 25 in the other) and different tables are given for different levels of probability. As with t-tests, it is possible to consider both one-tailed and two-tailed probabilities.

In this case, looking up $n_1 = 11$, and $n_2 = 11$, the tabulated ranges are:

10%	(5% in each tail) =	100–153
5%	in one tail =	96–157
2%	(1% in each tail) =	91–162
1%	in one tail =	87–166

Now our original hypothesis was that the afternoon patients would be more anxious: they would therefore have a higher pulse rate and therefore, a lower rank sum, (since the highest pulse rates are ranked 1, 2, etc.). We were therefore conducting a one-tailed test and would need to have found a sum *lower* than 96 to be significant at the 5% level. The difference we have found (lower sum, 111) is therefore not significant. Even if we had no preconceived views and merely wished to see if there was *any* difference between morning and afternoon cases, we should have needed one of the sums to be outside the range 100–153, and even that has not been achieved. (The same data are used for the worked example of a t-test in Appendix 3: the same conclusions are obtained, somewhat more laboriously!)

WILLCOXON'S TEST FOR PAIRED DIFFERENCES

In the above example, we were dealing with unpaired data from two different groups of patients. As with the t-test, Willcoxon's approach can also be used for dealing with paired data. Suppose the same data as that in Table 21.1 in fact referred to pulse rates in the same eleven individuals on two different occasions, say, before the first and second anaesthetics for the insertion of radium. The figures are laid out again in Table 21.2 with the new column, the actual differences $(A - B)$. These differences are again ranked in order of magnitude, but ignoring the sign. Differences of zero are ignored, since they contribute no information: furthermore, it would greatly influence the calculations which follow according to whether we gave the zero a positive or negative sign, and this is clearly nonsense. Once more, ties are given an average figure. Having ranked the data, the ranks are now given a sign according to whether the original difference was positive or negative.

This gives the fourth column of Table 21.2. Totalling positive and negative ranks, one derives the totals 16.5 and 38.5, with the negative ranks having the lower total. Again, we need to ask, 'Could these totals have arisen by chance with fair probability, or must we accept that the difference in

Table 21.2.

Group A	Group B	Difference	Rank
61	68	7	+6
66	64	2	−9
91	95	4	+7.5
84	92	8	+4
75	76	1	+10
72	80	8	+4
79	88	9	+2
69	69	0	(*)
74	70	4	−7.5
71	79	8	+4
72	88	16	+1

Sum of Positives   38.5
Sum of Negatives   16.5

* See text.

pulse rates indicates that the patients really have lower pulse rates before the second anaesthetic?'.

In this case, the number of pairs is only eleven. Looking up the limits in Table 4 in the Statistical Tables, we find that the relevant rank sums are:

10%	(5% in each tail)	= 13–53
5%	in one tail	= 10–56
2%	(1% in each tail)	= 7–59
1%	in one tail	= 5–61

Our values (16.5: 38.5) are again well within these ranges and we cannot reject the null hypothesis that there is no real difference.

Discontinuous variables

Previous discussion has centred around the analysis of data related to continuous variables, which are theoretically able to assume any value.

Some types of data, however, are discontinuous. For example, radioactive counts can never be other than whole numbers, and the proportion of patients who develop a sore throat following intubation will be based on a whole-number sample. There are mathematical distributions which can be used as models to represent most examples of discontinuous data.

THE BINOMIAL DISTRIBUTION

This is a special, simple case of a more general distribution, the multinomial distribution. If a population contains items or subjects which belong to one of two mutually-exclusive categories, it is a binomial population. The categories may be cured/not cured; awake/asleep; dead/alive; male/female, or any pair in which, if a variable is in one group, it is not in the other. Where there are three or more mutually exclusive categories, e.g. excellent, good, fair, poor, there is an appropriate multinomial distribution. If one wishes to describe the characteristics of such populations, there is only one parameter, namely the proportion of each component.

The experimenter is attempting, by categorizing a sample, to obtain an estimate of this parameter. The proportion he finds in the sample is the best estimate that can be made of this population parameter: however, to quantify such ideas as the confidence interval or the reproducibility of this estimate, one needs a variance estimate. It is not easy, at first sight, to see how to obtain this from such data. If one discovers from a sample that 15 out of a hundred times a fruit machine comes up with a winning line, there are no differences to square and sum. At the same time, one would not be surprised to find, on repeating the experiment, that twelve or eighteen winning combinations were obtained on a hundred attempts. Commonsense, in fact, dictates that the result is unlikely to be exactly repeatable, but also that it will not be very dissimilar. The sample means clearly do have a variance and therefore, a standard deviation. The size of the samples will also influence one's attitude as to how reproducible they should be. It turns out that the variance in the parent population is the product of the proportions of the components. Thus, a population of billiard balls which were half red and half white would not have the same variance as one containing 2% red and 98% white.*

* To try and get a mental picture of this, imagine a population of 10,000 billiard balls, of which only 2% are red, the rest white. In any random selection of one ball, there would be 98 chances of drawing white to 2 chances of drawing red. Suppose one were to draw samples of, say, 100 balls at random. We should expect to get 98 white and 2 red, but would on occasions get 99 or 97 white with 1 or 3 red. It would be distinctly rare to get 96 or 100 white and 95 white with 5 red would be most unusual: the variance of such sample means would be only one or two.

Suppose now, that the population is 50:50 white and red. In sample of 100 at random, one would expect to get 50:50 more often than any other proportion, but 45:55, or even 40:60 would not occasion great surprise. The spread of 'acceptable' answers is wider and therefore the variance is larger than in the case of the 98:2 population.

The sample variance depends on the size of the sample. Obviously, a sample of thousands could have a variance of dozens or hundreds, whereas a sample of dozens from the same population would have a variance of one or two. Thus, if the two proportions in a binomial population are p and q, the population variance is $p \times q$. In a sample of n items from such a population, the sample variance is $n \times p \times q$. The standard deviation is therefore $\sqrt{n \times p \times q}$. In the case of the two billiard ball populations referred to in the footnote* with samples of 100, the standard deviations are respectively $\sqrt{100 \times 0.02 \times 0.98} = 1.4$, and $\sqrt{100 \times 0.5 \times 0.5} = 5$. Thus, 96 per cent of samples out of a hundred taken from a 98:2 mixture would lie in the range 96:4 to 100:0 (± 2 s.d.) and from a 50:50 mixture in the range 40:60 to 60:40.

The billiard ball example also draws attention to another feature of this distribution. It would be impossible to get less than zero reds, so the sample distribution when the proportions are extremely disparate is markedly skewed. However, the amount of skewness is influenced by the sample size, becoming less so as the size of the sample increases.** When the proportions are reasonably balanced, the distribution is more symmetrical: furthermore, provided the samples are large enough, the distribution of the proportions approximates to a normal distribution.

** Again, to get a mental picture of this, suppose the proportions were 9:1 white to red. Then a sample of 10 could be 9:1 (most common), 10:0, and 8:2 (less common), 7:3 (increasingly rare) 11: −1 impossible. This is an obviously skewed distribution. If one increases the sample size to 100, but keeps the underlying population parameters the same, what happens? The most common sample would be 90:10, less common 89:11 or 91:9, less common again 88:12 and 92:8 and so on, but in a big sample like this it would be extremely uncommon to be outside the limits: 84–96 white.

(s.d. = $\sqrt{100 \times 0.1 \times 0.9} = 3$. Ninety-five per cent confidence limits $\simeq$ mean ± 2 s.d., i.e. $90 \pm 2 \times 3 = 84 - 96$). This has resulted in a virtually unskewed distribution.

As the relative proportions in the population differ more widely, it needs a larger sample to make the sampling distribution reasonably normal. As an approximation, the expected number of either category in a sample must be at least five if a reasonably normal distribution is to occur.

An exact comparison between sample data and proportions calculated from the binomial theorem is not very common. For one thing, it requires either knowledge of, or assumption about, the actual population proportions and this is usually the parameter one is trying to discover. When the conditions are appropriate, a normal distribution is assumed. It so happens that when one of the proportions is very small, the distribution approximates closely to that predicted by the Poisson distribution (see p. 296). When the proportions are not exact and sample size is large enough, the Chi-squared distribution (see below) can be used. These are all much easier than calculating binomial expansions which depend on sample size and assumptions about population parameters.

SEQUENTIAL ANALYSIS

This technique is an application of the binomial distribution and involves the use of specially-designed charts. These charts can be used only in an either/or situation. They have been most employed in comparing two drugs, or procedures, with regard to a single outcome. The assessment is based simply on a decision that the outcome of treatment A is better, or worse, than the outcome of treatment B, or that no difference can be detected. Matched pairs of patients are entered into the trial, and one receives treatment A and the other treatment B, according to a random selection process, such as tossing a coin. The chart is entered at the bottom left-hand corner, and after the first pair have received their respective treatments, a cross is drawn on the square vertically above the black square if treatment A is superior, and horizontally to the right if treatment B is superior (see Fig. 21.2). If there is no difference, no entry is made. A second pair is then entered into the trial and the process repeated. When the line of crosses so constructed passes over either of the lateral limits, that treatment is statistically superior to the other. The numbers of squares within the bounds are specific for the level of significance which is desired, and $P = 0.05$ and $P = 0.01$ charts are both available. If the middle boundary is crossed, no significant difference can be detected. A full analysis of the method can be consulted in Armitage (1960).

ASSOCIATION: GOODNESS OF FIT: THE CHI-SQUARED (χ^2) TEST*

There are many experimental situations in which it is possible to compare the *observed* results of an experiment with what might have been *expected*. Expectation in this

* Chi-squared is pronounced to rhyme with eye, preceded by a hard 'k' and written χ^2.

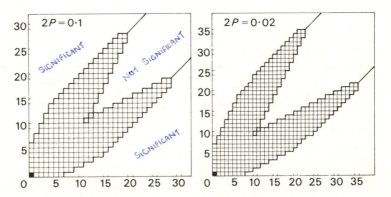

Fig. 21.2. Sequential analysis charts.

context may take various forms. It may, for instance, be calculable in advance on theoretical grounds. If one rolled a die 120 times, one would expect to get each face 20 times each. 'Expect', in this context, does not imply intense surprise if one got 19 fives or 22 ones, but one knows that if the trial was repeated often enough, the long-term value to which they would converge is 1/6 of the total, for each face. We could put it another way and say P for each face is 1/6. (Compare *this* expectation with the definition of probability on page 284). χ^2 can be used to test whether any particular departure from this theoretical distribution could have occurred as a result of chance sampling. Testing for deviation from these theoretical probabilities is a very rare situation in medical research.

However, as an extension of this idea, it can be used to compare the composition of the sample with what is known already about the population from which the sample has been drawn. The expected number in such a case is the one which would have been obtained if the sample was taken without bias. For example, suppose the age distribution of patients undergoing surgery in a particular hospital was known over several years. In a moderately large study on some other topic, the ages of the randomly-selected participants could be noted. The number of subjects falling into each age range could then be tabulated as in the second line of Table 21.3. Applying the percentage distribution already known, it would be also possible to tabulate how many patients could have been expected in

each group in that sample. These figures are given in the third line of Table 21.3. The question arises, 'Are these two sets of figures compatible with the belief that this sample is a representative one or are the differences sufficient to lead one to suspect bias in obtaining the sample?'.

In looking at this problem, one can follow very similar lines of reasoning to those used to introduce the Mean Absolute Deviation and the Mean Squared Deviation as measures of dispersion (pages 277–278). In the present case, one could also add up all the absolute differences between observed and expected; the higher the figure, the more suspicious one would be that the two sets of data were not compatible. The Mean Absolute Deviations so derived do not give, however, sufficient weight to the more extreme deviations so, as before, the differences are squared before being totalled. However, another step is necessary. Consider Table 21.4. Both groups A and B contain observed and expected values: the sum of the squared differences is 74 in both groups. Yet common sense tells us that a discrepancy of 7 when 13 are observed and 6 expected, is very much more significant than the same absolute discrepancy when the observed and expected numbers are 457 and 464 respectively. In the first case, the observed is twice as big as the expected: in the second, it is only a small fraction. To inject the necessary realism, it is necessary to divide the squared difference by the expected number. This produces a statistic whose size is influenced not only by the absolute magnitude of the discrepancies,

Table 21.3.

Age range	0–	10–	20–	30–	40–	50–	60–	70–	80–
Observed no. in sample	20	42	33	30	40	72	81	28	14
Expected no.	16	34	43	32	33	67	92	25	18
$[O-E]$	4	8	10	2	7	5	11	3	4
$[O-E]^2$	16	64	100	4	49	25	121	9	16
$\dfrac{[O-E]^2}{E}$	1.0	1.9	2.3	0.1	1.5	0.4	1.3	0.4	0.9

$$\chi^2 = \sum \frac{[O-E]^2}{E} = 9.8.$$

Table 21.4.

	Group A			Group B		
Observed (O)	13	7	12	457	496	303
Expected (E)	6	11	15	464	500	300
$[O - E]$	7	4	3	7	4	3
$[O - E]^2$	49	16	9	49	16	9
$\sum[O - E]^2$		74			74	
$\dfrac{[O - E]^2}{E}$	8.17	1.45	0.6	0.11	0.03	0.03
$\sum\dfrac{[O - E]^2}{E} = (\chi^2) =$		10.22			0.17	

but also by their relative importance. This is worked in full in Tables 21.3 and 21.4. χ^2 then, is the sum of all the squared differences between observed and expected frequencies when each has been normalized by dividing by the expected value. To return to the original problem, summarized in Table 21.3, χ^2 calculated in this way comes to 9.8. We can see that the more the observed numbers differ from the expected, the higher will χ^2 become and our question is now 'Has the value of χ^2 exceeded the value which might have arisen by chance?'. To answer this, we consult a table of χ^2 values, choosing the level of probability (certainty) which we think appropriate, $P = 0.05$ if we want only a 5% chance that the discrepancy would have occurred by chance, $P = 0.01$ if we want only a 1% chance and so on. Statistical Table 5, p. 313, is an example of a χ^2 table. We also have to determine the degrees of freedom which in this case is eight (one less than the number of categories). From this table, we can see that the critical values for $P = 0.05$ and $P = 0.01$ are 15.5 and 20.1. We have not found deviations which give rise to a value of χ^2 as great as this and can accept that it could be a random sample.

CONTINGENCY TABLES

If each member of the sample can be classified according to one of two or more mutually-exclusive criteria of classification, the results can be laid out in a table known as a contingency table. The criteria may be such things as cured/not cured, or treated/not treated, blood group, age group, sex, or a thousand others.

A common situation is where one criterion is treated/not treated and the other criterion classifies the outcome. Table 21.5 is an example of a 2×2 contingency table and displays the results of a clinical trial to evaluate the effectiveness of meprobamate in the prevention of suxamethonium pains.

Fifty patients were given the active drug and fifty a placebo. Each of the entries is the observed frequency (O) in the formula. In this situation, the expected frequency is derived from an assumption of the null hypothesis. If treatment had no effect, one would expect the number with and without pains to be equally distributed between the treated and untreated groups. In this instance, forty patients in all developed pain, so one could 'expect' twenty patients in each group to have pain and thirty to have no pain. These are the expected frequencies (E). To calculate χ^2,

$$\frac{[E - O]^2}{E}$$

is evaluated for each cell and added together. In consulting the table for the critical value of χ^2 for contingency tables, the appropriate degrees of freedom are obtained from the formula:

$$(\text{No. of columns} - 1) \times (\text{No. of rows} - 1)$$

which, in this case, reduces to 1 degree of freedom.

This can be confirmed by observing that once one entry is changed, the marginal totals fix all the other entries. Where there are only two categories, as in this example, a simple correction has also to be applied (the Yates correction—see Appendix 4). The calculation is worked in full in Table 21.5 which also gives the conclusion drawn.

Table 21.5. A 2 × 2 contingency table

	Pain	No pain	Totals
Meprobamate	10 (E = 20)	40 (E = 30)	50
Placebo	30 (E = 20)	20 (E = 30)	50
Totals	40	60	100

The observed number (O) is the figure entered in each square of the table. E is the expected number, on the assumption that as 40 patients had pain, there would be 20 in each group if the treatment had no effect.

$$\chi^2 = \sum \frac{[E - O]^2}{E}$$

$$= \frac{[(20 - 10) - 0.5^*]^2}{20} + \frac{[(40 - 30) - 0.5^*]^2}{30}$$

$$+ \frac{[(30 - 20) - 0.5^*]^2}{20} + \frac{[(30 - 20) - 0.5^*]^2}{30}$$

$$= \frac{9.5^2}{20} + \frac{9.5^2}{30} + \frac{9.5^2}{20} + \frac{9.5^2}{30}$$

$$= \frac{2 \times 9.5^2}{20} + \frac{2 \times 9.5^2}{30} = \frac{6 \times 9.5^2}{60} + \frac{4 \times 9.5^2}{60}$$

$$= \frac{10 \times 9.5^2}{60} = \frac{9.5^2}{6} = \frac{90.25}{6} = 15.04$$

Since this exceeds the tabulated value 10.8 (P = 0.001 for 1 DF), the result is highly significant (p < 0.001). See Statistical Table 5.

* Yates' Correction—see Appendix 4.

There is one important restriction, to the use of χ^2, namely, that the expected number of items in each category must be at least 5.

This test can also be used when there are more than two outcomes, or when, for example, one is comparing more than two treatments. In such cases a table is constructed in which each square or cell refers to one outcome, e.g. 'Treatment B no improvement'. $[E - O]^2 \div E$ is calculated for each cell and totalled to give χ^2. Such a table is a 2 × 3, or 3 × 3, contingency table, depending on its composition.

THE POISSON DISTRIBUTION

The data which have been handled in the previous section have been of the type that either an event occurred, or some alternative event occurred, or at least a recognizable 'non-event' occurred, i.e. the patient did *not* die. There are, however, situations in which events occur in which there is no meaningful measure of the non-events. In medical work, the most common example of this type of data is in the analysis of radioactive counts. One can count the number of disintegrations per minute, but no meaning can be given to the number of 'nondisintegrations'. If one makes replicate counts, there will be a tendency for the results to converge to a mean value, and there will be a variance of the individual counts about this mean. One can see that the greater the number of counts on any occasion, the more likely is the answer to approach the average count; it is not surprising, therefore, that the variance and hence the standard deviation are a function of the number of counts. It can be shown that the variance is equal to the mean and so the standard deviation equals the square root of the mean. Consequently the standard deviation becomes a progressively smaller *proportion* of the total counts as the number of counts increases. Provided that more than 100 counts are recorded, the confidence interval for the mean count can be estimated from a random sample count on lines familiar from the study of a normal curve, namely that the average count lies between the limits:

$$\text{sample count} \pm 1.96 \times \sqrt{\text{sample count}}$$

for a 95% confidence interval and,

$$\text{sample count} \pm 2.58 \times \sqrt{\text{sample count}}$$

for a 99% confidence interval.

Correlation

Many biological variables are interrelated. The height of children increases with age, the arterial Po_2 decreases with age, the blood volume increases with both height and weight. When the value of one variable can be predicted with greater accuracy when the value of another variable is known, the two variables are said to be *correlated*. If both tend to increase together, they are *positively* correlated and when one decreases as the other increases, they are *negatively* correlated.

There are two traps for the unwary that are particularly applicable to correlation data. The first is that a correlation is merely a mathematical relationship, and there is no certainty that a change in either variable is the cause of a change in the other. Many bizarre but mathematically quite sound correlations exist in which the two variables are both dependent on another factor, or the relationship may be entirely accidental. For example, it is highly likely that a significant positive correlation exists between the number of women doctors and the number of automatic dishwashers. Such correlations over time are extremely common, and usually fortuitous. In the case quoted, no one would be likely to proceed to argue that it has only been the washing-up which stopped women becoming doctors. However, when a biologically plausible 'explanation' exists, an unwarranted cause and effect relationship may be unjustifiably assumed. The second trap is unjustified extrapolation. One must not assume that the relationship between two variables exists outside the range of data that have been collected. For example, knowing the rate at which the height of children increases does not enable one to predict the height of 70-year-old people.

THE CORRELATION COEFFICIENT

When one makes two measurements on a random sample, the chief matter of interest is usually whether or not the measurements are related to one another. For each individual in the sample, two variables are measured which we can denote by x and y. The values of x and y may be thought of as the coordinates of points which would locate each individual on a graph such as Fig. 21.3, which is commonly called a

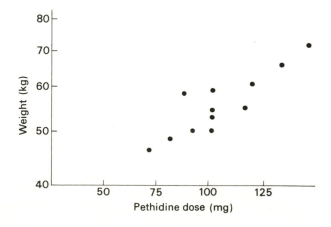

Fig. 21.3. A scatter diagram illustrating the relationship between weight and pethidine requirements.

scatter diagram. Such a diagram gives a rough visual impression of how the variables x and y are related. However, it is not sufficient to conclude that because half the points seem to be on a straight line, there is a linear relationship between x and y. At the same time, we cannot conclude that there is *not* a linear relationship. As always, we need a number whose magnitude tells us how much linear relationship there is between the two variables. This number is the (sample) correlation coefficient and is customarily denoted by r. The formula for calculating r is given in Appendix 5.

The value of r always lies between -1 and $+1$. A value of -1 indicates a perfect linear relationship between x and y, with the value of y decreasing as x increases—the larger x becomes, the smaller y becomes. A value of $+1$ likewise indicates a perfect linear relationship, but one in which increasing values of x are associated with increasing values of y. In both cases, a knowledge of the value of either variable allows one to predict the value of the other. When r is close to zero, there is no linear relationship between the two variables. Figure 21.4 illustrates three scatter diagrams and their associated r values.

Many people find the meaning of r confusing. It is a compound measure of two things: how nearly values fit a line and the likelihood that the line *is*, in fact, a slope. It does *not* give a measure of the slope itself in the units of the measurement. This is a function of the regression coefficient, which is discussed later. The relationship of r to the closeness of the fit of the points to a line has been illustrated by Fig. 21.4, where we saw that scattered points gave a lower r value. The relationship of r to the reality of the slope can be appreciated by approaching the matter from a different stand-point. It was stated earlier (page 278) that variances can be added. From this, it is a simple step to the concept that the total variance of data can equally be thought of as the summation of several variances which are attributable to various causes. Consider the variance of y in the different examples

of Fig. 21.4. If all the points fall exactly on the line, as in figure (a), all of the variance of y can be attributed to the fact that the points are on a slope. The fact that the various values of y are above and below the mean gives rise to a sum of squares, which is all attributable to the fact that the points lie on a slope. Let us call this the slope variance. Note that r is close to $+1$ or -1 In any real situation, however, there are additional experimental sources of variability which blur the relationship between x and y, causing the points to be scattered around the line, as in (b) and r is much less than $+1$ or -1. In this instance, one could calculate a sum of squares of the differences between the actual y values and the values predicted by the assumed relationship between x and y,

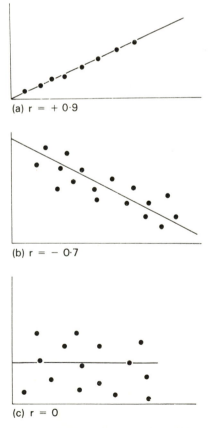

(a) r = + 0·9

(b) r = − 0·7

(c) r = 0

Fig. 21.4. Illustration of three values of the correlation coefficient.

i.e. the values on the line. (The values of y which are predicted by the line for various values of x are often designated $\hat{y}$, called y-hat.) This variance of the y value about the presumed line can be thought of as additional variance and is called the error variance. Added together, the error sum of squares $\Sigma(y - \hat{y})^2$ and the slope sum of squares $\Sigma(\hat{y} - \bar{y})^2$ make up the total sum of squares, $\Sigma(y - \bar{y})^2$.

In (c), there is no slope; all the variance is error variance and r is O. None of it can be attributable to slope. It should be clear now that r is really a ratio between the slope variance and the error variance. If there were no error variance (all the points on the line) then the regression (slope) sum of squares equals the total sum of squares and dividing one by the other would yield either $+1$ or -1, depending on the direction of the slope. Conversely, if there were no slope, all the variance would be due to error sum of squares and the ratio would approach O. (In fact, if the regression sum of squares is divided by the total sum of squares, one obtains r^2). With regard to the relationship between r and the actual slope, it is important to realise that, in any real relationship, the actual slope is entirely dependent on the particular units of measurement and the scale of the axes on which the data are plotted. One of the essential concepts in the computation of r is that the x and y values are standardized by being divided by their standard deviations. All slopes with the same correlation coefficients, therefore, have the same strength of correlation regardless of any apparent differences caused by the units or scales in which they are plotted.

SIGNIFICANCE OF THE CORRELATION COEFFICIENT

The correlation coefficient, r, is a sample statistic and as such, is only an estimate of the population correlation coefficient, ρ (Rho, pronounced Roe, the 17th letter of the Greek alphabet). What degree of confidence can we have in our sample statistic? Is there a 'significant' correlation? If we were discussing a sample mean, we would need the standard error to answer such questions and that is what we need in this situation also. If there are a large number of points in the sample, then it is reasonable to assume that estimates of r are normally distributed about ρ and the standard error can be computed from the formula:

standard error of the correlation coefficient

$$(s_\rho) = \frac{1}{\sqrt{(N - 1)}}.$$

As commonsense would indicate, the number of points has a significant influence: one is inherently more confident of a correlation based on more points in the same way as one is more confident of a mean based on more values. Thus, if $r = 0.5$ (say) and N is 26, the standard error is $1/\sqrt{25} = 0.2$. The null hypothesis is that there is no slope and that, therefore, r is really zero: values greater than twice the standard error for the correlation coefficient occur less than 5% of the time as a result of random sampling error. A value of 0.5 for r would thus indicate that the correlation is 'significant' in a sample of 26.

When the sample is small, as it so often is in medical work, this method of calculating significance becomes progressively inaccurate. As with the mean of small samples, we need to invoke the t-distribution; the calculation is very different, but the principle is the same. A formula for calculating t for small samples is given in Appendix 5.

REGRESSION ANALYSIS

For most practical purposes, problems in regression are handled in the same way as problems in correlation, although strictly speaking, there is a fundamental difference. Tests about the correlation coefficient assume that a random sample has been taken, and that the x values are as random as the y values. One is analysing two sets of randomly-obtained data from the population. In a regression problem, however, it is assumed that the experimenter has control over one set of variables. The experimenter may choose, say, age or weight, which is then the *independent variable*: the other, the *dependent variable*, is then measured at various values of the independent variable. The independent variable is usually plotted on the x axis and the dependent variable on the y axis. For example, the Pao_2 has been found to decline with age. In this case, although people of specific ages may not have been sought, it is logical to think of age as the independent variable and examine how the Pao_2 varies with age.

It is quite common for an experimenter to obtain several y values for each x value. It is thus possible to calculate the standard error of the mean of the y values at each x value, and this can be displayed as a vertical line of appropriate length for each value of x, on either side of the mean value (Fig. 21.5). It is easy to be misled by this. There is a natural tendency to think that the line of best fit will pass through each such line. In fact we know that one s.e. will include only about 68% of all large sample means. If the samples are *small*, the confidence interval will be even greater and related to the t-distribution rather than the normal (see p. 285). For example, if each point on a correlation graph is a mean of four samples, the length of line for 95%

confidence (see p. 286) should be more than three times the s.e. ($t = 3.18$ for 3 d.f.).

It is better therefore, to plot the mean value, and a vertical line corresponding to a 95% confidence interval for that sample. The line illustrating the correlation of the two variables (often called the *regression line*) will pass through nineteen out of twenty such lines. This, however, does not indicate the confidence limits for the line as a whole, for this depends on a statistic related to all the information. This statistic is the Standard Error of the Estimate which we will meet later.

CALCULATION OF REGRESSION LINES

In a regression problem one is not so much trying to ascertain whether two sets of observations are correlated but trying to find out the actual quantitative relationship. One is less concerned with questions such as 'is increasing age associated with increased operative mortality?' as 'how much of an increase in operative mortality is associated with a given rise in age?'

In tackling these questions it is best to start from the basic assumption that the correlation between the variables x and y (if it exists) is a *linear* one. If we suspect that it is not, it is usually more convenient to plot one variable on a different type of scale, so as to transform the relationship into a linear one rather than to attempt to work on a mathematically more complex relationship. This is of relevance in plotting drug dose–response curves where there is generally a linear response of some tissue to a logarithmic change in concentration of drug.

Figure 21.6 is a simple straight line graph showing a linear correlation. An equation that describes such a line is of the type:

$$y = bx + a$$

where a is the value of y when x is zero, and b is the slope. This tells us that each y-value is b times the appropriate x-value plus or minus a consistent increment. The value of b, the slope, is also known as the

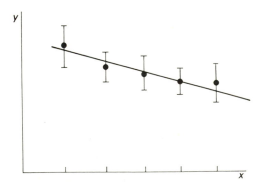

Fig. 21.5. Regression line with diagramatic illustration of the standard error of y at each value of x.

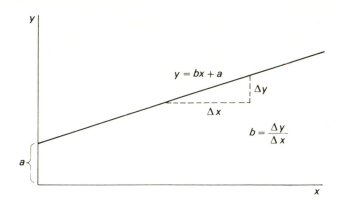

Fig. 21.6. The equation of a straight line.

regression coefficient. In any group of experimentally derived values, there will be a scatter of *y* values above and below the line. The line which fits the data best is the one that minimizes this scatter. It might be thought that it would be sufficient to place the line in such a way that the sum of the deviations of *y* from the line is a minimum. However, following the line of previous arguments, it is the sum of the squared *y* deviations which is minimized. This is the 'least squares line'. To show how the values of *a* and *b* in a linear equation are calculated to make this quantity a minimum requires differential calculus; however, the principle can be appreciated without it.

First of all, one can accept as reasonable that the line will pass through the value which represents the mean of *y* and the mean of *x*, i.e. the general mean. If it did not pass through this point, then clearly the sum of all the squared deviations would be larger. If this is accepted, the value of *a* in the regression line is immaterial since we now have a fixed point, and once the slope is calculated this will fix the whole line.

The slope is obviously some expression which relates an increase or decrease in *y* values to an increase in *x* values (Fig. 21.6). It can be thought of as the mean deviation of *y* divided by the mean deviation of *x*. It is actually calculated by the formula

$$b \text{ (Slope)} = \frac{\Sigma(x - \bar{x}) \cdot (y - \bar{y})}{\Sigma(x - \bar{x})^2}.$$

The denominator is the sum of squares (*SS*)

which is the basis of the calculation of the variance of single parameter variables, and which we have met earlier. The numerator is the sum of the product of the *x* and *y* deviations. Like the variance, it can actually be calculated on a calculating machine or pocket calculator more easily by an alternative formula (see Appendix 6).

ACCURACY OF THE REGRESSION EQUATION

The obvious purpose of calculating the regression equation is to enable one to make an estimate of *y* for any given value for *x*. Knowing that the PaO_2 is related to age enables one to predict what the value should be in any person whose age is known. However, the regression line is only the best fit on the data available and therefore it gives only the 'best estimate' of the quantity in question. Obviously the degree of uncertainty of both this estimate and the regression line are a function of *r*. The nearer *r* is to +1 or −1, the less the uncertainty about the line. One can assess the degree of uncertainty by calculating a statistic called the Standard Error of the Estimate (s_y) which depends on *r*. It is given by the formula:

$$s_y = \sigma y \cdot \sqrt{(1 - r^2)}$$

where σy is the standard deviation of the *y* values. This quantity is employed like any other standard error: in 95% of cases, the actual values will be within plus or minus two standard errors of the estimated values given by the regression equation: actual values will depart from the estimated value by three standard errors less than one in a hundred times. It may thus be useful to indicate the '95% confidence' of the regression line by drawing in parallel lines at two standard errors of the estimate. Ninety-five per cent of the true values will fall within this band.

CONFIDENCE INTERVAL OF A SLOPE

If the y values were not related in any way to the x values, there would be no correlation and the true slope would be zero. Any random sample of data, however, might yield either a positive or negative slope. If the confidence interval for the slope includes zero slope, then clearly the slope cannot be differentiated from a horizontal line and no true correlation exists.

This statistical procedure is analogous to estimating the significance of r by comparing it with its standard error as we did on page 299. If, however, r has not been calculated the necessary inferences can be drawn using regression methods. The quantity which indicates the degree of scatter of the value about the regression line is the error variance usually designated as $s_{y \cdot x}^2$ and the standard deviation of the y values around the regression line, therefore, is the square root of this ($s_{y \cdot x}$). This quantity can be calculated from formulae which can be obtained from standard textbooks (one form is included in Appendix 7).

Having obtained the error variance, one is in a position to calculate the confidence interval of the slope. The logic in this is exactly analogous to the logic in determining the confidence interval for the true mean from a sample of single parameter data discussed earlier. It is an equation of the type:

$$(\mu = \bar{x} \pm t(s_x)$$

in which we calculated the range in which the true mean (μ) lay, by reference to the sample mean ($\bar{x}$), the s.e. of the mean ($s_{\bar{x}}$), and the t value appropriate to the degrees of freedom. In the present case the formula is

$$\beta = b + t \cdot \frac{(s_{y \cdot x})}{\sqrt{SS_x}}.$$

β is the true slope, b the slope calculated from the sample data, $s_{y \cdot x}$ is the square root of the error variance, and $\sqrt{SS_x}$ the square root of the sum of squared deviations of the x values.

One can push the analogy between single parameter and correlation data even further. In the same way that it was possible to test for the significance between two sample means with a Student's t test, so one can test whether or not two slopes differ significantly. In this case, t is equal to the difference between two slope estimates, divided by a term which represents the standard error of the difference of the slopes. The standard error is computed by first estimating the population error variance by pooling the data, and the difference of slope is considered to be significant if a t value is exceeded (the formula is included in Appendix 9).

PERORATION

Statistics is a discipline which puts into numerical terms commonsense notions such as 'more likely', 'probable', 'confident' etc. The calculations required are simple, although tedious without electronic assistance, and rarely involve anything more complex than addition, multiplication, division and taking square roots.

The aim of these manipulations is usually to derive a number whose magnitude is a guide to the degree of 'probability', 'confidence' etc. For most doctors they need be only tools; it should be of interest to see the logic of the construction of the tools but not necessary to understand the detailed theory. However, no one can maintain proficiency with a tool merely by observing how it is used and how it is made. Only by using statistics as a tool, can one become familiar with them. As with most kinds of learning, the memory resides in the motor cortex.

References

ARMITAGE P. (1960) *Sequential Medical Trials.* Oxford: Blackwell Scientific Publications.

Further reading

BULMER M.G. (1967) *Principles of Statistics. 2nd edition.* Edinburgh and London: Oliver and Boyd.

DUNN O.J. (1967) *Basic Statistics: A Primer for the Biomedical Sciences.* London: John Wiley & Sons.

GOLDSTEIN A. (1964) *Biostatistics—An Introductory Text.* New York: The Macmillan Company.

HILL A.B. (1966) *Principles of Medical Statistics, 8th edition.* London: The Lancet Ltd.

MORONEY M.J. (1956) *Facts from Figures.* Harmondsworth, Middlesex: Penguin Books Ltd.

Appendices

1. Abbreviations used in Chapters 20 and 21

x — Any variable

$\bar{x}$ — The arithmetic mean of the x values

N — The number of observations in a sample

var (x) — The variance of a sample

s.d. — Standard deviation of a sample

SS — Sum of squared deviations from the mean

$\sum$ — Add up

μ — Population mean

σ^2 — Population variance ⎫ Theoretical

σ — Population standard deviation ⎭

s.e. $(s_{\bar{x}})$ — Standard error (of the mean)

s^2 — Estimate of population variance based on sample statistics

s — Estimate of population standard deviation based on sample statistics

d.f. — Degrees of freedom—the number of items of the data which are free to vary

$s_{(\bar{x}-\bar{x}')}$ — Standard error of difference between the means of two independent samples

d — A difference between two sequential observations in same patient

$\bar{d}$ — Mean of a population of differences

$s_{\bar{d}}$ — Standard error of differences

$\hat{y}$ — The value for y calculated from the regression equation

r — The correlation coefficient

s_y — The standard error of the estimate of y from the regression equation

2. A short-cut method for computing sum of squares variance and s.d.

$$\text{variance} = \frac{\sum (x - \bar{x})^2}{N} \qquad (1)$$

by definition. The term $\sum (x - \bar{x})^2$ is called the sum of squares (SS) and can be represented as:

$$SS = (x_1 - \bar{x})^2 + (x_2 - \bar{x})^2 \\ + \cdots (x_N - \bar{x})^2 \qquad (2)$$

Expanding each term gives:

$$SS = (x_1^2 - 2\bar{x}x_1 + \bar{x}^2) \\ + (x_2^2 - 2\bar{x}x_2 + \bar{x}^2) \\ \cdots (x_N^2 - 2\bar{x}x_N + \bar{x}^2) \qquad (3)$$

This may be shortened to:

$$SS = \sum (x^2) - 2\bar{x}\sum (x) + N\bar{x}^2 \qquad (4)$$

Now

$$\bar{x} = \frac{\sum (x)}{N}$$

Substituting for $\bar{x}$ in (4) gives:

$$SS = \sum (x^2) - 2\frac{\sum (x)}{N} \cdot \sum (x) + N\frac{(\sum (x))^2}{N^2}$$

Simplifying:

$$SS = \sum (x^2) - \frac{2(\sum x)^2}{N} + \frac{(\sum x)^2}{N}$$

$$= \sum (x^2) - \frac{(\sum x)^2}{N}$$

$\sum (x)$ is the total of the x values $= T$,

$$\therefore SS = \sum (x^2) - \frac{T^2}{N}$$

304

And therefore the population variance estimate from a sample:

$$s^2 = \frac{\sum (x^2) - (T^2/N)}{N - 1}$$

The standard deviation of the population from a sample is:

$$s = \sqrt{\frac{\sum (x^2) - (T^2/N)}{N - 1}}$$

The advantage of this formula is that T, the total of the values, and $\sum (x^2)$, the total of the squared values, can both be accumulated on a calculating machine. Note that the use of this formula does not involve subtracting values from the mean, or even calculating the mean. Additional values can easily be added without lengthy recalculation.

3. Detailed working of hypothetical examples of the use of the t test

EXPERIMENT 1

It is suggested that patients coming to afternoon surgery are more anxious than patients coming to morning surgery because of the longer period of waiting. Preoperative pulse rates are obtained for two matched groups of eleven patients.

$$N = 11 \qquad N' = 11$$

$$\bar{x} = \frac{\sum x}{N} = \frac{814}{11} = 74/\text{min}$$

$$\bar{x}' = \frac{\sum x'}{N'} = \frac{869}{11} = 79/\text{min}$$

$$\text{var}(x) = \frac{SS}{N} = \frac{690}{11} = 62.7$$

$$\text{var}(x') = \frac{SS'}{N'} = \frac{1124}{11} = 102.2$$

$$\text{s.d.}(x) = \sqrt{62.7} = 7.92$$

$$\text{s.d.}(x') = \sqrt{102.2} = 10.1$$

(The figures have been chosen to give easily managed whole numbers, so that the naturally derived formula for variance could be used as described on page 278. In a sample of natural data it is almost always quicker and easier to obtain SS— the sum of squared deviations, using the formula of Appendix 2).

Both groups can be used to estimate the

Group A—morning Pulse rates			Group B—afternoon Pulse rates		
(x)	$(x - \bar{x})$	$(x - \bar{x})^2$	(x')	$(x' - \bar{x}')$	$(x - \bar{x}')^2$
61	-13	169	68	-11	121
66	-8	64	64	-15	225
91	$+17$	289	95	$+16$	256
84	$+10$	100	92	$+13$	169
75	$+1$	1	76	-3	9
72	-2	4	80	$+1$	1
79	$+5$	25	88	$+9$	81
69	-5	25	69	-10	100
74	0	0	70	-9	81
71	-3	9	79	0	0
72	-2	4	88	$+9$	81
$\sum x = 814$	0	$SS_x = 690$	$\sum x' = 869$	0	$SS_{x'} = 1124$

theoretical population variance, by dividing SS by $N - 1$:

$$s^2 = \frac{690}{10} = 69 \quad \text{and} \quad s'^2 = \frac{1124}{10} = 112.4$$

The variance estimate derived from the afternoon cases is greater than that derived from the morning ones. Is this difference significant? It is possible to set up the hypothesis that the response to anxiety is very variable, and that this accounts for the larger variance. Alternatively, could random samples of eleven have variances such as these, quite by chance? Before we can go on to test for the significance of the difference between the mean pulse rates of the two groups, it is necessary to settle this point. This is tested by an F-test. The larger variance estimate is divided by the smaller:

$$F = \frac{112.4}{69} = 1.63$$

Reference to Table 2 of Statistical Tables with 10 degrees of freedom for each sample, shows that values of F greater than 2.98 occur less commonly than five times in a hundred (the table is constructed for $p = 0.05$). We can assume, therefore, that our value of 1.63 could easily arise by chance, and that there is no significant difference between the two variances.

Having established that the variances are effectively the same, we can pool the two samples to obtain the *best estimate* of the population variance:

$$\text{(pooled) } s^2 = \frac{SS + SS'}{(N - 1) + (N' - 1)}$$

$$= \frac{690 + 1124}{10 + 10} = \frac{1814}{20} = \underline{90.7}$$

The variance for each mean is found from the formula:

$$s_{\bar{x}}^2 = \frac{s^2}{N}$$

and the standard error for each mean can now be calculated if required:

$$s_{\bar{x}} = \sqrt{\frac{s^2}{N}} = \sqrt{\frac{90.7}{11}} = \sqrt{8.24} = 2.87$$

t is computed from the formula:

$$t = \frac{|\bar{x} - \bar{x}'|}{s_{(\bar{x} - \bar{x}')}}$$

The numerator we can do easily, i.e.

$$|74 - 79| = \underline{5} \text{ (absolute)}$$

The denominator is the square root of the sum of the two sample mean variances:

$$s_{(\bar{x} - \bar{x}')} = \sqrt{\frac{s^2}{N} + \frac{s^2}{N'}}$$

As the samples are of equal size, this can be simplified to

$$s_{(\bar{x} - \bar{x}')} = \sqrt{\frac{2s^2}{N}} = \sqrt{\frac{2 \times 90.7}{11}}$$

$$= \sqrt{16.4} = \underline{4.05}$$

Therefore

$$t = \frac{|\bar{x} - \bar{x}'|}{s_{(\bar{x} - \bar{x}')}} = \frac{5}{4.05} = 1.23$$

Looking up the critical values of t in Table 3 of the Statistical Tables at 20 d.f., we find that t must exceed 2.09 for the difference to be significant at the 5% level. We cannot reject the null hypothesis, therefore, and must accept that a mean difference of five could have occurred by chance.

Actually, our original hypothesis was that the afternoon patients would be more anxious and have a *higher* pulse rate. A one-tailed test is therefore appropriate, but even so the critical value (1.73) is not reached, and we cannot even assert that the second mean is significantly greater.

Note, that if our mean values had been based on a total of 220 values instead of about 20, the SS would have been about 20,000 instead of 2000 and the best estimate of the variance about

$$\frac{20000}{220} \simeq 90,$$

i.e. almost the same. But the standard error of the difference would have been:

$$\sqrt{\frac{2 \times 90}{218}} = \sqrt{0.82} \simeq 0.9,$$

instead of 4.05. This would make

$$t \simeq \frac{5}{0.9} \simeq 5.5$$

which would be significant at the 1% level. Our earlier result is not necessarily an indication that our hypothesis is valueless; it can be regarded as an indication to increase the numbers of cases in the trial. It also brings out the mathematical basis for the fact that we are more inclined to believe in the reality of a relatively small change in mean pulse rate, when the means are based on a large number rather than a small number of observations.

EXPERIMENT 2

Suppose now that the same data apply to an experiment in which the x-values are pre-operative pulse rates in patients undergoing a first insertion of radium, and the x'-values are the pre-operative pulse rates of the same patients undergoing a second insertion of radium 1 week later. We would like to know whether there is any evidence that patients are more, or less anxious facing the second operation. This is a situation in which the differences between the patients is not relevant, and only the difference in each patient between one occasion and another is of interest.

The first step is to derive these differences:

x	x'	$x - x' = d$	d^2
61	68	+7	49
66	64	−2	4
91	95	+4	16
84	92	+8	64
75	76	+1	1
72	80	+8	64
79	88	+9	81
69	69	0	0
74	70	−4	16
71	79	+8	64
72	88	+16	256
		$\sum d = +55$	$\sum d^2 = 615$

$$N = 11$$

$$\bar{d} = \frac{\sum d}{N} = \frac{+55}{11} = +5$$

$$\mathrm{var}(d) = \frac{\sum d^2}{N} = \frac{615}{11} = 55.9$$

$$\mathrm{s.d.}(d) = \sqrt{55.9} = 7.48.$$

The next step is to estimate the variance of the theoretical population of differences from the sample of differences. (As there is only one sample of differences an F-test is neither possible nor necessary).

$$s_d^2 = \frac{\sum d^2}{N - 1} = \frac{615}{10} = 61.5$$

The standard error of the mean differences is the square root of the population variance divided by N.

$$s_{\bar{d}} = \sqrt{\frac{s_d^2}{N}} = \sqrt{\frac{61.5}{11}} = \sqrt{5.59} = 2.36$$

$$t = \frac{\bar{d}}{s_{\bar{d}}} = \frac{5}{2.36} = 2.12$$

Entering Table 3 of Statistical Tables with 10 d.f. (one less than the number of differences) the critical values for t are found to be 1.81 for one tail and 2.23 for both tails. In the experiment as planned, it was not possible to say whether the patients would be more or less anxious, and a two-tailed test should be used. The calculated value (2.12) does not exceed the critical value (2.23) and so the difference is not significant at the 5% level.

However, as a result of the experiments it is now possible to suggest that the first experience of radium insertion is unpleasant, and that patients are likely to be more anxious the second time. The calculated figure of t exceeds the critical value for a one-tailed test, and one can say that there is a significant *increase* ($P < 0.05$). However, it is a very marginal result, and the acquisition of further data would be wise.

In general, the hypotheses which underlie experiments most commonly imply an expectation of change in some measurement in a specified direction, and one-tailed tests are much more commonly correct than two-tailed tests.

4. Yates correction: Method of rapid calculation of chi-squared

YATES CORRECTION

χ^2 is a continuous distribution: when it is applied to a 2×2 contingency table, however, it is being utilized with data which are binomially distributed. To meet this objection, Yates Correction increases by 0.5 units the observed number in cells in which the observed numbers are less than the expected and decreases by 0.5 units those in which observed exceed expectation. (The same result is, of course, achieved by subtracting 0.5 units from all the differences as has been done in the worked example on page 296.) If, as a result, any difference is reduced to zero or a negative quantity, that term is eliminated from the computation.

RAPID CALCULATION OF χ^2 FOR 2×2 CONTINGENCY TABLES

Calculations are speeded up by using a formula which does not require the computation for each cell. If a 2×2 contingency

table is laid out symbolically in the following way:

	Affected	Not Affected	
Treatment 1	a	c	e
Treatment 2	b	d	f
	g	h	k

$$\chi^2 = \frac{(bc - ad)^2 k}{efgh}$$

Using the data from page 296, we get:

$$\chi^2 = \frac{(29.5 \times 39.5) - (10.5 \times 20.5)^2 \times 100}{50 \times 50 \times 40 \times 60}$$

$$= \frac{(1165.25 - 215.25)^2 \times 2}{50 \times 40 \times 60}$$

$$= \frac{950^2 \times 2}{120,000} = \frac{90.25}{6} = 15.04$$

5. Correlation Coefficient (r)

$$r = \frac{\sum [(x - \bar{x})(y - \bar{y})]}{\sqrt{[(x - \bar{x})^2] \cdot [(y - \bar{y})^2]}}.$$

For easy machine computation, this can be algebraically rearranged as follows:

$$r = \frac{\sum xy - \frac{(\sum x) \cdot (\sum y)}{n}}{\sqrt{\left[\sum x^2 - \frac{(\sum x)^2}{n}\right] \cdot \left[\sum y^2 - \frac{(\sum y)^2}{n}\right]}}.$$

SIGNIFICANCE OF THE CORRELATION COEFFICIENT

$$t = \sqrt{\frac{r^2(N - 2)}{1 - r^2}}$$

Tables are entered to find the critical value of t for $N - 2$ degrees of freedom. If this value is exceeded, the slope is significant at the chosen level.

6. Calculation of Regression Slope (b)

$$b = \frac{\sum (x - \bar{x})(y - \bar{y})}{\sum (x - \bar{x})^2}$$

The numerator is called the *covariance* of x and y and can be designated SP_{xy} (sum of products). The denominator is familiar as SS_x (sum of squares). For machine computation the above formula can be redrawn as follows:

$$b = \frac{\sum xy - \left[(\sum x)(\sum y)/N \right]}{\sum x^2 - \left[(\sum x)^2/N \right]}$$

7. The Error Variance

If $\tilde{y}$ is the 'true' value of y as given by the regression equation for each value of x, the error variance ($s_{y \cdot x}^2$) is given by the formula

$$s_{y \cdot x}^2 = \frac{\sum (y - \tilde{y})^2}{N - 2}$$

Note, division by $N - 2$ makes $s_{y \cdot x}^2$ an unbiased estimate of $\sigma_{y \cdot x}^2$, just as division by $N - 1$, made s^2 (sample variance) an unbiased estimate of σ^2 (population vari-

ance). There are $N - 2$ degrees of freedom because two parameters are being estimated (mean *and* slope).

8. Confidence Interval for the True Slope (β)

$$\beta = b \pm t \left(\frac{s_{y \cdot x}}{\sqrt{SS_x}} \right)$$

Where $s_{y \cdot x}$ is the square root of the error variance ($s_{y \cdot x}^2$) and $\sqrt{SS_x}$ is the square root of the sum of squared x deviations. t, being related to two parameters, has again, $N - 2$ d.f.

9. Difference between Two Slopes

$$t = \frac{b - b'}{s_{y \cdot x} \sqrt{\dfrac{1}{SS_x} + \dfrac{1}{SS_{x'}}}}$$

b and b' are the slope estimates. A pooled error variance ($s_{y \cdot x}$)^2 is computed by combining the data and dividing by $(N - 2) + (N' - 2)$. t has $(N - 2) + (N' - 2)$ d.f.

Statistical Tables

1. Areas of the Normal Curve

The probability (P) that the value of any observation will lie outside given limits is proportional to the area under the curve lying outside these limits. Values of the number of s.d. are tabulated for various fractions of the total area. This area is found by adding a P value in the left-hand column to one in the top horizontal column e.g. $P = 0.47$ yields a value of 0.722. Thus 47% of values would be more than ± 0.722 s.d. from the mean: conversely, 53% would be within ± 0.722 s.d., that is, there is a probability (P) of 0.47 that a value will be outside the limits ± 0.722 s.d. Similarly, the limits which contain 95% of the observations are those which exclude 5% of the observations: these limits are given by $P = 0.05$ and the corresponding value is therefore 1.96. A value $> 1.96 \times \sigma$ accordingly has a probability of occurring less than 5 times in 100.

Since the means of large samples are distributed normally the table can also be used to predict the range within which any sample mean is likely to lie at any desired level of probability (*see* page 278). In this case, when $p = 0.05$ is chosen, it means that 5% of sample means lie outside the limits μ (population mean) $\pm 1.96 \times$ s.e.m.

Since any given fractional area is equally divided between both tails of the curve, the value of a particular area in one tail is found by entering the table at twice the desired value of P. Thus $P = 0.05$ in both tails is the area outside ± 1.96 s.d.; but $P = 0.05$ in one tail when $P = 0.10$ in both tails, i.e. beyond either $+1.64$ s.d. or -1.64 s.d. in the relevant specified direction. Likewise, $P = 0.01$ in both tails at 2.58 s.d., in one tail at 2.33 s.d.

P	0.00	0.01	0.02	0.03	0.04	0.05	0.06	0.07	0.08	0.09
0.00	∞	2.58	2.33	2.17	2.05	1.96	1.88	1.82	1.75	1.70
0.10	1.64	1.60	1.55	1.51	1.48	1.44	1.41	1.37	1.34	1.31
0.20	1.28	1.25	1.23	1.20	1.17	1.15	1.13	1.10	1.08	1.06
0.30	1.04	1.02	0.994	0.974	0.954	0.935	0.915	0.896	0.878	0.860
0.40	0.842	0.824	0.806	0.789	0.772	0.755	0.739	0.722	0.706	0.690
0.50	0.674	0.659	0.643	0.628	0.613	0.598	0.583	0.568	0.553	0.539
0.60	0.524	0.510	0.496	0.482	0.468	0.454	0.440	0.426	0.412	0.399
0.70	0.385	0.372	0.358	0.345	0.332	0.319	0.305	0.292	0.279	0.266
0.80	0.253	0.240	0.228	0.215	0.202	0.189	0.176	0.164	0.151	0.138
0.90	0.126	0.113	0.100	0.0878	0.0753	0.0627	0.0502	0.0376	0.0251	0.0125

2. The F-distribution

The F-distribution arises when two independent *estimates* of a variance are divided one by the other. If the values in the Table are *exceeded* for the appropriate sample size, the variances are too dissimilar to have come from the same population (95% probability*).

	d.f. = 1	2	3	4	5	6	7	8	10	12	24
d.f.' = 2	18.5	19.0	19.2	19.2	19.3	19.3	19.4	19.4	19.4	19.4	19.5
3	10.1	9.55	9.28	9.12	9.01	8.94	8.89	8.85	8.79	8.74	8.64
4	7.71	6.94	6.59	6.39	6.26	6.16	6.09	6.04	5.96	5.91	5.77
5	6.61	5.79	5.41	5.19	5.05	4.95	4.88	4.82	4.74	4.68	4.53
6	5.99	5.14	4.76	4.53	4.39	4.28	4.21	4.15	4.06	4.00	3.84
7	5.59	4.74	4.35	4.12	3.97	3.87	3.79	3.73	3.64	3.57	3.41
8	5.32	4.46	4.07	3.84	3.69	3.58	3.50	3.44	3.35	3.28	3.12
9	5.12	4.26	3.86	3.63	3.48	3.37	3.29	3.23	3.14	3.07	2.90
10	4.96	4.10	3.71	3.48	3.33	3.22	3.14	3.07	2.98	2.91	2.74
12	4.75	3.89	3.49	3.26	3.11	3.00	2.91	2.85	2.75	2.69	2.51
15	4.54	3.68	3.29	3.06	2.90	2.79	2.71	2.64	2.54	2.48	2.29
20	4.35	3.49	3.10	2.87	2.71	2.60	2.51	2.45	2.35	2.28	2.08
24	4.26	3.40	3.01	2.78	2.62	2.51	2.42	2.36	2.25	2.18	1.98
30	4.17	3.32	2.92	2.69	2.53	2.42	2.33	2.27	2.16	2.09	1.89
40	4.08	3.23	2.84	2.61	2.45	2.34	2.25	2.18	2.08	2.00	1.79
60	4.00	3.15	2.76	2.53	2.37	2.25	2.17	2.10	1.99	1.92	1.70

d.f. and d.f.' are the degrees of freedom of numerator and denominator respectively.
* Another table would need to be consulted for 99% probability.

3. The *T*-distribution

If the values in the table are *exceeded* at the appropriate degrees of freedom, the result is significant at the stated level of probability.

Degrees of freedom	Two-tailed test		One-tailed test	
	$P = 0.05$	$P = 0.01$	$P = 0.05$	$P = 0.01$
1	12.7	63.7	6.31	31.82
2	4.30	9.93	2.92	6.70
3	3.18	5.84	2.35	4.54
4	2.78	4.60	2.13	3.75
5	2.57	4.03	2.02	3.37
6	2.45	3.71	1.94	3.14
7	2.36	3.50	1.90	3.00
8	2.31	3.36	1.86	2.90
9	2.26	3.25	1.83	2.82
10	2.23	3.17	1.81	2.76
12	2.18	3.05	1.78	2.68
15	2.13	2.95	1.75	2.60
20	2.09	2.85	1.73	2.53
25	2.06	2.79	1.71	2.49
30	2.04	2.75	1.70	2.46
40	2.02	2.70	1.68	2.42
60	2.00	2.66	1.67	2.39
120	1.98	2.62	1.66	2.36
∞	1.96	2.58	1.65	2.33

4. Willcoxon's Test for Pair Differences

n = number of pairs. Tabulated values are the rank sums *outside which* the sample values must lie if the difference is significant at the desired levels of probability shown. Columns 1 and 3 are for a two-tailed hypothesis: columns 2 and 4 are for a one-tailed hypothesis.

n	5% in each tail	5% in one tail	1% in each tail	1% in one tail
5	0–15	—	—	—
6	2–19	0–21	—	—
7	3–25	2–26	0–28	—
8	5–31	3–33	1–35	0–36
9	8–37	5–40	3–42	1–44
10	10–45	8–47	5–50	3–52
11	13–53	10–56	7–59	5–61
12	17–61	13–65	9–69	7–71
13	21–70	17–74	12–79	9–82
14	25–80	21–84	15–90	12–93
15	30–90	25–95	19–101	15–105
16	35–101	29–107	23–113	19–117
17	41–112	34–119	28–125	23–130
18	47–124	40–131	32–139	27–144
19	57–137	46–144	37–153	32–158
20	60–150	52–158	43–167	37–173
21	67–164	58–173	49–182	42–189
22	75–178	66–187	55–198	48–205
23	83–193	73–203	62–214	54–222
24	91–209	81–219	69–231	61–239
25	100–225	89–236	76–249	68–257

5. The Chi-squared distribution

This table gives the values of χ^2 which must be exceeded for a significant result at; $P = 0.1, 0.05, 0.01$ and 0.001. The values of χ^2 are tabulated in degrees of freedom (one less than the number of categories).

Degrees of freedom	$P = 0.1$	$P = 0.05$	$P = 0.01$	$P = 0.001$
1	2.71	3.84	6.64	10.8
2	4.61	5.99	9.21	13.8
3	6.25	7.82	11.3	16.3
4	7.78	9.49	13.3	18.5
5	9.24	11.1	15.1	20.5
6	10.6	12.6	16.8	22.5
7	12.0	14.1	18.5	24.3
8	13.4	15.5	20.1	26.1
9	14.7	16.9	21.7	27.9
10	16.0	18.3	23.2	29.6
12	18.5	21.0	26.2	32.9
15	22.3	25.0	30.6	37.7
20	28.4	31.4	37.6	45.3
24	33.2	36.4	43.0	51.2
30	40.3	43.8	50.9	59.7
40	51.8	55.8	63.7	73.4
60	74.4	79.1	88.4	99.6

Index